PSYCHOLOGICAL THERAPIES FOR SURVIVORS OF TORTURE

A HUMAN-RIGHTS APPROACH WITH PEOPLE SEEKING ASYLUM

Edited by

Jude Boyles

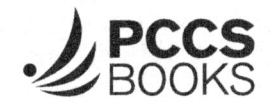

PCCS BOOKS

First published 2017

PCCS Books Ltd
Wyastone Business Park
Wyastone Leys
Monmouth
NP25 3SR
United Kingdom
contact@pccs-books.co.uk
www.pccs-books.co.uk

This collection © Jude Boyles, 2017
The individual chapters © the contributors, 2017

All rights reserved.
No part of this publication may be reproduced, stored in a retrieval system, transmitted or utilised in any form by any means, electronic, mechanical, photocopying or recording or otherwise, without permission in writing from the publishers.

The authors have asserted their right to be identified as the authors of this work in accordance with the Copyright, Designs and Patents Act 1988.

**Psychological Therapies for Survivors of Torture:
a human-rights approach with people seeking asylum**

British Library Cataloguing in Publication data: a catalogue record for this book is available from the British Library.

ISBN 978 1 910919 33 0

Cover design by Graeme Armstrong, Greyswood Art and Design – www.greyswoodart.com
Typeset in-house by PCCS Books using Minion Pro and Gill Sans
Printed by Lightning Source

Contents

	Preface	*v*
	Glossary	*viii*
	Introduction	*1*
1	Assessing survivors of torture for psychological therapy Jude Boyles	*11*
2	'The door to my garden': Kevin, me and the clock Norma McKinnon	*36*
3	Recovery and reconnection Kirsten Lamb	*56*
4	Talking about racial and ethnic differences with torture survivors Rajita Rajeshwar	*76*
5	Treat us like people Prossy Kakooza, in conversation with Jude Boyles	*97*
6	Working with women survivors of torture and gender-based abuse: a woman-focused approach Katie Whitehouse	*109*
7	Alone in the world: therapy with separated young people Ann Salter	*135*
8	Understanding shame with survivors of torture Colsom Bashir	*156*
9	The application of cognitive behavioural therapies with survivors of torture Colsom Bashir	*187*
10	Queering the pitch: sexuality, torture and recovery Ashley Fletcher	*223*
11	You are here with us now (we have changed): systemic therapy with families who have survived torture Emma Roberts	*246*
12	Creating a safe haven: a community-based, creative approach to working with refugee and asylum-seeking families and young people affected by torture Carl Dutton	*271*
13	Trauma, attachment and development: the impact of torture on children and young people Ann Salter	*288*

14	Be there but don't be there: working alongside interpreters with survivors of torture in exile *Jude Boyles, Desiré Kinané and Nathalie Talbot*	*307*
15	The strength and stress of triangles: training and supervision for interpreters and therapists *Beverley Costa*	*331*
16	Holding hope: the challenge for therapists working with survivors of torture *Jess Michaelson*	*350*
17	Walking a journey alongside a survivor: therapeutic social work with survivors of torture *Anna Turner*	*370*
	Postscript	*396*
	Contributors	*397*
	Index	*401*

Acknowledgements

With thanks to Hermione McEwen for checking the legal input in the chapters. Thank you to Beate Dasarathy, who is the editor on my shoulder!

Thanks to Kevin and Reza, Prossy Kakooza, Abdelaziz Mousa and Jonathan Kazembé for sharing your experiences with us.

And finally, thank you to Graeme Armstrong at Greyswood Art and Design for creating a cover image that so powerfully captures the themes of the book.

Publisher's note

Some clients have given their permission for their stories and words to be published in this book. In all other cases, the client stories are anonymised amalgamations drawn from the caseloads of the authors and are not identifiable to any individuals.

The views expressed in this book are those of the authors and are not those of any organisations for which they work or have worked.

Preface – Keep the door open

Jude Boyles

I first started working with survivors of torture in 1999, during the Kosovo conflict. Leeds offered refuge to large numbers of Kosovars fleeing the war, some of whom had been tortured. In that same year, following the dispersal of people seeking asylum to West Yorkshire, the statutory crisis service where I worked began to receive referrals from people fleeing torture, gender-based abuse, conflict and persecution.

Much has changed since then. At that time, people seeking protection in the UK were not referred to as 'asylum seekers', and every passing year I wonder if the context within which survivors seek protection could get any worse. As an activist, I can celebrate the successful campaigns in the asylum and human rights sector and am inspired and reassured by the work being done with/by survivors in the face of such hostility, often with few resources. However, I write this knowing that torture survivors are still being detained in immigration removal centres, left destitute and denied access to food and shelter, and forcibly returned by the UK government to countries where they are at risk of further torture or even death.

When I first began working with survivors of torture, over 18 years ago, I had many years' experience of working with women survivors of male violence. My supervisor reassured me that my approach would be readily transferable to working with survivors of torture. In many ways, she was right; there was much I could draw on. But the work was different, and I knew that I needed to make changes in my therapeutic approach. I tried to be flexible, to adapt my model, and I sought training in trauma, but nonetheless I often felt quite lost. I looked in vain for a practical book that would help me explore these differences and prepare me for the challenges of therapy with survivors who are living in poverty and under threat of return.

The idea that I would, one day, edit such a book began to form – not an academic book, but a practical guide, written by therapists working with survivors in a range of settings, as well as those of us working specifically in the refugee field.

The first torture survivor I worked with was called Reza, and he kindly consented to my writing about our work together. In our second session, he arrived disturbed and frightened, as his house had been attacked by a group of racist youth. He was too frightened and shocked to go home and just sat and shivered in the clinical room. Reza was my last client of the day. My colleagues looked on in confusion as I kept the centre open late to provide immediate assistance. The only helpful thing to do at that time was to ring the housing provider and get Reza moved to a place of safety. Reza did not have the language, information and power to do this for himself. I could sense my colleagues' disapproval, but it felt the right and only thing to do.

This was the first occasion that I picked up the phone for a survivor, and, of course, I have done it many times since. Reza said, many years later, that this had been the turning point for him, not just in relation to his committing to the therapy, but in giving him hope about his situation. Until this point, the world had felt harsh and humiliating. A capable and skilled man, he was confused and undermined by a set of chaotic systems that treated him like a criminal. He felt believed and listened to for the first time.

Therapy organisations can provide welcoming and helpful services to survivors of torture who approach them for assistance. When therapists are asked to keep the door to the clinical room open by a survivor who is terrified of being locked in, we can do that easily. Sadly, we are not always willing to make these small changes that can make such a difference to a client, as they fall outside what we would normally do. We must keep the door to our organisations open, and ensure we do everything we can as professionals to make our services accessible and responsive to people who have experienced such profound abuses of their human rights in their country of origin and in exile.

Jonathan Kazembé, a former colleague at a torture rehabilitation centre and a survivor of torture from the Democratic Republic of the Congo, reminds us why therapy can be so important in the face of such brutality:

> When I started therapy, I had no idea what therapy meant. I came from a country where, if you are traumatised, you either ignore your feelings or you have to be delivered from the evil spirit. You are seen as being weak if you show your feelings, especially if you are a man. You cannot complain if you are physically hurt. When I look back on the time when I first arrived at the centre receiving therapy, I feel like I have been attending a school of life.

Therapy gave me the time and the space to understand what I was and what I could be. It was a great opportunity for me to explain and understand many things that could take many years to explain. Through therapy I am able to accept myself and am now able to cope better with my past experiences.

I must admit that there were many moments during my therapy sessions when I felt like I was being stabbed by a knife. I was at times very scared and ashamed of my own story. I am so delighted that therapy helped me to develop a different relationship with pain. I have learned that there is only so much pain one can have. Telling my story again and again made me realise that sometimes I feared the unknown. After pain, there is nothing. I know now that therapy was not to take away my experiences, but to help me be in control of my future. It gave me the future I never thought I had.

Therapy continues to happen in my life in many different ways, and I feel proud of all the progress I have made over the years. The voice I felt I had lost can now reach so many places, more than I could have imagined. I have been given so many opportunities to be heard in the community I can now call home.

Glossary

The jargon and language of the asylum process can be confusing to those unfamiliar with, and new to, working with refugees. I have outlined below the key terms and legal frameworks referred to in the book.

Torture

The definition of torture referred to in the book is in Article 1 of the United Nations (UN) Convention Against Torture (UNCAT): the Convention Against Torture and Other Cruel, Inhuman or Degrading Treatment or Punishment (the Torture Convention). The Convention was adopted by the General Assembly of the United Nations on 10 December 1984. The Convention entered into force on 26 June 1987. As of October 2016, the Convention has 160 state parties signed up to it (or state signatories).

Article 1.1 of the Torture Convention defines torture as:

> Any act by which severe pain or suffering, whether physical or mental, is intentionally inflicted on a person for such purposes as obtaining from him, or a third person, information or a confession, punishing him for an act he or a third person has committed or is suspected of having committed, or intimidating or coercing him or a third person, or for any reason based on discrimination of any kind, when such pain or suffering is inflicted by or at the instigation of or with the consent or acquiescence of a public official or other person acting in an official capacity.

This, and the other conventions and laws, are intended to refer equally to men and women, of course. Women suffer disproportionately from gender-specific torture, sexual violence and abuse, including rape, deliberate infection with HIV, enforced impregnation, sexual slavery, disfigurement, mutilation of sexual organs and enforced nakedness or sexual humiliation during questioning or detention. It must be remembered that our work with women survivors takes place against a backdrop in which, in every conflict zone, either during a conflict or in its aftermath, sexual violence is inflicted against women on a widespread and systematic scale.

Article 2 of the Torture Convention prohibits torture and requires parties to take effective measures to prevent it in any territory under their jurisdiction. This prohibition is absolute and there are no exceptional circumstances whatsoever. The writers of this book believe that torture can never be justified as a means to protect citizens or prevent emergencies.

Related to our work with survivors of torture is Article 3 of the Torture Convention, which prohibits parties from returning or extraditing individuals to a country where there are 'substantial grounds for believing that he would be in danger of being subjected to torture'.

The right to rehabilitation

Article 14 of the UNCAT states:

> Each state party shall ensure in its legal system that the victim of an act of torture obtains redress and has an enforceable right to fair and adequate compensation, including the means for as full rehabilitation as possible. In the event of the death of the victim as a result of an act of torture, his dependants shall be entitled to compensation.

Refugees and people seeking asylum

I have not summarised the asylum process in the UK as asylum law and processes are constantly changing.

An individual who has left their country of origin to seek safety is referred to as a **person seeking asylum** throughout the book. The term most commonly used in the UK media is 'asylum seeker'. Contributors have chosen not to use this term, as it is commonly used to define the person, rather than describe a legal process in which that person is engaged. A number of contributors have used the term **refugee/s** to refer to both people seeking asylum and those granted asylum.

Under the 1951 United Nations Convention Relating to the Status of Refugees and the 1967 Protocol, a refugee is defined as:

> A person who, owing to a well-founded fear of being persecuted for reasons of race, religion, nationality, membership of a particular social group or political opinion, is outside the country

of his nationality and is unable or, owing to such fear, is unwilling to avail himself of the protection of that country; or who, not having a nationality and being outside the country of his former habitual residence as a result of such events, is unable or, owing to such fear, is unwilling to return to it.

In the UK, a person is considered a refugee when they have had their claim for asylum accepted by the Home Office. A person given refugee status is normally granted leave to remain in the UK for five years.

A person seeking asylum can register their asylum claim in any country that is a signatory to the Refugee Convention. In European countries, people seeking asylum can also register their asylum claims under Article 3 of the European Convention on Human Rights 1950 (ECHR). Where the term 'seeking asylum' is used in this book, the person's claim for asylum has not yet been determined and a grant of status made.

Article 3 (of ECHR) Prohibition of Torture states: 'No one shall be subjected to torture or inhuman or degrading treatment or punishment.'

A person can make a claim for protection based directly on Article 3 of ECHR, as states are prohibited from returning a person to a country where s/he may suffer a violation of their rights under Article 3. A person given protection under Article 3 is normally given humanitarian protection status and granted leave to remain in the UK for five years.

Language of the asylum process

The **Asylum and Immigration Tribunal** or **Asylum Tribunal** is part of Her Majesty's Courts and Tribunals Service (HMCTS), and considers appeals against decisions made by the Home Office in relation to claims for asylum. An **immigration judge** is appointed by the Lord Chancellor to decide appeals made to the Asylum and Immigration Tribunal.

An asylum interview is referred to as a **substantive interview**, and is a fully recorded interview (either by audio or in handwriting) with the person seeking asylum, which is conducted by a Home Office official, normally using a Home Office interpreter. It seeks to establish a person's reasons for claiming asylum in the UK.

The substantive interview follows a **screening interview**, which usually takes place at the point of entry. This is a shorter interview, to establish the person's identity, nationality, route to the UK, liability to return to a third country, eligibility for support, liability to prosecution, and liability to detention. The screening interview is conducted by immigration officers at an asylum screening unit. At this interview, the person will have their photo and fingerprints taken and be issued with an asylum registration card (ARC) as proof that they have registered an asylum claim.

The **Istanbul Protocol** (IP) is the first set of internationally recognised guidelines on the documentation of torture (OHCHR, 1999). It was developed to support the prevention of torture and to hold perpetrators to account in torturing states. It became an official United Nations (UN) document in 1999. In the context of this book, it is the framework in which expert report writers document the physical and psychological evidence of an individual's account of torture. Professional report writers are also informed and guided by the protocol.

Asylum caseworkers at the Home Office make the initial decision on an individual's claim for asylum. They are not required to have any clinical or law qualification.

Asylum support refers to the accommodation and financial support given by the Home Office to people seeking asylum. In the UK, it was previously known as National Asylum Support Service (NASS) support. People in receipt of this support will be placed on a no-choice basis to a dispersal area in the UK, where they are offered accommodation and a weekly cash allowance or card payment to buy food at named supermarkets. Unless they have dependent children, they lose their accommodation and financial support when their asylum claims are rejected and they have no outstanding legal challenges against the negative decision.

The term **Home Office** is used throughout the book to denote the official government immigration agency. The Home Office is the UK government department responsible for immigration, security, law and order. UK Visas and Immigration (UKVI) is currently the department of the Home Office responsible for these matters.

Family reunion is the policy enabling people granted refugee status, or other forms of protection such as humanitarian protection, to apply to bring to the UK people who were part of their family unit before they claimed asylum. Spouses, partners and dependent children are all eligible.

A fresh claim is a new asylum claim made by someone who has had their initial claim rejected. A fresh claim can be prepared and submitted by a legal representative when significant new evidence becomes available that has not been submitted in the initial claim and creates a real prospect of the claim now succeeding. The claimant should not be removed from the UK while the fresh claim is being considered by the Home Office. The claimant should also become eligible for asylum support while their fresh claim is under consideration.

Legal representative is the term used throughout the book for an asylum lawyer, solicitor, barrister or qualified caseworker. Legal representatives providing legal services funded by the Legal Aid Agency (LAA) in the UK are regulated by the Law Society Immigration and Asylum Accreditation Scheme. Other legal representatives providing immigration/asylum advice are regulated by the Office for the Immigration Services Commissioner (OISC).

People seeking asylum in the UK have a right to access legal advice. Because most people seeking asylum are not entitled to work and do not normally have access to any capital they may have held in their home country, most are eligible to receive free advice and representation through the Legal Aid Agency (in Scotland, through the Scottish Legal Aid Board).

An **initial accommodation centre (IAC)** is the initial accommodation where people seeking asylum are placed while they wait for the decision on their application for asylum support. Once support is offered, they are moved to accommodation in a dispersal area.

An **immigration removal centre (IRC)** refers to the detention centres where people are detained under Immigration Act powers, which can happen at any stage in the asylum process. People should only be detained if there are plans to remove them and there is a risk they will abscond, but in the UK they can be detained for long periods of time, including in prisons, under Immigration Act powers. **Removal** is the term used to describe the enforced return to another country of someone whose asylum claim has been rejected in the UK.

An **immigration reporting centre** is where people seeking asylum are expected to report to the immigration authorities in order to maintain contact. People are required to report at their nearest centre at frequencies determined by the Home Office. Some centres are in police stations.

An **age-disputed child** is a young person who has applied for asylum claiming to be a child under 18 years and whose claimed date of birth is not accepted by the Home Office and/or the local authority that has been approached to provide them with support.

Immigration Law Practitioners Association (ILPA) is a membership organisation established to 'promote and improve the advising and representation of immigrants' (www.ilpa.org.uk).

References

OHCHR (1999). *Istanbul Protocol: manual on the effective investigation and documentation of torture and other cruel, inhuman or degrading treatment or punishment.* New York and Geneva: UNHCR.

Introduction – Everyone should know what happens to us

Jude Boyles

My first ever client who was a survivor of torture was an Iranian man called Reza. Two pictures from Tehran that his mother sent me still hang on the wall of my therapy room, and I have thought of him often while editing this book. I read through some of his quotes before writing this introduction – they provide its title and the last words of the book – and was reminded just how overwhelmed and deskilled I felt when we first met. I remember wishing then that there was more guidance for therapists embarking on this work.

Reza once said the following to me, and, in many ways, he is describing the overarching theme of this book – the importance of adopting a holistic and flexible approach:

> One time you helped me with my housing. One time you listened to me about my prison. One time you helped me find peace inside as I was so fear[ful] and panicky, and one time we talked about the politics of my country. But every time you cared for me and were like a sister.

Survivors often tell us that what helps is not just the caring, human presence of a therapist who listens and wants to hear their story, but a therapist who can directly offer help when they need it to manage overwhelming responses to trauma. Our clients also tell us that it is important that we are willing to engage with them in conversations about their home country's politics and the UK government policies that deliberately keep people seeking asylum in poverty: '… torture survivors living in exile in the UK are pushed into poverty by government systems' (Mendez, 2013: 2). They tell us that sometimes we need to act – by writing a letter, chasing the housing provider or ringing their legal representative.

Reza said to me in one of our early sessions: 'Do you know what they do to us in my country? You would not believe it if I tell you.' Sadly, in the UK, survivors are frequently not believed. The UK Parliament's Home Affairs Select Committee (2013: 11) reports that there is a 'tendency of those evaluating asylum applications to start from the assumption that the applicant is not telling the truth'. Following the refusal of his asylum claim, Reza said: 'They say I have lied, but I have not told them most of what they did to me.' He was devastated, and found it almost impossible to find the words to describe the agony of not being believed, and the humiliation of being portrayed 'as a liar'.

Without exception, all the survivors I have worked with have found the process of seeking asylum distressing and humiliating, and many have fared badly within it. I have witnessed how the stress of a badly administered system, long delays and poor decision-making creates high levels of anxiety. I have seen even the most resourceful and resilient survivors worn down by the process, as each year passes. Most survivors live with an inherent dread of their claim being refused and/or being returned to the country from which they fled. The fear of detention is exacerbated when survivors have to report to the UK authorities. An ex-client described to me how the threat of reporting hung over her for most of the month between reporting dates, and she felt safe only for a few days immediately afterwards. Boyles and Shaez (2015: 13) write: '... he has only one or two days after reporting when he feels a sense of relief or safety. Then his anxiety begins to build again towards his next reporting date.' The process of seeking asylum can take from three months to seven or more years, and many people will be separated from their immediate family during that time.

As human rights therapists, we bear witness to these abuses, whether they occur in the country of origin, a third country in transit, or in the UK. We name them as human rights violations. We know that, alongside responding to psychological distress, we need to act to ensure a survivor's basic needs are met and they are made aware of their rights in their country of exile.

Too often, survivors living in poverty or who are homeless and under threat of return are denied access to psychological therapies because of their circumstances. They are told that they cannot 'use treatment effectively' until their life is stable or they have been granted refugee status. This can be a very long wait for most people. Survivors have a right to treatment wherever they are positioned in the asylum process, and they can benefit from therapy at all stages. Therapists must be willing to be flexible and to adapt their models and their sometimes fixed approaches to working with trauma in order to provide help to survivors for whom the trauma is not yet over.

The appalling treatment of people seeking asylum in the UK comes as a shock to many therapists. As a supervisor, I have seen the impact on therapists when they come up against the cruelty of the asylum process for the first time. It is painful for therapists to sit with a client's distress when a full and painfully given disclosure is dismissed in a few lines in a Home Office refusal. We in the west work in a context of racism, xenophobia and anti-migrant feeling, and I have consistently witnessed first-hand the impact this has on clients, therapists and interpreters from refugee and ethnic minority backgrounds.

I have worked in the refugee field for nearly two decades and always knew that any one of my clients could be detained. But one of my worst moments was when it happened for the first time. I felt powerless and outraged, and deeply saddened to witness the mental stability for which he had worked so hard in therapy dissolve in a 'cell' in an immigration removal centre. Sometimes, when we spoke on the phone during his detention, it was evident that the experience was retraumatising him and he was finding it hard to distinguish between his cell in the Democratic Republic of the Congo (DRC) and the one in the UK.

> I am still shocked… I will never forget it. You ask yourself, 'Why am I in prison, I have not done anything?' It is the same. (Boyles & Shaez, 2015: 14)

Reza asked me in our early work together if I knew what torture was. I can't remember my response to him, but I remember we talked of his fear that I could not possibly understand what it is to be tortured, not knowing if you will live or die, day after day. It is daunting to try to summarise the range of experiences and forms of torture I have come across in my working life, but it also feels important that I try, as the details of torture are easy to avoid. Survivors are imprisoned by the state or organised groups, and may be tortured for weeks, months or years. Some are held in camps, brutally beaten and raped, and escape after a few weeks. Many live in such camps for years. Survivors are beaten, whipped, burned, electrocuted, suspended, have nails removed or limbs chopped off, and are sexually violated in numerous, cruel ways. They are held in packed, stinking cells, naked with no facilities to wash. They are subjected to sexual violence by other prisoners and repeated rape by their guards. Some are held in solitary confinement. They may have to urinate and defecate in their cell. The smells are unbearable and can haunt a survivor for years after. Prisoners hear the screams of others being tortured, or are made to witness or take part in torture or other atrocities, or they see family members or colleagues killed. It is not just adults who are tortured, but children and young people too.

Many survivors describe mock executions and other forms of humiliation that are hard to bear and leave them feeling ashamed and defeated. Food and/or water are often given just once a day, and can be foul or contaminated. Survivors are made to lie in the sun or drink urine. Women are forced to become sexual slaves to soldiers, and both women and men are forced to undertake hard labour. They are threatened, mocked and stripped of all dignity. They are forced into painful positions and kept awake by water being repeatedly thrown into the cell or by continuous loud noises. For some, imprisonment with others may provide some comfort and a sense of solidarity. For many, the cell is also a place of violence.

I have worked with activists who were detained and tortured several times and who had some expectation of being imprisoned and/or harmed. Others were not political activists, but were attending their first demonstration, or were lesbian or gay or from a persecuted minority tribe. Some had a family member who was active or involved in politics. Many women describe sexual violence that began in childhood and continued into marriage, as well as repeated rape in conflict: 'Many states exhibit a societal acceptance of widespread and systematic violence perpetrated against women, where abuse forms part of women's daily lives' (Smith & Boyles, 2009: 8).

Some survivors leave quickly following their release or escape from prison; others plan their journey into exile with their political party and/or family over many months. Many do not remember how they got to the UK, or describe long and traumatic journeys. Some leave with family; others leave their family behind, hoping to be reunited soon. Some planned to come to Europe; many did not know their destination until after they arrived.

All leave behind their culture and homeland, and a known way of life. They leave behind their family, community, work, political life, home and friends. Some survivors have left developing countries and/or countries in conflict, where access to food, education and healthcare is limited. Others have left countries and lives where they had established careers as engineers, lawyers, farmers, and have lost their professional identity, their business and their land.

The UNHCR, the United Nations refugee agency, estimates that there are 59.5 million forcibly displaced people in the world. Women and girls will make up 50% of these. Around 86% of all refugees are displaced within the developing world, not to industrialised countries (UNHCR, 2017).

I approached the contributors to this book because they all have significant experience of working with survivors and share a commitment to human rights. Some are based in NHS primary or secondary care psychological therapy services; others work in third-sector specialist or refugee therapy services. A number work or have worked in rehabilitation centres for survivors of torture. What we all have in common is a commitment to work holistically, from a rights-based approach.

Our aim is to share what we have learnt with therapists who are working in a range of settings. We are aware that most therapists do not have access to in-house services, such as advocacy or physical therapies, to support their work with survivors, who may have multiple, complex social and medical/health needs. It is our hope that this book will inform and give confidence to practitioners that there is much they can offer in their day-to-day work with survivors of torture.

As human rights practitioners, we believe in the right of survivors of torture to rehabilitation and justice. Article 14 of the UN Convention Against Torture (UNCAT) (OHCHR, 1984) entails a duty on member states to provide effective rehabilitation to survivors. Rehabilitation is an 'important component of reparation', and the UN Basic Principles on remedies for victims require that 'rehabilitation should include medical and psychological care as well as legal and social services' (Mendez, 2013: 2).

Rehabilitation may hold a different meaning for therapists working in the torture field than for those in social care. For the purposes of this book, we define rehabilitation as the right to physical and psychological care that supports a survivor to recover from their experiences, as well as access to a range of services that meet their multiple needs, including legal, medical, social and educational.

It is important to remember that not all survivors are traumatised, and not all need or want therapy. Many survivors I have met have been saddened and distressed by their experiences of torture, but their difficulties have been to do with living in exile and being separated from their family and homeland, as well as the stress of the asylum process. Therapy is not for everyone, and many survivors would not choose a talking therapy. Many will recover or choose to seek support from within their families, communities, in women's groups or with fellow activists and survivors, friends and allies. When asked, many would probably put other concerns or issues first, before therapy: the right to work, to be treated with dignity and respect, to fairness and not to be kept waiting endlessly in the asylum process, and to an asylum process that is itself independent of the government agenda. Survivors often say that they just want to be allowed to rebuild their lives in safety, with community support, and access to education and training.

I once asked a survivor, Amy, who came from Burundi and had been waiting for four years for a decision on her claim for asylum, what she wanted from therapy. I suspect the question held little meaning for her. She said:

> I want to go home and be safe, if you don't want me here, and if I can't do that, I want them [the Home Office] to let me stay, leave me in peace so I can rebuild my life. I don't need your help; I just need my visa [grant of refugee status] so I can live.

Therapists in this book reflect on how hard it can be at times to remain confident that the very practice of therapy and the ways in which we understand trauma will not further oppress and undermine those we are seeking to help. Many of us struggle daily with the fear that we are applying individualistic approaches to working with trauma and distress that do not respect 'the complexity of how different human beings living in different cultures respond to terrifying events' (Bracken, 2002: 80). As a white therapist practising in the refugee field in the racialised context of the UK, I am very conscious of the considerable power I hold as a professional. I am reminded daily of my ability to oppress, influence or harm people through my belief system and frameworks for understanding and 'treating' distress. Working self-reflexively is at the core of the work, and of this book, as is ensuring we are properly supported and trained to undertake this work.

Many of the writers refer to Judith Herman's wonderful book, *Trauma and Recovery* (1992). The first three chapters of this book reflect Herman's three-stage approach to working with survivors of atrocity. In the first chapter, I explore my experience of assessing survivors holistically, and emphasise the importance of providing direct help where possible in early sessions, to instil hope and support engagement. I advocate for an assessment process that gives both client and therapist time to fully explore the full range of difficulties, and thereby ensure that we establish a sense of safety before trauma work is undertaken. In Chapter 2, Norma McKinnon reflects with her client, Kevin, a survivor of torture from Darfur, what made the difference for him in his therapy and his experience of processing his painful history in Sudan. In chapter 3, Kirsten Lamb draws on her work in both an NHS secondary care service and a torture rehabilitation centre to explore the final phase of work with survivors, that of reconnection.

Next Rajita Rajeshwar considers how therapists might facilitate conversations about racial and ethnic differences in therapy and shares her own experiences of working with survivors, as a second-generation British Tamil.

In the next chapter, we are given a first-hand account of torture by Prossy Kakooza, a lesbian survivor of torture from Uganda. Prossy was imprisoned and tortured because of her sexuality, and describes vividly the benefits and challenges of having counselling in the UK. Prossy reminds therapists to learn about the asylum process, in order to better understand the context in which survivors are living. Linking with this, in Chapter 6, Katie Whitehouse shares her work with women survivors in a women-only setting in Leeds, and reminds us of the limitations of the international legal framework to protect women from gender-based abuses. Katie emphasises that psychotherapy cannot be undertaken without attention to the social, cultural and political context of women's lives, and an understanding of the discrimination women have lived with in their home country and continue to live with in the UK. Her chapter explores how women's experience of torture is very different to that of men, and how they are also exposed to other forms of gender-based abuse, such as female genital mutilation, domestic violence and forced marriage.

Next, in Chapter 7, Ann Salter shares her work with separated young people, and encourages therapists to be mindful of the impact on young people of being separated from their family and the risks they are exposed to in exile, as well as the challenges they face in the asylum process.

Colsom Bashir worked for many years as a specialist clinical psychologist for refugees within the NHS in a deprived area of Greater Manchester. In the first of two chapters, Colsom addresses the very central issue of shame, which features in many survivors' narratives, and encourages us to ensure we place these narratives in the context of the wider narratives and social purposes of shame.

The NHS in England offers few choices to people seeking psychological help, and CBT is currently the model offered by most providers. In chapter 9, Colsom provides guidance for CBT therapists on working from a human rights framework in a setting where therapists may be working within significant time constraints and other limits imposed by their organisation.

Next, Ashley Fletcher, a gay activist and psychotherapist from Manchester, describes his work with gay men who have been tortured because of their sexual orientation. He emphasises the importance of the commitment to supporting survivors' applications for asylum, by writing professional reports and letters. He points out that the therapist is in a powerful position to document and testify to the impact of torture on a survivor, but also to provide the decision-maker with an understanding of the experience of being gay in the survivor's country of origin.

In chapter 11, Emma Roberts turns the focus on a very important aspect of the work – the needs of survivors who have come as a family, or have been reunited in the UK. Emma came to train in systemic family work through having had to manage situations where women survivors with no access to childcare arrived at therapy sessions with their child. Her chapter describes vividly the difficulties and dilemmas facing the therapist when seeking to hold the distress of families where the roles of the parents have been reversed and their children have abandoned cultural and religious beliefs and practices deeply held by their parents.

Next, Carl Dutton describes his work with survivors at the Haven project, in Liverpool, which is now closed – a casualty, along with so many other wonderful projects, of the last decade of austerity. Carl argues for a creative and community-based approach to supporting survivors and shares some of the groupwork that was at the core of the Haven's approach.

In her second chapter, Chapter 13, Ann Salter examines the issue of trauma and attachment in her work with young people, and the impact of torture on development. Ann's chapter is relevant for those working with children and young people, as well as therapists working with adults who may have been tortured as children or young people.

Working with interpreters is a skill with which most therapists will not be familiar. It can provoke anxiety, and the therapist can experience the interpreter as an intruder. There can be an assumption that having a third person in the room negatively impacts on the client, and inhibits the therapist in developing a therapeutic alliance. In Chapter 14, the first of two chapters on working with interpreters, I, with my former colleagues Desiré Kinané and Nathalie Talbot, argue the need for therapists to regard the interpreter as a partner in the therapy triangle, and we share our experience of developing those working relationships to benefit survivors. We argue that the skilled interpreter also bears witness to the survivor's narrative, alongside the therapist, and can be a warm and affirming presence that supports a survivor's recovery.

The chapter offers practical advice on how to engage suitable interpreters and on good practice in joint working. In the following Chapter 15, Beverley Costa, from the groundbreaking Mothertongue project, explores the training and supervision needs of interpreters, and unpacks some of the common dynamics in the triadic relationship.

In Chapter 16, Jess Michaelson examines the impact on the therapist of working with survivors. She shares her own experience of finding a place of internal safety in which to practise safely and offers guidance on how we can mitigate against vicarious trauma. Importantly, she also writes about how the work with survivors can help therapists to grow professionally and build personal resilience.

Our final chapter is by social worker Anna Turner, who provides an insight into social work with survivors. She emphasises the key role of social work in the refugee sector and outlines the core principles underpinning social work today and its potential to bring about social change and the empowerment and liberation of people. Anna argues that social justice, human rights, collective responsibility and respect for diversity are central to social work practice, and highly applicable to working with survivors of torture and their families in exile.

This book doesn't claim to be a comprehensive or definitive picture of work with survivors of torture in exile. It is a snapshot of these individual practitioners' experience, and the stories of some of their clients. Kevin speaks for so many people like him when he asks (Chapter 2): 'Do I not have a right to live? Do I not have the rights of a human being?' The chapters that follow describe how these authors have sought to answer those questions.

References

Boyles J, Shaez M (2015). In the shadow of detention. *Therapy Today* 26(4): 10–16.

Bracken P (2002). *Trauma: culture, meaning and philosophy.* London: Whurr Publishers.

Herman JL (1992). *Trauma and Recovery: the aftermath of violence – from domestic abuse to political terror.* New York: Basic Books.

Home Affairs Select Committee (2013). *Asylum: seventh report of session 2013–14.* London: Stationery Office. https://publications.parliament.uk/pa/cm201314/cmselect/emhaff/71/71.pdf (accessed July 2017).

Smith E, Boyles J (2009). *Justice Denied: the experience of 100 torture surviving women of seeking justice and rehabilitation.* London: Medical Foundation for the Care of Victims of Torture

Mendez JE (2013). Foreword. In: Pettitt J (ed). *The Poverty Barrier: the right to rehabilitation for survivors of torture in the UK.* London: Freedom from Torture.

OHCHR (1984). *Convention Against Torture and Other Cruel, Inhuman or Degrading Treatment or Punishment (UNCAT).* Geneva: OHCHR.

UNHCR (2017). *Global Trends: forced displacement in 2016.* Geneva: UNHCR. www.unhcr.org/uk/statistics/unhcrstats/5943e8a34/global-trends-forced-displacement-2016.html?query=global%20trends%202016 (accessed July 2017).

1. Assessing survivors of torture for psychological therapy
Jude Boyles

> What constitutes a broken spirit? What does it mean when the core of the self and identity begins to fragment and unravel, like a tightly wound ball of string that gets dropped and loses its layers of thread nicely wound together? (Wilson, 2004: 110)

This chapter aims to share my experience of undertaking assessments with survivors of torture who are refugees or seeking asylum in the UK. As a human-rights therapist, my approach to assessment reflects my commitment to bear witness to the atrocities a person has survived, with the responsibility that carries. Working from a human-rights framework means that I am required to take action both inside and outside the therapy room, as well as stand alongside survivors in the struggle to prevent torture and achieve justice, protection and rehabilitation for survivors.

Torture is a sustained and gross abuse of a person's human rights, defined as 'any act by which severe pain or suffering, whether physical or mental, is intentionally inflicted on a person' (OHCHR, 1984). Elsass states: 'The aim of torture is not always to make the victim confess and give information. The primary aim is more to break down the identity of the victim. The pain consists in particular in this breaking down and in the destruction of the personality' (1997: 10).

Therapists worldwide have reported varied approaches to working with traumatised survivors, but, at the time of writing, no one model has emerged as the most effective. This is hardly surprising, as Aroche and Coello point out, 'given the diversity of refugees and asylum seekers as a group and the variety of clinical presentations encountered' (2004: 70).

Prevalence of depression, anxiety and post-traumatic stress disorder (PTSD) is higher among people seeking asylum than in the general UK population (Turner & Gorst-Unsworth, 1990; van der Veer, 1998; Lavik et al, 1996; Fazel, Wheeler & Danesh, 2005).

The asylum system itself can be experienced as retraumatising and dehumanising, and many survivors describe living in constant fear of detention and/or removal to their own or a transit country, and that this fear is exacerbated by the requirement to report to the authorities on a regular basis.

In the UK, most cities and towns accommodating people seeking asylum do not have refugee therapy services, let alone torture rehabilitation services. This means that therapists are not usually working alongside a team of colleagues who can attend to the medical, physical, social, legal and welfare needs of survivors. Kira (2002) has developed a model of torture rehabilitation called the Wraparound Approach, which is delivered by community treatment teams and involves community support, networking and family work, as well as individual therapy for the survivor. Most torture rehabilitation services across the globe apply this holistic, multidisciplinary approach, where psychosocial and physical rehabilitation sit alongside medico-legal documentation, torture prevention, legal and welfare advocacy and survivor activism.

In this chapter, I will explore how therapists can apply a holistic and human-rights framework to working with torture survivors that is applicable in any clinical setting. A holistic approach aims to attend to the whole person:

> A shattered life needs multiple levels of intervention in striving to become whole again, especially in a situation in which real-life tragedy continues and can never be reversed, can never be made whole again. (Graessner, Gurris & Pross, 1996: xxi)

We know that survivors of torture benefit from early access to psychosocial support, but many will not be referred for therapy until they are in crisis. 'Early psychosocial support is a decisive factor in the development and severity of PTSD symptoms' (Drožđek & Wilson, 2004: 245).

Survivors will be referred for assessment at all stages of seeking asylum. They may be referred on arrival to the UK, unaware of the difficult challenges ahead and relieved to be safe. Others may be referred after several years of failed asylum claims, and present with chronic difficulties and little trust in helping services, having lost hope that they will ever be granted protection. Many therapists ask if it is ethical, appropriate and/or safe to offer therapy to traumatised survivors who are still in the asylum process, when their future is still unclear and the trauma is not yet over for them. It is my experience that, following a thorough assessment and a period of stabilising work, many traumatised survivors can and do process traumatic experiences effectively while still in the asylum process. Many survivors may choose not to narrate the trauma story, and it is not always a therapeutic necessity. Therapy that aims to stabilise psychological health as well as attend to the physical and social context can be profoundly helpful. The 'assumption that asylum seekers should "survive" migration and a long application procedure before treatment is potentially pathogenic' (Drožđek & Wilson, 2004: 245).

At whatever stage the assessment takes place, be prepared to offer a longer assessment; two to four sessions provide enough space to fully explore the range of difficulties experienced by the survivor, and their impact.

My work is guided by Judith Herman's three-phase approach to working with trauma, as is that of many of the contributors to this book. Here, the 'central task of the first stage is the establishment of safety, before reconstructing the trauma story' (1992: 3).

The case studies used are fictional and based on amalgamated examples from my practice over the last 18 years.

Survivors in exile

Torture survivors seeking asylum in the UK are accommodated on a 'no-choice' basis, usually in deprived areas and in multiple-occupancy housing. They are denied the right to work or to claim welfare benefits, and are given Home Office financial support amounting to some 54–70% of Income Support. 'Torture survivors living in exile in the UK are pushed into poverty by government systems' (Mendez, 2013: 2).

Most survivors will be feeling stressed and overwhelmed by the asylum process. They may be feeling exhausted or defeated by the bureaucracy, long waits and poor decision-making inherent in the UK asylum system (Amnesty International, 2004).

Separation, multiple losses and the sudden or violent death of family members and friends are endemic in the experiences of refugees. Even when a family is able to seek asylum together, there may be loved ones left behind: immediate family members, and others, such as nieces and nephews, who were part of their family life. For many refugees, relatives, friends or colleagues may be missing or disappeared.[1]

---

1. In international human rights law, a person who is 'disappeared' has been abducted or imprisoned by the state, or by an organised political group with the authority of the state or a political organisation. Their disappearance is not acknowledged.

Survivors will have lost not just their home but their homeland and community, their political identity, job, career, and their hopes for their future and that of their family. They may have lost land and farm stock, or it may have been seized. They may have lost ancestral places, social ceremonies and rituals. Their traditional skills may have no place in their country of exile. The loss of social structure and culture can cause a profound grief reaction, described by Eisenbruch as cultural bereavement (1990).

Papadopoulos argues that an important function of 'home' is that it anchors and gives coherence to a family's story and that, 'regardless of the shape or style of home, all human beings have a sense of home... which often evokes powerful feelings, be they positive or negative' (2002: 10). Home may have been a loving and close family in a war-torn country with limited access to food, water and healthcare, or home could be a hidden world of violent oppression amid relative privilege.

Women survivors are likely to come from societies where they have experienced profound oppression and violence as part of daily life, and will describe long histories of abuse that preceded the torture. Some may be unaccustomed to having any say or control in their lives, and may have been excluded from public life; some may have been activists. As Summerfield writes, women refugees are frequently portrayed as victims and 'this has tended to obscure the extent to which women made significant contributions to political struggles' (1996: 4). The Freedom from Torture report *Rape as Torture in the DRC* found that the most common reason for women's imprisonment and torture was political activism – their affiliation to or perceived membership of groups opposed to the state (2014: 35).

The context of the asylum process, the status in the west of people seeking protection, and the denial of their basic human rights mean that survivors may come to an assessment needing more practical support than most therapists would normally expect to offer. In addition, survivors are likely to be unfamiliar with the UK's social, legal and cultural systems, and may ask the therapist for advice and information. This can create an unfamiliar challenge for therapists new to working with refugees. Gurris advises that the therapist can become a representative of the country for the client, and so our role is to 'educate patients about this alien culture in a manner that is enlightening, sensitive and neither injurious or condescending' (2001: 41).

Establishing safety

> The feeling of trust in the world, both human and natural, which is essential to ordinary life, has been broken apart, and people describe living in a meaningless void. (Bracken, 2002: 142)

Establishing safety is part of the assessment process and should start the minute a survivor is welcomed into the clinical space. The therapeutic assessment will be more accessible if the therapy room is comfortable, welcoming and non-clinical, and survivors can recognise art or objects from their own and other cultures. Survivors have described feeling reassured when they have recognised a picture from their country, and that this suggested to them that the organisation was both welcoming to refugees and culturally diverse. As van der Veer emphasises (1993), every contact with the agency is important, from the initial phone contact with the receptionist to the welcome in the building and the waiting room. 'For most of us, putting the client at ease, perhaps offering them a cup of tea, or talking about the journey, is more important at the very beginning than anything else' (Chaplin, 1988: 25).

It can be helpful to assume that the survivor will have little experience of therapy and of talking to strangers as a way of resolving personal difficulties. It is important to establish trust and rapport before you start asking questions about very personal and sensitive issues. The dynamic of the professional helping relationship may be new to the survivor, and much of what a therapist usually says and does might be culturally inappropriate and incomprehensible. Even an open, gentle, enquiring approach may be unfamiliar to some, and may feel a bit disconcerting and uncomfortable. Herman writes that, when working with survivors of trauma, the 'single most common therapeutic error is avoidance of the traumatic material', but she argues that the 'second most common error is premature or precipitate engagement in exploratory work, without sufficient attention to the tasks of establishing safety and securing a therapeutic alliance' (Herman, 1992: 155–156).

The usual seating arrangement, where a therapist sits across from a survivor and makes eye contact, 'can function in a way that diminishes and that harbors a danger of retraumatising torture victims' (Graessner, Gurris & Pross, 1996: 39). Put simply, it may remind them of past interrogations. Pace the intensity of your gaze, and allow the client to adjust to your attentiveness. Bryant-Jefferies talks of inviting the client back 'into a human relationship, not forcing' (2005: 15). Elsass emphasizes the importance of creating a 'therapeutic space in which the torture survivor can feel safe and prepared' (1997: 89).

Survivors describe how they are made to feel like criminals and frequently face hostility, xenophobia and racism in the communities where they are accommodated, and barriers to services when they seek help. The harsh realities of a survivor's life in exile can lead many to lose hope and anticipate a hostile or indifferent response when approaching a service or meeting a professional for the first time. Malloch and Stanley describe how '[m]edia and political representations of asylum seekers and refugees have been infused with language denoting images of "danger", "criminality" and "risk"' (2005: 1).

Therapy may be familiar to survivors who have sought help from health professionals in the past, either in the UK and/or before they fled their country of origin. However, it can still be useful to assume that there are few shared understandings about the therapeutic relationship: '... human action takes place in a reality of understanding that is created through social construction and dialogue. From this position, people live, and understand their living, through socially constructed narrative realities that give meaning and organisation to their experience' (Anderson & Goolishian, 1992: 2).

In my experience, it can be helpful for the therapist to introduce themselves to a new client in the waiting area, separately from the interpreter, so that the therapist is the first point of contact for a survivor. If the interpreter is introduced by the therapist in the therapy room, it can help establish the therapist and interpreter as a partnership (good practice in working with interpreters is covered in Chapter 14).

Every assessment starts with introductions, but take more time to do this: it will help the survivor adjust to this new environment and enable them to evaluate the skills of the interpreter. Survivors may be assessing what the therapist can offer, whether the interpreter can be trusted, and whether the agency is benign. Tell them who made the referral and explain how the agency relates to the healthcare system and, if relevant, the voluntary sector structure. Share what you already know about the survivor.

Ask how they like to be addressed. It shows respect and illustrates your approach of seeking their consent throughout the assessment and therapy process. In many cases, survivors' names have been misspelt, or they are referred to by their family name rather than their first or preferred name. Names may have been shortened to make them easier to pronounce, or the survivor may have used a false name to travel to the UK. It is rare that anyone official has taken the time to find out their full name, its meaning for them, and what they prefer to be called, let alone attempted to pronounce it properly.

After a few minutes, pause and check that the client is understanding the interpreter. If the survivor launches straight into talking about their problems, gently slow their narrative and remind them that it is helpful if they can just speak in two sentences at a time, so the interpreter can capture and translate everything they say in the way that they say it. How well you work in the therapist–client–interpreter triad at assessment can influence the success of the rest of the therapy, so you need to identify and address poor practice by the interpreter or misuse of the interpreter by the client as soon as you can.

Explain the confidentiality policy of the agency in a way that the client will understand, and make sure they have understood when you might need to break confidentiality. In most clinical settings, therapists are required to use self-report questionnaires to assess the client's mental health. The practice is to apply questionnaires developed in the west and translated from English. These tools are often diagnosis- or symptoms-based. Given the diversity in the refugee population, it is not easy to find tools that are appropriate for a survivor's reading skills (if they are able to read) and cultural and educational background. The development of torture-specific tools is at a very early stage internationally, and there is no space to expand on this work here. Whatever tool is being used, spend time explaining it to the survivor. Clients may find it distressing and invasive to be asked direct questions about their private thoughts and feelings. Be prepared to put the questionnaire aside if it is distressing the client – it could harm engagement or lead to over-arousal. 'The use of standardized instruments for psychological assessment of torture victims must be done with great care. For some victims, the test-taking situation may be too evocative of the torture situation' (Pope & Garcia-Peltoniemi, 1991).

Explain the purpose of the assessment, what will be discussed and over how many sessions. Tell the survivor how long each session will be and why. Try to limit unpredictability and be alert to cues from the survivor. Notice if they react to a particular movement or noise, so they know they have your full attention and that you are familiar with torture and its impact. Explain that you are a qualified practitioner and briefly outline how therapy can help. If appropriate, talk to them about therapy, and how it is a western construct. Find out if they have anything similar in their home country. Ask gently what they would call a particular mental health problem in their language, or how a symptom is understood in their culture. Try to find out how people seek help for these kinds of problems in their home country and what has helped them in the past.

Be clear about how you can help, and what you can and cannot do for them; this will establish your credibility. Be prepared to give time to explaining your approach; it may need revisiting several times during the assessment. Try to avoid asking too many open questions, as survivors may misinterpret a non-directive approach: 'Many refugees are unfamiliar with this approach, misinterpreting it as a sign of inadequacy or lack of interest' (van der Veer & Waning, 2004: 187).

'Their bodies re-experience terror, rage and helplessness, as well as the impulse to fight or flee, but these feelings are almost impossible to articulate' (van der Kolk, 2014: 43). Survivors who are traumatised and want to avoid feeling overwhelmed or exposed may give short, anxious answers, to keep themselves intact, and only later are able to articulate the terror and humiliation of torture. 'It may be a therapeutic mistake to provoke an exploration and identification of the feelings due to torture. In this stage, the survivor has a primary need for control and safety' (Elsass, 1997: 78). Pacing is vital to minimise the risk of over-arousal in the early stages of engagement.

Van der Veer and Waning describe safety as 'including protection from the maltreatment of others and care for basic needs such as safe living quarters, eating and sleeping properly, medical care, financial security and a supportive social network' (2004: 188). You will therefore need to gather information well beyond what is usually sought in assessments, so you can gauge the stability of a survivor's living situation and the full range of stressors to which they may be exposed. You will need to get details of their legal representative, asylum status, financial and housing support arrangements and date of arrival. If you work for a specialist refugee therapy service, you may also want to record how often they have to report to the immigration reporting centre.

Asking for these details may help survivors feel reassured that the therapist understands the asylum context. Therapists need to know how the asylum process works and what housing and financial support arrangements are in place for people seeking asylum. If therapists are unfamiliar with the process, they may find it difficult to provide a containing environment in times of crisis, when any of these systems breaks down. The Refugee Council provides information in several languages about the UK asylum process and support arrangements (www.refugeecouncil.org.uk).

In my first few weeks of working with refugees, a survivor from Afghanistan brought a Home Office refusal to therapy. He was devastated, and terrified of being returned. At the time, I knew little of the asylum process and felt overwhelmed and frightened too. I thought he might be detained and returned to Afghanistan immediately. If I had known at the time that his legal representative would appeal this decision and it wasn't 'the end', I would have been able to provide a more containing space for him to explore his outrage, and ensured that he was able to consult his legal representative quickly.

You are very likely to find yourself acting as an advocate for a client, or referring them to community support networks. This can make a real difference to a client's circumstances, and be actively therapeutic. A client may not have the information, language and/or power to act for themselves in many situations. Linking survivors to social support can be enormously helpful in the immediate and long term. Find out if they have ever attended English classes, or if they attend a church or mosque or other faith group – all these factors will help you find out about their wider sources of support and resources. Communities can be a powerful aid in the rehabilitation process: 'Survivors are often psychologically and physically isolated from community life, by their torture and by their need to flee for safety' (Bothne & Keys, 2016: 4).

The assessment process itself has the potential to revictimise a survivor when they are already feeling diminished and ashamed for not being able to manage. This, alongside the intimacy and exposure of the therapeutic encounter, can feel very confusing and uncomfortable. Keep finding opportunities throughout the assessment to recognise and validate the fact that they have survived; notice and point out the positive strategies they are using day to day, to remind them of their resilience and strengths. Survivors may feel ashamed about seeking help, and so it can be useful to 'reframe accepting help as an act of courage' (Herman, 1992: 159). Survivors may even regard asking for help as a sign that the torturers have successfully broken them.

Responding to crises

In our second assessment appointment, Reza, a survivor from Iran, arrived frightened and distressed: the night before, his house had been surrounded by young people, and bottles had been thrown at him. He was newly arrived, didn't speak English, and didn't know who to contact at the housing provider, or how to get in touch with them to request an urgent relocation. He was not sure what his rights were and didn't expect his complaint to be heard, given his negative and hostile experiences of the authorities in the UK. I picked up the phone and he was quickly relocated to a safer house. 'Empowerment is claimed to be at the heart of therapy. But the ability of a person to change his/her personal circumstances through therapy is dictated, limited, or moulded by social power' (McLeod, 2004: 375).

It is inevitable, when working with survivors of torture seeking asylum, that crises in their daily life will enter the therapy room. McFarlane argues: '... there are few situations that are more challenging than the assessment of the individual caught in the midst of a life and death struggle for survival' (2004: 83).

The assessment period is very likely to be interrupted with crises related to the asylum process. Therapists in most settings will not see it as their role to advocate or undertake practical tasks, but you can provide information, refer the survivor to other agencies, write letters or just check that another service is providing advocacy and support. Simply signposting survivors can be unhelpful, and many will not follow up suggestions to attend services they do not know or trust. This is particularly the case when the survivor is signposted to non-refugee services.

It is always shocking, even to therapists experienced in this work, when financial and housing support are withdrawn from a client who is appeal rights exhausted (ARE). It is impossible to overestimate the impact on clients. Sitting with someone when they have received the news (I've found myself having to explain to survivors what the letter means when they have brought it to the session) is one of the hardest things I have done in my working life. The collapse of a survivor's claim for asylum is a frightening time and confronts them with the likelihood of detention and/or removal to the country they have fled. 'The threat of detention and/or removal hangs over our clients from arrival and can last many years' (Boyles, 2015: 12). Ethically and therapeutically, imminent homelessness cannot be ignored; putting aside this immediate, pressing need is likely to rupture any therapeutic alliance. However, while a practical response to the crisis is immediately reassuring, it must sit alongside an assessment of the survivor's mental health. Responding to a housing crisis so early on in a developing relationship may establish a dynamic that can be difficult to return from, so careful negotiation with the survivor about when you will advocate on their behalf is vital as therapy progresses.

That the survivor has asked for help should also be seen as a strength: 'Their perception that the therapist's intervention will enable greater access for them is (also) reasonable, especially given the current political climate, with its consequent growth of prejudice. By using what they know and asking for help, they are not relinquishing autonomy but acting with autonomy' (West, 2006: 12).

Psychological assessment

> ... human suffering is not always synonymous with psychological trauma and discerning the delicate balance between therapeutic intervention and therapeutic witnessing is not easy.
> (Papadopoulos, 2002: 39)

It almost goes without saying that, in order to provide therapeutic assistance a traumatised survivor of torture, one of the therapist's tasks must be to assess whether the survivor is traumatised by their experiences. Not all survivors are traumatised by the torture; they may be distressed or experiencing what Papadopoulos refers to as 'ordinary human suffering' (2007).

Trauma cannot be worked with if it has not been diagnosed or named. However, working with trauma may be new for some therapists, and training in trauma work is essential if you are to work effectively and safely with survivors. Whatever words we use to describe how someone responds to a traumatic event, or events – PTSD, complex PTSD or continuing traumatic stress (CTS) – understanding our response to extreme events can help survivors 'recognise the harmful nature of the abuse and provides a reasonable explanation for the patient's persistent difficulties' (Herman, 1994: 158).

Therapists working from a human-rights framework may be anxious that we are pathologising a survivor's responses by adopting a diagnostic framework, and worry that this will invalidate the refugee experience and obscure the social injustice. Some therapists in the refugee field consider that the diagnostic label of PTSD 'does not recognise the shattered individual, familial and communal lives of torture victims – a shattering that goes far beyond the specific clinical syndrome of a single individual' (Laub, 2001: xix). Afuape writes: 'The PTSD diagnosis cannot take account of the magnitude, depth and complexity of refugee people's experience in its entirety' (2011: 53). Summerfield argues that using what he regards as a narrow, diagnostic approach 'risks creating inappropriate sick roles and sidelines a proper incorporation of people's own choices, traditions and skills into strategies for their creative survival. It also aggrandizes the role of western experts and their mental health technology, which is assumed to be universally applicable' (1996: 4).

In my experience, not naming and failing to provide a framework for understanding a survivor's response to horrific events can leave them feeling frightened, confused and overwhelmed by symptoms they do not understand or know how to manage. Survivors describe the relief of understanding why they have these symptoms and are reassured that there are established ways of helping people manage these responses. Psychoeducation can provide both hope and reassurance: 'It is difficult enough to deal solely with the symptoms of trauma without the added anxiety of not knowing why we are experiencing them or whether they will cease' (Levine, 1997: 46). Alongside this, naming the injury acknowledges that a crime/s has been committed, that it has a consequence, and that, with this acknowledgement, comes a right to rehabilitation.

Most survivors will describe sleeplessness, nightmares, flashbacks, anxiety, panic attacks and intrusive thoughts. Many will struggle to concentrate, worry that they cannot remember dates and times, and have a sense of dread and hopelessness about the future. When exploring a survivor's psychological health, it can be reassuring if you don't appear overly concerned or deeply affected by what the client tells you; it may reduce a survivor's feelings of shame and anxiety. Techniques to help manage their symptoms, such as breathing, grounding, mindfulness or relaxation methods, can be introduced at assessment and built on in the early stages of your work together. It can be useful to share what other survivors have found helpful, and to offer some suggestions for self-care. Be careful not to undermine a survivor's understanding of their health crisis, and always be clear that what is happening may be a rational, normal response to the extremity of their current situation. Pace your explanations about trauma, and work towards a culturally congruent, shared framework of understanding: 'If the client's problems are conceptualised in a manner that is incongruent with the client's belief systems, the credibility of the therapist is diminished' (Elsass, 1997: 124).

Bear in mind that hearing the voices of the torturer and other auditory and visual hallucinations are common and disturbing aspects of complex trauma. A survivor may find it particularly hard to disclose that they are hearing voices. However, it may be culturally unexceptional for others. Pay attention to the meaning of the voices from a cultural perspective.

Elssas argues that the therapist working with survivors of torture must attend to existential dilemmas in their work: 'Meaninglessness, alienation and shame are some of the all-important and very specific sequelae of torture' (1997: 37). Be prepared to engage with feelings of separation, alienation and loneliness, and loss of meaning and purpose in life. Some clients will come up with these questions the moment you sit down together; others will turn to the search for meaning as the therapy progresses. 'The individual knows how fellow human beings can act towards one another, people who, as is often the case, will have been living side by side with each other. There is something about this knowing of the capacity of the human being to inflict pain and suffering that has a significantly traumatising effect' (Bryant-Jefferies, 2005: 15).

If a survivor is traumatised and highly symptomatic, recommend that they make an appointment with their GP to discuss if pharmacological treatment might be helpful, alongside psychological therapy.

Assessing suicide risk

> It is important to consider what a man must have suffered and endured in order to feel glad at the thought of his impending execution. (Grossman, 2006: 200)

People seeking asylum are at high risk of suicide, as Juliet Cohen's study, *Safe in Our Hands?* (2008), reveals. Most therapists will be familiar with assessing suicide risk. However, many survivors will be reluctant to talk about their suicidal thoughts, for religious or cultural reasons. Developing a plan to keep a survivor safe can be difficult when the person is isolated, has no family and few friends in the UK and may not be known to their GP. It is harder still if the survivor has little or no English, no credit on their mobile telephone and no cash to pay for transport to visit friends or relatives in the UK, or to access support services,

Increased risk of suicide is strongly linked with fears of being forcibly returned to their country of origin. If a person has received bad news about their claim for asylum, the risk can escalate. For many survivors, it is at the point of detention, or on the day of the forced return, that the risk becomes acute.

A therapist's role is to instil and hold hope for the client at this point, and ensure that all possible support and advice is in place to help them manage. 'What clients need from us is hope, reassurance and a calm determination to do all that we can to help within our role' (Boyles, 2015: 53). It may seem a hopeless situation, but there may be other challenges a legal representative can make following a lost appeal. Clients facing destitution and homelessness can be put in touch with voluntary sector and other organisations offering shelter, food parcels and small amounts of money to buy phone cards or weekly bus tickets.

Having a safe and welcoming place to go when feeling suicidal can be important. Being alone day after day can exacerbate a survivor's sense of isolation and powerlessness, and may feel like they are back in prison. Survivors may have friends and faith-based resources they can access, such as prayer groups, and social/community networks that can provide support. Checking-in calls from the therapist/agency can help a survivor feel less alone too.

The therapist must find a balance between responding to an asylum crisis and completing the risk assessment. Those of us familiar with this work know we can become too practical when an asylum claim is refused. Our need to rescue at such times can be overwhelming, but the risk assessment process might be compromised if we immediately turn to practical interventions, like contacting a new lawyer or finding the client somewhere to sleep that night. Sometimes, however, you may need to intervene to help keep a survivor safe. I have accompanied torture survivors to hospital for mental health assessments when they have been at risk of serious self-harm. Sometimes the assessing mental health professional has been thoughtful and skilled, but on many occasions the gap between the survivor's experience and the comprehension of the mental health professional has been so huge that I have wondered if the mental health assessment has become a harmful process in itself. I have witnessed a client's humiliation when questioned, and have watched their demeanour change as the exchange begins to feel like an interrogation. Crisis and home treatment teams may become involved, but as most individuals seeking asylum are accommodated in multi-occupancy settings, it can stigmatise the survivor if they are visited at home by a mental health team. Therapists can play a crucial role in explaining to a survivor's GP or to mental health professionals the nature of torture and its effects, and the impact of the asylum process on mental health.

Survivors' lives in exile are by definition unpredictable, and so predicting an escalation of suicide risk is not always straightforward. 'Chronic stress causes a slow wearing on our minds and bodies that can compound underlying trauma-related issues' (Emerson & Hopper, 2011: 23). Your knowledge of the survivor's past and present life, of any previous suicide attempts and upcoming asylum decisions, are important elements in planning how to minimise serious self-harm collaboratively when there is any sudden increase in risk.

I assessed a Kurdish survivor, Mohsen, who told me he often thought of suicide and hated the UK, and that only the thought of his family in Iran kept him alive. He had two brothers, who were in prison, and he was in constant contact with the rest of his family. I was aware, as our assessment progressed, that any bad news from home would significantly escalate his risk of suicide. One of his best friends had died just before Mohsen was referred for psychological therapy and he had made a serious attempt on his life in response to this news. A further risk factor was that he saw no point to his life in the UK, and felt estranged from the political struggle he had been engaged in at home. He missed 'everything about his life' in Iran, and was aching for the familiarity of home. His family were all activists and regarded imprisonment and torture as part of the life of any Kurd, and this only exacerbated his guilt that he wasn't coping in a safe, democratic country, when his community was at risk 'at home'. Mohsen was clear what his tipping point was: 'If they kill the youngest, that will be it.'

The way we managed the risk in our early sessions together was by talking about the meaning of what had happened to him, and his faith, and reconnecting him with a political purpose and with other Kurds in the UK. As Papadopoulos writes: '... [people] retain more resilient functions if they secure a collaborative and reciprocal support with others rather than when they struggle to overcome adversity on the basis of their own personal strength' (2011: 4–5).

Mohsen stayed safe, and the core of our work following on from assessment was helping him find a new community in the UK from which he could draw strength and support. It was important to him that he was well enough to contribute and that he had a role. To abandon the Kurdish struggle in pursuit of his personal safety could have undermined his identity as a resistance fighter.

Our role, as human rights practitioners, is to collectivise the atrocities our clients survive. It was important to Mohsen that together we honoured and remembered the lives lost in the Kurdish resistance, and that he was still a part of the struggle that had been his life. This was not a personal assault, with a personal recovery. It was a collective assault, and his pathway to rehabilitation was through connection with other Kurdish activists and communities. If I had not sought, in the assessment, to understand Mohsen's world here and in Iran, we would not have been able to help him identify the means to live 'for now'. Mohsen was never interested in exploring his past experiences of imprisonment and torture; his goal was to function well enough to 'become part of the world again'.

> Social support is not the same as merely being in the presence of others. The critical issue here is *reciprocity*: being truly heard and seen by the people around us, feeling that we are held in someone's else's mind and heart. (van der Kolk, 2014: 79)

Family and cultural background

Taking the history of a client's family, cultural and religious background is a fundamental part of any assessment. Did they grow up in conflict? Were they a child soldier? Did they suffer neglect and abuse, or live in a persecuted community where oppression and exclusion from mainstream society was the norm? This knowledge will help you get a fuller picture of the person they were before the torture. The survivor may find it painful to talk about their family, but it's important to know who has been lost or left behind, and who, if anyone, has accompanied the survivor into exile. Is the family in the country of origin still at risk? Are they still in touch, or has communication broken down or been severed?

It is always useful to do some background reading about the culture and history of the torturing state. Some brief research into the current political climate and its human rights abuses will also prepare you and help with engagement with the client.[2]

Survivors frequently describe feeling alone and alienated, and talk about their fear that they could die and no one would know or care. Sharing their family history can reduce this sense of isolation and alienation and help survivors connect with the person they were before torture. It can also help the therapist identify resilience and hope. Often such explorations enable the therapist to identify a survivor's resources, skills and interests.

Some therapists prefer to use an unstructured model of assessment. An open invitation is given to clients to share what has led them to therapy, and the therapist may choose not to ask for a family history and to let the client give this information in their own time. However, many survivors will not talk about those memories and histories if the therapist doesn't create the opportunity and give them time, permission and encouragement to do so. Our clients tell us that, at the beginning of therapy, they 'did not know where to start or what to say'.

Physical health assessment

Torture is likely to cause acute and chronic physical health problems that require assessment and treatment. 'Torture always happens at both the psychological and the physical level, which is why psychological and somatic complaints can hardly be separated from each other' (Karcher, 2001: 72). Also, it is widely recognised that 'traumatic symptoms not only affect our emotional and mental states, but our physical health as well' (Levine, 1997: 164).

Survivors are likely to suffer from headaches, skin rashes, weakness, sexually-transmitted diseases (STDs), neck and back pain and other physical health problems, alongside the psychological distress. Poor physical health will also be influenced by stress and the impact of living in poverty, with a poor diet, no meaningful activity, and little sunlight. The therapist needs to check that the survivor is getting medical help for their physical health needs. The torture may have involved the breaking or pulling of teeth, as well as the

---

2. Information about a country's history and human rights record can be found from Amnesty International www.amnesty.org.uk or Human Rights Watch www.hrw.org

long-term damage caused by prolonged malnourishment while in captivity, so dental care may be needed too.

'Among the multitude of problems presented by torture survivors referred for treatment, persistent pain in the musculoskeletal system is recognised as one of the most frequent physical complaints' (Amris & Williams, 2007: 1). GPs may dismiss these symptoms as purely somatic, or the survivor may not even get to tell the GP about them, when appointments offer so little time. There may also be a problem with diagnostic overshadowing: 'Overemphasizing the importance of psychological problems may result in insufficient recognition of the value of medical assessment and in failure to recognise and treat physical pain' (Amris & Williams, 2007: 1).

Survivors often report that their bodies are broken and permanently damaged, and may perceive themselves as physically weak, and so avoid walking or any movement that causes discomfort. Amris and Williams argue that this may 'contribute to the development and maintenance of persistent musculoskeletal disorders after injury' (2007: 3). In many cultures, physical pain is seen as a sign of damage and decline. Western pain management approaches may not fit with a survivor's personal or cultural beliefs about the meaning of pain. Survivors may want to be cured of pain and may find it difficult to accept working towards a reduction in pain, rather than its cure. For some, the pain signifies that the torturers have been successful in perpetrating long-term damage.

Most therapists do not have access to in-house physical and occupational therapy teams, but you can ensure appropriate investigation is undertaken by the client's GP and encourage physical movement, if recommended by the treating clinician or GP. A pain assessment, including a comprehensive musculoskeletal examination and a neurological evaluation, are advised for survivors of torture. Pharmacological treatment may have a role in the management of pain.

Sadly, the management and treatment of pain in survivors of torture remains highly specialised, despite the numbers of survivors presenting with chronic pain conditions. There is a need for more research into chronic pain conditions and their treatment among survivors of torture.

Bearing witness to a survivor's history of torture

> Man's capacity to dig himself in, to secrete a shell, to build around himself a tenuous barrier of defence, even in apparently desperate circumstances, is astonishing. (Levi, 1979: 62)

Bearing witness to a survivor's history of torture and abuse is fundamental to a human-rights approach, and can be central to the assessment process, depending on the psychological health of the survivor and their need to share their story.

'A human rights standpoint moves us from arbitrary conjecture about who might be enlisted to meet client needs to identifying "duty bearers" who hold the responsibility to ensure refugee rights are honoured' (Bowley & Bashir, 2015: 16). Bowley and Bashir emphasise the responsibility of healthcare professionals to ensure our clients' rights are recognised, which might require us to advocate, bear witness to and document the abuses our clients have experienced, in order to support their asylum claim.

Every service will have its own protocols for record keeping. Accurate and detailed note-taking is vital. If you are required to write a clinical letter or report following the assessment, or at some other stage during therapy, you may find it helpful to refer to the *Istanbul Protocol*, the UN manual on the principles of the effective investigation and documentation of torture and other cruel, inhuman or degrading treatment of punishment (OHCHR, 1999).

Taking a history at assessment is a matter for the therapist's clinical judgment. In my experience, many survivors will want to tell their story, but there are likely to be significant gaps. Traumatised survivors may have no words to describe their experiences. They may have just fragments of memories that only later can be formed into a narrative, once the therapeutic work is under way. 'The imprints of traumatic experiences are organised not as coherent logical narratives but in fragmented sensory and emotional traces: images, sounds and physical sensations' (van der Kolk, 2014: 176).

In my experience, many survivors choose not to disclose their experiences of torture until trust has been established and they feel safe enough and are invited to do so. Sadly, many survivors I have worked with have only had an opportunity to give a history of their torture in situations where they have had no choice: they have been required to give an account to the authorities, for example, or to their legal representative. Therapists will need to ensure that, if survivors choose to give a history, it is given freely, rather than because a survivor thinks it is required or because they need to prove they have a right to care and support. Many survivors say that the context of seeking asylum can lead them to feel as if every encounter is linked to the all-encompassing process of trying to gain protection and proving their credibility.

Before taking a testimony, it is useful to know what the survivor's previous experience of telling their torture story has been, and what they think the consequences will be of sharing their history in full. Survivors often think that the worst of their experiences cannot be shared or tolerated, by them or others. Speaking in a normal tone and being curious while ensuring our own horror or shock is carefully managed can reduce a survivor's guilt about causing distress. It is always helpful to explain the potential impact of the telling. These histories are often deeply disturbing, and you need to be careful not to either silence the survivor or make them feel they are responsible for upsetting you.

Parviz came to assessment with an urgent need to share his story, but was worried about its impact on me, as I would be a future source of support. He watched me intently as he talked, searching for shock and vulnerability, and was anxious to tell me that he never gave up any information to the torturers and that he was *strong*. As therapy progressed, Parviz realised that he had buried some memories that he couldn't tolerate when we first met, including the occasions when he gave up information about political colleagues 'to make it stop'. I suspect that if, at assessment, I had expressed admiration for his strength, it would have been harder for him to disclose this. Living with the guilt of what has been said, seen or done to others in these brutal and extreme situations is part of the horror of torture. In crowded, hot cells, when people are hungry and thirsty, kept naked, and forced to urinate and defecate where they lie, they may be driven to act in ways that they later find hard to live with. Such histories are excruciating to share and so it is important to always be aware of what is not being said, and to remain measured in your responses.

Naming as human rights abuses the appalling conditions in which people have been kept is important and reminds the survivor that they sought and deserve protection and that they have a right to rehabilitation. The therapist's role at these times can be to remind the client of the intention of torture – that its aim is to induce shame and silence its victims. It is deliberate, and it is political.

I remember taking a torture history at assessment from a young Iraqi man, Ahmed, who wanted me 'to know' what had happened to him. He was distressed and outraged by his imprisonment and torture, but was not traumatised. During the narrative, I asked him gently how he was suspended. Ahmed jumped up and went to the wall and showed me how he was tied. The more he talked, the more relief he appeared to feel. The look of anger on his face as he showed me was powerful. Thereafter, he would often refer back to this moment. It was as though both I and the interpreter were bearing witness to this painful act of cruelty. He would point at the place in the therapy room where he had stood and shake his head. He later told me that what made a difference was that I was trying to understand exactly what had happened in the cell; I wanted to know. It made him feel less alone. He had a witness.

Naming the differences and exploring power

Our sense of self and identity is socially and culturally embedded. In all therapeutic settings, there are cultural and racial differences, as well as other power differences, whether they are based on gender, disability, race, class or caste, sexual orientation or other oppressions or personal experiences. 'Deeply embedded "whites only" constructs of thought and ideology... permeate our culture, largely outside of ordinary awareness' (Ryde, 2009: 43). Therapists will be familiar with the process of opening up conversations with clients about difference, and exploring the structural power of the therapist's role. Naming, exploring and being curious about cultural differences and understandings are vital if the therapy is to be genuinely helpful to a survivor. 'Acknowledging and being prepared to address this diversity and its complexity is crucial to connecting to the individual' (Aroche & Coello, 2004: 55).

'Mental health professionals who presume that they are free of racism seriously underestimate the social impact of their own socialization and the inherited, in some instances unintentionally covert, racism' (Bemak, Chung & Pederson, 2003: 47). In a racialised context, and as a white therapist, I hold considerable power in the therapy room, and so a commitment to practising self-reflexively is vital. Self-reflexivity emanates from systemic theory (Dallos & Stedmon, 2009) and requires us to consider from moment to moment how our position, reactions and assumptions influence how we practise, both in the moment and after the session.

The power of the therapist's position can be amplified for survivors in exile. People are often so profoundly disempowered by the asylum process and the lack of autonomy that they come to therapy feeling worthless and deskilled. It can be uncomfortable when a capable and thoughtful client says 'You know best' when exploring a dilemma together, when you first meet. When survivors are overwhelmed and bewildered by confusing systems, they can lose confidence in their ability to assess a situation and make decisions. At such times, I have found it helpful to share the dilemma of being asked to decide the way forward when it is not my decision to make, and to slow down the pace of the assessment so that survivors have time to explore their choices and examine potential ways forward. It is important to remember that, at the same time as they are managing all this, traumatised people 'have more general problems with focused attention and with learning information' (van der Kolk, 2014: 245).

So, when does the treatment start?

> I saw this nice man for a few months [in a primary care team], but the treatment never began; we just talked about my problems.

This is how a former client, Chandra, described to me what was a 16-week course of therapy. Assessing survivors in exile is complex, given the huge range of difficulties people face. The first step after assessment is generally to contract with the client. How you do this will depend on your model of therapy and your organisation's protocols. Profoundly traumatised clients are unlikely to be able to grasp the significance of the contract until they have developed a relationship of trust with the therapist, have regained some sense of control and stability and can understand what therapy is. Therapists new to refugee work frequently make the mistake of contracting with a survivor before they genuinely understand and have freely chosen to engage with therapy, and survivors can feel intimidated and anxious when written contracts are produced.

As the assessment comes to an end, it can be helpful for the therapist and survivor to revisit what therapy is and how it differs from the assessment. For therapists working in brief intervention settings, this process may be quite focused and task based. In other settings, the therapist may be able to offer an open-ended contract and can explore with the survivor how they will work together and what they will focus on.

It is important that you explain to the survivor at assessment that any therapy that follows is likely to be time limited, but how and when you tell them will need to be carefully managed. Giving an impression that the relationship is never-ending can be damaging in the long term; many therapists new to working with refugees will avoid mentioning endings at all, given the scale of a client's losses and concerns about the impact this may have on engagement.

The therapist may be the only constant person in a survivor's life in the early stages of therapeutic work. The responsibility of being the *only one* can be quite a shock, but it can also be seductive. It is important that the therapeutic relationship is realistic, can be sustained, and is one of many helping relationships and resources in a survivor's world. 'Restoring relationships and community is central to restoring wellbeing' (van der Kolk, 2014: 38)

Not knowing

As each year passes in my work with refugees, I have found myself becoming more comfortable with not knowing. Social constructionists Anderson and

Goolishian talk of adopting a 'not-knowing approach' in their work: '... the therapeutic question is the primary instrument to facilitate the development of learning, by curiosity and by taking the client's story seriously, the therapist joins with the client in a mutual exploration of the client's understanding and experience' (1992: 30).

At the core of any assessment must be a holistic approach to hearing and attending to the range of difficulties with which the survivor presents, however challenging that can be in the limited time available. We must attend to the whole person, and remember that the process of recovery belongs to the survivor. 'The initial aim, surely, is to put ourselves as close as possible to the minds of those affected, to maximise our capacity for accurate empathy and enrich our ways of seeing' (Summerfield, 1996: 21).

Supporting survivors to achieve a sense of control and hope is at the core of assessment, as well as what Summerfield describes as endeavouring to understand people when they express themselves in their own terms (1996: 21). 'We need an environment sensitive to our situation before we can be expected to feel safe to talk, or to listen and take in information and advice' (Women Asylum Seekers Together, 2008: 6).

Naming the injustice our clients have survived and honouring the histories we witness form the basis of our human-rights approach to working with survivors. These testimonies, either written to validate an account of torture or held by us, as activists, can challenge those who seek to deny human rights atrocities. Action alongside survivors to achieve social justice for them in the UK is equally important, as there may come a time when the UK government will seek to deny or minimalise the appalling treatment of people who sought protection in the UK.

There is no quick fix to the brutality of torture, and no one intervention that works for all. Sometimes, in the face of such extreme distress, I have wondered how my therapeutic approach can possibly provide any relief. Sephora, a survivor from the Democratic Republic of the Congo (DRC), disclosed the following history to me several months after our assessment. She witnessed the rape of her mother and one of her sisters when their bus was stopped by rebels. She was kidnapped and became a 'rebel wife' and was repeatedly raped in a camp over a period of seven months. As our work progressed, we talked about the use of rape in war, and Sephora reflected on this and its meaning for her own experience and her sense of shame and responsibility. She later found validation in a refugee women's project, where many of the women had been raped in conflict. 'Wartime rape will stop when the status of women changes and the shame lands on the perpetrators, not the victims' (Baker, 2016). Sephora went on to volunteer in the project and, by the time therapy ended, she had refugee status and planned to train as a nurse.

When I reached the end of Sephora's assessment, I wondered whether the young woman in front of me was even aware of my presence. Many agencies might have considered Sephora 'inappropriate for therapy', given she said very little over those four sessions and told me she 'didn't want to talk'. Sephora, alongside so many of my clients, taught me that sometimes all that is needed is compassion and patience, and everything else can wait.

References

Afuape T (2011). *Power, Resistance and Liberation in Therapy with Survivors of Trauma: to have our hearts broken.* London: Routledge.

Amnesty International (2004). *Get it Right: how Home Office decision-making fails refugees.* London: Amnesty International.

Amris K, Williams AC (2007). Chronic pain in survivors of torture. *International Association for the Study of Pain; Clinical Updates XV*(7): 1–6.

Anderson H, Goolishian H (1992). The client is the expert: a not-knowing approach to therapy. In: McNamee S, Gergen KJ (eds). *Therapy as Social Construction.* London: Sage Publications (pp25–39).

Aroche J, Coello MJ (2004). Ethnocultural considerations in the treatment of refugees and asylum seekers. In: Wilson JP, Drožđek B (eds). *Broken Spirits: the treatment of traumatised asylum seekers, refugees, war and torture victims.* Hove: Brunner Routledge (pp53–80).

Baker A (2016). The secret war crime: the most shameful consequence of conflict comes out into the open. [Online.] *Time Magazine* 10 March. http://time.com/war-and-rape/ (accessed January 2017).

Bemak F, Chi-Ying Chung R, Pedersen PB (2003). *Counselling Refugees: a psychosocial approach to innovative multicultural interventions.* Westport, CT: Greenwood Press.

Bothne N, Keys CB (2016). Creating community life among immigrant survivors of torture and their allies. *Torture Journal* 26(2): 3–18.

Bowley J, Bashir C (2015). Working with people seeking asylum. In: Tarrier N, Johnson J (eds). *Case Formulation in Cognitive Behaviour Therapy: the treatment of challenging and complex cases.* London: Routledge (pp322–351).

Boyles J (2015). In the shadow of detention. *Therapy Today* 26(4): 10–14.

Bracken P (2002). *Trauma: culture, meaning and philosophy.* London: Whurr Publishers Ltd.

Bryant-Jefferies R (2005). *Counselling Victims of Warfare: person-centred dialogues.* New York: CRC Press.

Chaplin J (1988). *Feminist Counselling in Action.* London: Sage.

Cohen J (2008). Safe in our hands? A study of suicide and self-harm in asylum seekers. *Journal of Forensic and Legal Medicine* 15(4): 235–244.

Dallos R, Stedmon J (2009). Flying over the swampy lowlands: reflective and reflexive practice. In: Stedmon J, Dallos R (eds). *Reflective Practice in Psychotherapy and Counselling.* Maidenhead: Open University Press.

Drožđek B, Wilson JP (2004). Uncovering trauma-focused treatment techniques with asylum seekers. In: Wilson JP, Drožđek B (eds). *Broken Spirits: the treatment of traumatised asylum seekers, refugees, war and torture victims.* Hove: Brunner Routledge (pp243–276).

Eisenbruch M (1990). The cultural bereavement interview: a new clinical research approach to refugees. *Psychiatric Clinics of North America* 13(4): 715–735.

Elsass P (1997). *Treating Victims of Torture and Violence: theoretical, cross-cultural and clinical implications.* New York, NY: New York University Press.

Emerson D, Hopper E (2011). *Overcoming Trauma through Yoga: reclaiming your body.* Berkeley, CA: North Atlantic Books.

Fazel M, Wheeler J, Danesh J (2005). Prevalence of serious mental disorder in 7000 refugees. *The Lancet* 365(9467): 1309–1314.

Freedom from Torture (2014). *Rape as Torture in the DRC: sexual violence beyond the conflict zone.* London: Freedom from Torture. www.freedomfromtorture.org/feature/drc_report/7878 (accessed July 2017).

Graessner S, Gurris N, Pross C (1996). *At the Side of Torture Survivors: treating a terrible assault on human dignity.* Baltimore, MD: John Hopkins University Press.

Grossman V (trans Chandler R) (2006). *Life and Fate.* London: Vintage Books.

Gurris N (2001). Psychic Trauma through Torture – Healing through Psychotherapy. *At the side of torture survivors: treating a terrible assault on human dignity.* Baltimore, MD: John Hopkins University Press (pp29-56).

Herman JL (1992). *Trauma and Recovery: the aftermath of violence – from domestic abuse to political terror.* New York, NY: Basic Books.

Karcher S (2001). 'In my fingertips I don't have a soul anymore': body psychotherapy with survivors of torture – insights into work with concentrative movement therapy. In: Graessner MD, Gurris N, Pross C (eds). *At the Side of Torture Survivors: treating a terrible assault on human dignity.* Baltimore, MD: John Hopkins University Press (pp70–94).

Kira IA (2002). Torture assessment and treatment: the Wraparound approach. *Traumatology* 8(2): 54–86.

Laub D (2001). Survivors' silence and the difficulty of knowing. In: Graessner MD, Guris N, Pross C (eds). *At the Side of Torture Survivors: treating a terrible assault on human dignity.* Baltimore, MD: John Hopkins University Press (ppxxvi-xxii).

Lavik NJ, Hauf E, Skrondal A, Solberg O (1996). Mental disorder among refugees and the impact of persecution and exile: some findings from an outpatient population. *British Journal of Psychiatry* 169: 726–732.

Levi P (1979). *If This is a Man/The Truce* (trans. SJ Woolf). London: Abacus.

Levine PA (1997). *Waking the Tiger: healing trauma.* Berkeley, CA: North Atlantic Books.

Malloch MS, Stanley E (2005). The detention of asylum seekers in the UK: representing risk, managing the dangerous. *Punishment and Society* 7(1): 53–71.

McFarlane AC (2004). Assessing PTSD and comorbidity: issues in differential diagnosis. In:

Wilson JP, Drožđek B (eds). *Broken Spirits: the treatment of traumatised asylum seekers, refugees, war and torture victims*. Hove: Brunner Routledge (pp81–103).

McLeod J (2004). *An Introduction to Counselling* (3rd ed). Maidenhead: Open University Press.

Mendez JE (2013). In: Pettitt J (ed). *The Poverty Barrier: the right to rehabilitation for survivors of torture in the UK*. London: Freedom from Torture.

OHCHR (1999). *Istanbul Protocol: the UN manual on the principles of the effective investigation and documentation of torture and other cruel, inhuman or degrading treatment or punishment*. Geneva: OHCHR. www.ohchr.org/Documents/Publications/training8Rev1en.pdf (accessed July 2017).

OHCHR (1984). *Convention against Torture and Other Cruel, Inhuman or Degrading Treatment or Punishment (UNCAT)*. Geneva: OHCHR.

Papadopoulos RK (2011). *A Psychosocial Framework for Work with Refugees*. Seoul, Korea: NANCEN Human Rights for Refugees Center. www.southeastsafenet.eu/sites/default/files/3.pdf (accessed July 2017).

Papadopoulos RK (2007). Refugees, trauma and adversity-activated development. *European Journal of Psychotherapy and Counselling* 9(3): 301–312.

Papadopoulos RK (2002). *Therapeutic Care for Refugees: no place like home*. The Tavistock Clinic Series. London: Karnac Books.

Pope KS, Garcia-Peltoniemi RE (1991). Responding to victims of torture: clinical issues, professional responsibilities, and useful resources. *Professional Psychology: Research and Practice* 22(4): 269–276.

Ryde J (2009). *Being White in the Helping Professions*. London: Jessica Kingsley Publishers.

Summerfield D (1996). *The Impact of War and Atrocity on Civilian Populations: basic principles for NGO interventions and a critique of psychosocial trauma projects*. London: Overseas Development Institute. www.files.ethz.ch/isn/97846/networkpaper014.pdf (accessed July 2017).

Turner S, Gorst-Unsworth C (1990). Psychological sequelae of torture: a descriptive model. *British Journal of Psychiatry* 157: 475–480.

van der Kolk B (2014). *The Body Keeps the Score: mind, brain and body in the transformation of trauma*. London: Penguin Books.

van der Veer G, Waning AV (2004). Creating a safe therapeutic sanctuary. In: Wilson JP, Drožđek B (eds). *Broken Spirits: the treatment of traumatised asylum seekers, refugees, war and torture victims*. Hove: Brunner Routledge (pp187–219).

van der Veer G (1998). *Counselling and Therapy with Refugees and Victims of Torture: psychological problems of victims of war, torture and repression* (2nd ed). Chichester: John Wiley & Sons.

van der Veer G (1993). *Psychotherapy with Refugees: an exploration*. Amsterdam: Stichting voor Culturele Studies.

West A (2006). To do or not to do – is that the question? *Therapy Today* 17(6): 10–13.

Wilson JP (2004). The broken spirit: posttraumatic damage to the self. In: Wilson JP, Drožđek B (eds). *Broken Spirits: the treatment of traumatised asylum seekers, refugees, war and torture victims*. Hove: Brunner Routledge (pp109–157).

Women Asylum Seekers Together (2008). *WAST recommendations for good practice for agencies working with women asylum seekers*. Manchester: WAST. www.wast.org.uk/new/admin/wp-content/uploads/2012/03/A4 Booklet-RECOMMENDATIONS.pdf (accessed July 2017).

2. 'The door to my garden': Kevin, me and the clock

Norma McKinnon

> You answer the questions you are asked, but the answers to these questions do not tell our full stories. Our lives are complex... all the questions they asked – 'How did you not die?' 'Why do you live?' All these questions were hard and made me think, 'Do I not have a right to live? Do I not have the rights of a human being?' But I also remember coming here at first for therapy and I was not approached in this way, but still, the first time I came, it was just so difficult, you know, just difficult... phhheww... just difficult. My life was a disaster, it was just a disaster. I had problems of a big kind, and in the end, it was all about the therapy, because without that therapy I would have lost my, you know, I would have lost my life, I would just have lost my life. I mean, you also asked me difficult questions, but you asked in an OK way. (Kevin)

The UNHCR estimates that there are some 65.6 million forcibly displaced people worldwide, of which 22.5 million are refugees and 40.3 million are internally displaced (UNHCR, 2016). A small number make the perilous journey to the UK to seek protection. As a psychological therapist working with torture survivors, I bear witness daily to the impact of traumatic events, both past and present. I work with people from across the world. They speak different languages, practise different faiths, are from diverse educational backgrounds and of different ages and genders, with different sexual orientations and different political opinions. I believe that, if we can be open and reflexive as therapists, we can learn a lot from the clients who seek us out, improve and enrich our practice and learn how to tolerate the 'not knowing', which I now recognise is essential to working with such diversity.

I have worked in the refugee sector for almost 20 years. I started this journey as a community worker, interested in working alongside refugees to build on their strengths and improve their personal and community wellbeing. I currently work as a psychological therapist and for the past 10 years I have specialised in working with survivors of torture.

My understanding of trauma and approach to my clinical work have been informed and shaped by my experience in both community and clinical settings. I see a place for both: for both clinical and community interventions to contribute to healing and rehabilitation. My therapeutic training is culturally bound to the context I live in; however, my practice needs to be responsive and meaningful to people from all over the world. I acknowledge that my clinical practice alone will not support healing and recovery: survivors of human rights abuses also need justice, redress, a sense of meaning and connection, to support their healing. I also believe it is essential to adopt a human-rights approach in this work. I believe it is my role as a therapist not only to support clients to achieve the internal changes they seek, but also to seek to change their social context when and where I can.

This chapter offers some personal reflections, written in collaboration with a former client, Kevin, on the therapeutic process of working with one survivor of torture. Kevin now finds himself one of the 22.5 million refugees worldwide, which is how we met, but he was not always so.

I originally started writing a different chapter, advocating that survivors' voices should be included when writing about our clinical work. I felt a sense of discomfort in advocating but not acting on my own advice. I had sought consent from Kevin to include excerpts from a clinical case study I had written about previously, and what started as a conversation about that became this collaboration. Kevin was interested in having a means to reach other therapists; he hoped that, by sharing his experiences, we could all learn something. Kevin did not want to be co-author of this chapter; he just wanted to deliver some key messages he felt were important, to add his reflections on the therapy process, and to review the finished piece.

We could not cover everything that happened during the therapeutic journey, so we focused on the key moments in our therapeutic process that illustrated for Kevin some of the barriers he has faced in trying to get support for his recovery. This includes some of our early work together, and also Kevin's attempts to access support elsewhere. This was important to Kevin: he hopes it will support other survivors to access therapy by ensuring therapists are better prepared for what they may encounter.

We did not enter into this endeavour lightly. We explored the possible impact on Kevin of including some of the material about his experiences, and the painful memories it could ignite, given that the chapter focuses on a time when Kevin was physically, psychologically and socially in a very different place from where he is now. Writing this chapter would also involve me being open about my experiences of the work.

So, what advice would Kevin like to give therapists should we meet a torture survivor who describes their life as a disaster, like Kevin did at the point he sought therapy? 'Don't stress yourselves,' he says, laughing, and then points out a key principle to be followed if adopting a human-rights approach – that of non-discrimination: 'When two people are stressed, there is no way out, mainly the therapist helps the stress come down and then the therapist is the guide to help the other party feel OK. We are all different… You need to welcome everyone and not think, "Oh, this one is green, this one is white." You need to just be open to people… most refugees come from here and there, our traditions are different from yours.'

'My life was a disaster'

There is laughter now, but for a long time there was not. When I first met Kevin, he was just about to become street homeless, following the refusal of his asylum claim.

The details of Kevin's life were unknown to me at the start, and only emerged slowly, over the course of therapy, to form a coherent narrative. Indeed, it was his inability to construct this coherent narrative that caused his asylum claim initially to be refused.

Kevin was born into slavery in a small village in Darfur, Sudan. He speaks five tribal languages, in addition to Arabic and English. He was excluded from school and made to work on a farm, with his mother, father and two brothers. His sisters were married and lived in another part of Darfur. He is married with two children, but the whereabouts of his wife and children were unknown until recently. Kevin's mother was murdered by the family that his family served, and Kevin was witness to the beating that led to her death. His father and two brothers were killed by the Janjaweed.[1] Kevin was sent to retrieve his brothers' mutilated bodies following the attack and was injured, suffering bullet wounds and burns. Before the attack on his village, Kevin had been arrested, detained for three months and tortured in prison.

---

1. The Janjaweed is a militia that operate in Darfur, western Sudan, and eastern Chad.

His decision to share these experiences here was both painful and purposeful. It is important to acknowledge the traumatic history that led Kevin to seek protection and become one of the 22.5 million people in the UNHCR statistic. Kevin spoke about his application for protection being refused:

> A judge told me I am not from Darfur. When he says this, he is telling me I am not from my mother, not from where she was born, or where she gave birth to me, or where she died and where she rests in the ground. If the judge is correct, then my mother lied to me, and her mother lied to her. A lot of the time I feel hungry and angry.

I believe it is important to recognise that, despite having sought protection from those experiences, Kevin was unable to explain them coherently enough to get help through the asylum system. Kevin's traumatic experiences began in infancy and continued into his adulthood. They included extreme human rights violations and torture, and they were compounded by what happened to him when he sought asylum in the UK. Kevin and his experiences do not fall easily into a simple medical model diagnosis. I know from my experiences of working with other people seeking asylum who are street homeless that therapists may question what therapeutic work can be undertaken when a survivor's social context is so insecure. However, Kevin strongly advocates not being too quick to judge a survivor's initial ability to engage, as this is one of the hurdles that he found difficult to overcome when he was first seeking support.

'Get the basics right'

I thought Kevin's initial assessment appointment was disastrous. The session had ended with me sitting on the floor, surrounded by the 30 packets of medication he had brought, trying to help him to organise them into bundles that made some kind of sense. My countertransference to finding myself in this position was to question my own competency. This was not exactly what I had planned for that first session. I had forms to fill in, questions to ask, consents to be sought, but I was sitting on the floor tying rubber bands around packets of pills. I could see in front of me that Kevin was involved in a very personal struggle that I was yet to understand. He was sitting hunched over, silent, making no eye contact; within my own cultural framework, I might have understood these behaviours as avoidant. I might have even decided that Kevin was not engaging with the assessment. I would have been wrong.

Kevin did not respond to most of the questions I asked, leaving me bereft of the information I sought. However, I recognised that there was engagement: first, Kevin was here, clutching an appointment letter and a bag of medication; second, he had given me this bag. When I asked Kevin what he knew about the medication, he said he had no idea what they were all for. I sensed that, despite his withdrawn demeanour, he was watching and listening intently to me.

I decided that, to have any chance of doing something meaningful for Kevin in that moment, I would need to attune to his rhythm and his timing. Kevin had obviously come with expectations that I did not know how to meet. My form-filling would have to wait, and this caused me some anxiety, as it meant I would not meet the expectations of the organisation I was working for. I asked if it would be helpful to sort through the medications, and Kevin said it would. I later learned that, by taking the plastic bag of medications, discussing with Kevin what we should do with them, and offering to contact his GP and ask him to review the prescriptions and how they were administered, I had responded in a way that was 'good enough' for him.

I did not know at that point that Kevin had had a previous negative experience of therapy elsewhere, and had stopped attending. Kevin later explained why he decided to come back for his next appointment with me:

> I kept coming here because in this place you treated me like a human being and I felt safe, and when I had gone to the other place they made me feel very tense and stressed, because of the way they tried to approach me. OK, I was alone in my life, and those people just told me that 'You are doing this,' and they seemed to accuse or blame me for who I was and what I was suffering. And then I came here. You were warm and you did not limit me in what I could do or say. I never went home from an appointment with you thinking, 'Why did she talk to me like that?' The difference between here and there was that you tried to get the basics right and get inside me as a human being. The other therapist just did not get it.

So, even in the very first appointment, there had been a risk of my 'not getting it'. My reflections were that it had been a difficult encounter where I had failed as a therapist. But Kevin had left feeling respected. He told me later the significance for him of my response that day: my decision to abandon my usual assessment process and to focus instead, with his agreement, on the medication.

You helped me change my medicine and arranged for me to have it in weekly dosages. My memory at the time was poor. Every day I was taking more and more medicines. I had 30 different packets. I had so much medicine at one point I thought it could have killed me. I was so confused. Now I don't take so much and I know what I have to take.

Kevin still credits this intervention with saving his life.

'Therapists need first to listen to what's going on'

From that point onward, Kevin attended regular weekly sessions, hardly ever missing appointments, even when he was street homeless. The therapy did not follow a straightforward trajectory, where my interventions had the kind of immediate impact we, both therapist and client, would all hope for. It did not move seamlessly along a continuum of safety, remembrance, mourning and reconnection as a pathway to rehabilitation following trauma, as proposed by Herman (1992).

Kevin has very clear views on what therapists need to offer in order to be helpful to people in his situation:

Most therapists are probably good, but some are crap and can make your life hell. Therapists first need to listen and have an understanding before trying to help. At the beginning of therapy, in my brain, I was angry. I thought you could hurt me, but you didn't; you sought to understand me. Therapists need to first listen to what's going on inside, and then work in a way where decisions about care and treatment are made together. I want therapists to know that the scars I have on my body can be treated, but inside my brain, it's not for therapists to try and treat this, but if the therapists work alongside me, together we can work on resolving this pain and sadness. The first time a torture survivor comes to therapy, they need to understand what the therapists is on about, why they want certain information, what they are going to do. Both therapist and client need to understand each other. In the main, I am happy to try to keep away from people, but the therapist can build your trust, first in them, and then towards others.

Kevin is also illustrating another principle of a human-rights approach, that of the therapist being accountable to our clients, and properly explaining our processes. Therapists see the root causes of suffering every day in our consulting rooms. Part of our role is, perhaps, to bear witness to this. However, we can do more. If we regard trauma as situated in a social context, we should recognise that most treatment planning takes a reductionist approach that sees trauma and its effects in terms of symptoms and diagnosis. If we focus our therapeutic interventions solely on symptom reduction without acknowledging the injustices our clients have experienced, we may be contributing to the oppressions they experience and serving to silence them again. Kevin wanted something more from his therapeutic encounter.

I work with many people who would rather spend some of their therapy hour focusing on the situation of people in the country they have fled before talking about any personal difficulties they may be having. Kevin needed to use some of the therapeutic hour to talk about the political crisis that led him to be here. He needed to analyse what was happening, consider its impact, and make meaning of it. I did not think it was my role to direct him away from this exploration and back to his inner world. He told me: 'Every time I asked myself why? It takes weeks for me to try and answer this question. Sometimes this feels just like torture but I could share this trauma in therapy and move through it.'

I became a minor expert on the International Criminal Court through Kevin. Our conversations would start at the global and filter down to the personal. This seemed to help Kevin think about his own needs and acknowledge them and his feelings.

We therapists also need to acknowledge our power. We are often involved in deciding who can access treatment, what kind of treatment it should be, how long the treatment will be and when someone is considered to no longer need it. Sometimes our decision-making powers are limited by the procedures and rules of the organisations for which we work. Some decisions will be framed by the expectations of funding bodies or service commissioners. We may need to balance what we think is a moral and ethical response to our client at any particular moment with the demands of policies and procedures. A human-rights approach advocates the principles of participation and empowerment.

The interventions that we decide have (or do not have) therapeutic value, and who we decide to offer them to, could be influenced by our own psychological responses to witnessing the intensity of the suffering the survivor is experiencing. Kevin frequently gave feedback about what worked for him and what did not work, and the therapy needed to be guided by that.

'They think it makes you feel better'

There is a wealth of studies on working therapeutically with refugees, and numerous theories of trauma, too many to cite here. As a practitioner witnessing daily how trauma manifests in human distress, I sometimes feel overwhelmed by the different arguments in the research. Some argue that our understanding of trauma and human rights is rooted in western liberal traditions, and therefore lacks cultural validity; others strive to establish evidence of cross-cultural validity. Our training as therapists rarely specifically covers work with refugees,[2] or cross-cultural working and working with language support. We are not taught to consider trauma within a wider socio-political context.

Working with refugees confronts us with all these elements. Therefore, it is our responsibility to equip ourselves with a basic understanding of the circumstances that cause people to flee their home country and seek international protection elsewhere. We need to understand the systems and processes that affect our clients' lives now. In addition to the difficulties created by their insecure immigration status, survivors who are in the process of applying for asylum have no right to work, and those who do have refugee status or UK citizenship may experience poor physical or psychological health that prevents them working or engaging in other purposeful activities. Many live in poverty, rendered passive by the removal of authority to make decisions about their lives while the state provides support. All of this is likely to affect their psychosocial wellbeing and will impact on the therapeutic work. As Kevin says, therapists need to 'listen to what's going on and then work in a way where decisions about care and treatment are made together'.

Social networks and connections can be severely disrupted and difficult to re-establish. Survivors may want to fill the therapeutic hour by talking about their profound loneliness and hopelessness, the pain, grief and loss caused by family separation, and any news, or the absence of news, from home. Many therapists, and some trauma models, would consider Kevin unsuitable for 'trauma' work because his social context was too insecure: he was street homeless and at constant risk of removal from the UK.

For the first six months, Kevin spent most of our sessions sitting in silence, with his head bowed. I focused on building a therapeutic alliance, as the basis for sessions. I felt I was being 'tested', but did not know the criteria I was being

---

2. For ease I have used the term 'refugee' in this chapter. I use this term to cover people who are seeking asylum and those who have been granted refugee status in the UK, as well as people living outside their country of origin in other parts of the world.

tested against. Kevin later told me he was sounding out my consistency of character. Occasionally he would make a vivid disclosure or a rapid outburst of dislocated statements about a traumatic event. Neither Kevin nor I could place them in a context that we could both understand.

I tried to find ways to help Kevin manage the symptoms that disrupted his life. I tried bi-lateral stimulation, a well-known tool that can help people establish a 'safe' or 'sacred' mental space. This was met with, 'Don't bother ever trying that again.' I knew that Kevin had not lost his capacity to make decisions about his care and circumstances, even when his suffering appeared overwhelming. I knew my inner rescuer was activated, I wanted to be able to fix things and for Kevin to experience the interventions as positive – for them to do what I thought they should – but I knew I needed to be guided by Kevin's feedback. Of the use of some therapeutic tools, Kevin said: 'Some people try to push you around, force you into things, make you do things. They think it makes you feel better, and it actually makes things worse.'

The trauma narrative evolved in unexpected ways. For example, on one occasion I gave Kevin a calendar to mark his appointments, as he liked to have them written down and sometimes worried about his forgetfulness. I noticed that he kept opening and shutting it. He did not tell me what was going on and I thought he seemed confused. He looked at each month and then put the calendar face down on the table, then picked it up and went through the same process again. This was repeated six times. Kevin then shook his head, and showed me some scars on his wrists: 'They are from Darfur,' he said, 'when they drove nails through my wrists.' He would not say more. Kevin was redefining our exchange, in a perhaps unconscious way, to support the emergence of his story, moving from questions about appointments to a disclosure.

'You helped with my past and my future'

Erskine and Trautmann (1996) explain how severe and cumulative denial of human relational needs results in a severing of personal and interpersonal contact. The person loses touch with their own feelings, needs, memories and thoughts, and cuts off contact with others, in order no longer to experience the feelings of loneliness and pain. This can result in a denial of relational needs – needs for security and validation in relationship; for dependability and consistency in others, and shared experience; for the capacity to have an impact in relationship; for another to initiate and the person to experience gratitude and appreciation. Erskine's thinking influences my own, contact-orientated approach, with its focus on the importance of the therapeutic relationship. With Kevin, we would need to rely on the strength of the therapeutic relationship, as Kevin rejected all the tools and techniques I was trying. He later said:

> Yeah, so these meetings with you, at this time I was having a massive terrible time, and we spoke about these things, and about different things as well, you know. It helped me with the way things are, because, you know, some people had made my life hell, and I would get upset and aggressive, and at the end of the day I would speak to you and you would try and help me to feel that something in life could be OK, and I didn't focus on the crisis and the horrible things I was seeing [flashbacks] that were terrible, terrible, and sometimes I would come here, and on the way I would think about harming myself but I would talk to you and you would calm me down. I used to walk past that river and it would come to my mind just to jump in, but talking to you in therapy really helped, and I could pass the river and just go on my way. Talking in therapy helped me decide, no, I will not jump in, how could I jump in? I would lose the things that have helped me.

Creating a safe space is considered essential for stabilisation work. This is part of a stage-oriented treatment first described by Pierre Janet over 100 years ago (van der Hart, Brown & van der Kolk, 1989), when he wrote about the need for the therapist to build 'rapport', which we now call the therapeutic alliance. Trauma specialists such as Herman (1992) advocate a three-stage approach: safety, remembrance and mourning, and reconnection. Therapists have tools and techniques they can use to facilitate this, and I was trying them all, with little impact. For example, I tried to teach Kevin some relaxation techniques (visualisation, muscle tension releasing, breathing exercises) in the sessions, but Kevin wouldn't try them. He simply told me he did not want to 'fuckin' relax', He then asked, 'Why are they killing people on the road to Zalinge?' and abruptly left. I didn't know what the road to Zalinge was at that time. So it was important to find out.

An unexpected thing happened that supported the therapy. Kevin came to the office one day and noticed a box in my room with arts materials in it, including cross-stitch. He took some away with him, and when he brought them back to the following session, asked me if I could cross-stitch and offered to teach me. I was rubbish at it. After this, he stitched a beautiful 'Thank you' in cross-stitch to go on the office wall. This was the start of his gift-giving, to which I will return later. Having previously learned cross-stitch in Sudan, Kevin had lost touch with this kind of activity in his current context. Kevin now credits his rediscovery of cross-stitch as an effective therapeutic tool.

In ways such as this, Kevin set the pace for therapy and found his own solutions.

> Well, you know where the cross-stitch comes from [laughs]. I came here and got some materials and when I sit down at night and I am having massive thinking, I said to myself, well, let's do some cross-stitch, and this helped me to keep myself [in the present moment] and adapt my thinking [stop himself from ruminating].

Our work at that time was focused on creating a coherent narrative of Kevin's experiences, which was necessary (as explained above) for Kevin's asylum application. Stutheridge (2006) believes this to be essential in trauma work. It was a painful process. Kevin had survived both genocide and torture. His family, culture and language were lost to him. His grief was profound and he coped by withdrawing. Reconstructing the narrative revived a series of shocking images. Kevin brought a letter he had received from the Home Office via his legal representative, and his name had been spelt wrongly. We spoke about it in the session – not the content of the letter, but simply the spelling of his name. Kevin wrote his name down, and then the variations that had been used to spell it. Then he scrubbed out some spellings to indicate they were wrong and, without prompting, wrote down the names of his family: his mother, two sisters, two brothers, his father, his wife and two children.

Kevin then described how his father was shot and about his mother's murder. He told me what happened to his two sisters, saying the same phrase over and over again to describe it. Kevin then marked the names of those who had died. In these ways, I learned what Kevin had survived. I held it all in mind, session after session, and eventually worked with Kevin to create a timeline, based on all the dislocated statements he had made over time. Kevin also made some pictures and we created maps, and then we brought it all together. Then we both knew what he had survived.

It felt at this point that we had made some therapeutic progress. I could see a difference, but Kevin was still struggling to manage some of his experiences. Sometimes our clients will not 'heal' in the way we want and can easily measure. Recovery needs to be meaningful for the client. Kevin has strong views on what he calls 'therapy bureaucracy' – the tools we use to measure progress. He freely admits to saying 'stuff just to make you get on with it so we can talk about the real stuff'.

On the occasions when I tried to measure some therapeutic outcomes, Kevin felt I was missing the point:

> You ask me, how did I sleep this week, how did I sleep last week, and you totally miss the point. You helped me to remember my past when I could not. You helped me focus on things here when I could not. You helped with my past and my future. There have been things that have happened that, if it was not for you, I would not have come back from. You have always treated me with respect and dignity. You have helped me to be capable and function at times when I couldn't. You have helped me to write the story of my life when I could not.

'I was both sick and well at the same time'

Our understanding of trauma is evolving. There have been recent revisions to the diagnosis of post-traumatic stress disorder (PTSD), and there are likely to be more. Fassin and Rechtman (2009) chart the development of our clinical understanding of trauma from its early formulations to the inclusion of specific diagnostic criteria for PTSD in the *Diagnostic and Statistical Manual for Mental Disorders* (DSM-III) in 1980 (APA, 1980). They make an argument that PTSD was developed in response to the wider socio-political context in the aftermath of the Vietnam War. PTSD is probably the most commonly used diagnostic criteria relating to trauma, and the one that is probably most recognisable to the wider public.

Kevin was diagnosed with PTSD, but this diagnosis did not explain all he experienced. There are other formulations, some validated and some not, such as Herman's concept of Complex PTSD and Disorders of Extreme Stress Not Otherwise Specified (DESNOS) (Herman, 1992). ICD-10, the World Health Organization's diagnostic manual, also offers the diagnosis of enduring personality change after a catastrophic experience (World Health Organization, 1992).

I believe it is a mistake to use solely diagnostic criteria as our main source for understanding trauma. The profound psychological disturbances some people experience cannot be divorced from their situational context. It can also lead to the mistaken belief that the same set of techniques that work with one client will achieve the same outcomes with others, simply because they share the same immigration status and experiences of human-rights abuses.

There are some therapies that are viewed as effective in treating trauma and achieving recovery quickly, such as bilateral stimulation and somatic reprocessing. I question whether these treatments, which are designed to treat the individual, can address the wider context of trauma. In the 2010 documentary *5 Broken Cameras*, cameraman and co-director Emad Burnat says: 'Healing is a challenge in life. It is the victim's sole obligation. Healing is resistance to oppression.' I watched this film shortly after a trip to Palestine. Throughout that trip, people had explained to me that the people of Palestine were experiencing a collective trauma, not an individual one: a trauma that was caused by the situation in which they lived, and that the trauma was not in the past but ongoing. I thought about what Kevin had told me about his previous experience of therapy, where he felt he was blamed for what he was suffering and for the way he was coping within that suffering. It had also been so important to Kevin to use therapy to explore what he called the 'why' questions, which 'felt just like torture'. Some of those questions, as I remember, were about the sociopolitical landscape that contributed to the suffering of people Kevin met, but they were also about how Kevin experienced the world around him: how he felt negatively judged as an 'asylum seeker', as a man who was homeless, as someone whose human rights had been abused.

I am not questioning the validity of these interventions in treating trauma; however, my own perspective is not to view trauma as solely an intrapsychic response, but to consider it also as a relational one. Therapists are uniquely placed to understand the impact of social contexts on trauma and recovery; we could use this experience and knowledge outside the therapy room to inform and contribute to social change.

Kevin engaged with 'talking therapy', but he had no time for some of the other techniques I tried:

> I need to see my therapist as a human being, and be received as one, not judged on how I look. Life can change at any time, and people can change too. If you see someone who has been thrown onto the street, we are sometimes judged. My advice is this: our situations cause this; I do not cause this. My body experienced a beating and my mind ran away from it, but it didn't make me a bad person. I was both sick and well at the same time. Therapists, you can't treat the person unless the person trusts you.

Herman views trauma as existing somewhere between remembering and forgetting: 'The conflict between the will to deny horrible events and the will to proclaim them is the central dialectic of psychological trauma' (Herman, 1992: 1). Kevin's therapeutic journey did, in part, address this dialectic, and this was part of the healing. At the start of therapy Kevin was silent, but didn't want to be; he had frequently been silenced. In the beginning, he could not find a way to explain his experiences to others.

'They didn't ask me about any of this real stuff'

At a certain point, my response to our work together was to begin questioning if I was a good enough therapist. I thought things had improved, but that Kevin might need additional support, as some of the symptoms causing him distress had reduced but he was still enduring others. Over several months of careful negotiation, Kevin agreed to an onward referral to another mental health service. I felt relieved that he was going to get more support, but Kevin's experience at the other service was not the positive one we had, in different ways, hoped for.

Non-discrimination recognises sameness and difference while striving for equity and fairness. In our work, we must recognise the structural inequalities that impact on a survivor's ability to heal. Kevin was highly suspicious of health services. This was rooted partly in his experiences in Sudan, and partly in his perception of people's reactions to him in the UK. He felt at times that he was being blamed for his experiences; he often felt culturally misunderstood and that he was sometimes treated poorly, or even, from his point of view, with hostility and aggression. It was a priority for Kevin to include this here.

When he went for an initial assessment at another facility where we both hoped he would get additional support, he described walking into a room lit by a flickering fluorescent light. The reception desk was partitioned off with a screen; the furniture was bolted to the ground; the windows had grills on them. Kevin reported feeling distressed and disturbed by the environment; he experienced a sensitivity to the flickering light and said he started blinking rapidly before 'seeing everything again' in front of his eyes. Not feeling safe, he asked how to get out of the building, and then, when he finally got to see the mental health professional, asked for the door of the consulting room to remain open. Kevin did not feel these requests were responded to in a positive way. He remembered trying to explain his circumstances and talking about scavenging for food when he was destitute, and explaining that the Janjaweed had killed his family. Although the assessment was undertaken in English, which Kevin can speak, something was lost in translation: Kevin was left with the impression that the mental health professional thought the Janjaweed was some kind of street drug, and he felt that the assessment had focused on the possibility that he had a problem with substance misuse or addiction.

The mental health professional seemed to have got the impression that Kevin's presentation was histrionic. Kevin later received a letter discharging him, even though he had had no treatment other than the assessment appointment:

> I mean, how could they ask me about buying cocaine or marijuana when I did not have anything even to put in my stomach or even a small roof to go over my head – what were they thinking? Here was different. You did not try to bully me, and those people are bullies. Bullying means when a person is in disaster and you ask him stupid fucking questions. I mean, why did they not ask me, 'How do you eat?' No, they didn't ask about any of this real stuff.

It was disappointing that Kevin had been treated in this way, and it deterred him from taking up some of my other suggestions for putting more support in place.

Alongside the therapeutic work, I was working with many other professionals towards improving his living conditions, with his consent. They included social workers, housing support workers, housing lawyers, welfare advisers and an asylum legal representative. This was my attempt to change his social context, which was clearly causing him suffering. Each intervention required careful planning and negotiation, and all had to be attuned to Kevin's pacing. A human rights approach to trauma looks at all the factors that impact on the person's life. This may mean the therapist needs to think creatively about their work and expand their remit to include working on issues related to the right to health. In Kevin's case, I did this by working with others to ensure his basic needs were met, such as adequate housing, food and water, and by supporting Kevin to maintain contact with other health professionals when he found that problematic. He preferred to keep them at arm's length. We would often 'fight' about my repeated attempts to keep him in touch with his GP. Kevin needed his GP's support to be able to access other health professionals. Over time, his engagement with health services improved, which was fortunate when a serious and potentially life-threatening physical illness was diagnosed, years after the event that caused it.

'The most painful thing we did'

Now that Kevin could explain his past; his legal representative saw an opportunity to present new evidence that would help his asylum claim. This was a forensic, medico-legal report by a doctor, documenting evidence of his torture. Kevin would not undergo the necessary examination without my presence. He had more than 50 scars to document, as well as a soul seared by psychological ones. The doctor had to document Kevin's past now that he was able to put a narrative to his body's map.

For days, I sat next to him while he lay on a medical examination bed and gently negotiated with him the removal of his clothing so the doctor could measure the scarring. Hours seemed to pass before he would release an arm from a sleeve, the doctor would make pen marks on his body, measure the scars and document them, and Kevin would quickly recover the arm, and the process to uncover another area of his body would begin. It is one of the most profound experiences I have ever shared with another human being. Technically, it was not therapy, but the process became part of the therapy. I was on hand to support Kevin when a helicopter flying overhead triggered a flashback. In that moment of terror, Kevin's primary concern appeared to be my safety and that of the doctor.

The medico-legal report provided the evidence that enabled the Home Office to reconsider Kevin's asylum claim. He was given refugee status, or 'Sod Off Heaven' as he calls it. He was no longer homeless. This was less important for Kevin than that he would not have to undergo the medico-legal report process again:

> That, what's it called, that medical report, that made me feel terrible... I mean, it was the most painful thing we did. I don't think you could have done anything differently but I would not do it again. I know it helped... but the pain... I don't remember much about doing it but I know I would not do it again, no matter what.

The report helped his legal and social circumstances, but Kevin felt he had only just recreated a narrative about his experiences, and it was too soon to be exposed to a doctor's examination. Kevin warns against asking the same questions over and over, but there was a system of asylum support around him that required Kevin to answer questions about past events.

'I started changing'

Kevin developed rituals in the therapy sessions, especially around how they ended and how he interrupted them. Once, he got up, left the office and returned with a bowl of fruit from the reception area. He took some oranges from his bag, put them in the bowl, and returned it to reception. Then he left the room. I did not understand what was happening. He returned five minutes later and was silent for 20 minutes. I was bemused and remember reflecting a lot about the meaning of dignity. This was a continuation of the gift-giving that began with the cross-stitch picture, and also the beginning of Kevin's need to reach out to support other survivors who were using the reception area. Kevin always tried to find ways to give something back, perhaps as a way to fulfil a 'need to express love' (Erskine & Trautmann, 1996).

We have at different times received a variety of unusual gifts, some of which Kevin has told us he found in skips outside supermarkets. They included onions (you can imagine what an office of therapists made of that), 60 mince pies, a collection of cuddly toys, a sleeping bag and rucksack and £13.13. One Christmas he donated a clock. I commented that I was interested in its significance and pointed out that he seemed to find the constraints of the therapeutic hour and 'time up' difficult. He was silent, thinking, for a while, and then erupted into laughter. He looked directly at me and said: 'Bloody clock. I have totally set myself up, haven't I?'

Kevin would end sessions in ways that I found difficult to understand, and they were always changing. Sometimes a session would end with Kevin standing, facing the corner of my office, and muttering at the wall. I recognise how difficult it must have been to leave a place that felt safe and venture out into an environment that he experienced as hostile. Kevin agrees when he looks back on this behaviour. He would then rush from the office without looking back or saying goodbye. Then he changed the ritual: 15 minutes before the session was due to end, he would start trying to argue with me. More recently, at the 15-minute point before the end, he has started to wrap things up before I 'sack' him, as he likes to call it. He has developed the same instinctive awareness of the passing of an hour as many therapists.

He found breaks in our weekly sessions difficult, and blamed them for the occasional outbreak of what he called 'cold wars' between us. He stills talks about me 'disappearing' when I went on leave. We laugh about this now, but I also understand just how frightening this felt to Kevin, and the significance of people 'disappearing' from his life.

However, he has also said:

> We were having cold war because, in my opinion, sometimes we did not understand each other, and sometimes what you said was right and sometimes what I said was right, but cold wars could start from misunderstandings. These civil wars we had, you were patient with me, and I with you, and we worked on them, and I started changing. Sometimes I would create a civil war because I was pissed off with you. It's the trauma inside. Sometimes I am terrified and the therapeutic relationship was challenging.

The important thing is we always tried to sort out these wars; it was part of our therapeutic agreement with each other.

'I can open the door to my garden'

Kevin has a list of skills that he says are imperative for therapists working with refugees and survivors of torture. At first glance, they seem to be the core professional skills of any therapist. However, Kevin can point to a hundred examples of exchanges with caring professions where these skills were neglected, and only a handful of encounters where he felt he experienced them, so I dare say sometimes we are getting things wrong.

Kevin asks that we listen and seek to understand; that we explain what we are doing in a way that clients can easily understand; that we recognise the complexity of the therapeutic relationship and work to build it; that we involve clients in making decisions about their own care; that we are consistent; that we recognise that we have to earn our client's trust through our behaviours and actions, and don't expect it to be handed to us just because of our professional status, and that we acknowledge that, despite all our training, we are not the experts and we have no easy answers. Kevin does not want us to force our therapy models, tools and techniques on survivors. He asks that we negotiate each intervention, offer choice, and are flexible. He asks us not to rush into things, or expect instant results, or make irrelevant judgments about progress. Kevin asks that we learn something about the people we are working with, about their background and culture, their ideas, beliefs, and what formed them. He asks that we do not decide a survivor's mental competency from our first observations and how we interpret them. He points out that, even if they are undergoing the most major crisis, survivors deserve our respect, and that they have the right to make informed decisions, even if those decisions don't always suit the therapist. He views therapy not as something that is done to, but done with:

> Therapy is working inside the brain. Good therapy helps us move forward; it helps us make connections; it helps us want to get up, open the door, go into the garden. However, the therapist should invite you out slowly; they should not pull you out forcefully. I don't need my life to be any harder. I almost died, and I want to live. I don't want someone to force me into things. When I am in lockdown and there is no sleep, I want the therapist to help me work out my problems. I need to trust them. If I don't feel better at times, I don't want to feel it's my fault. Trust can be broken. You know, therapists can take the people who are in the grave and make them alive again, because some people, they look alive, but they are dead inside. Therapy helps us become alive again, step by step. It's true, and it is very important.

Kevin concludes that all survivors of torture should have access to therapy, and all therapists should be equipped to respond. He recognises that this may require investment:

> Resources are needed to build a survivor's confidence and trust and make them feel comfortable. It is not the place you go for therapy that counts, it is the person you see as a therapist. If the therapist changes, trust can be broken, and sometimes it can't be rebuilt. I didn't have to experience that, but some people I know did. Resources are important to keep therapists what they are, therapists, and where they are. Different people can impact you in different ways. At least I could judge you on your actions over time. I sometimes go to a garden. It helps me as well, it keeps me busy, but the garden is my hobby and I am happy doing it, and I can talk to other people there and sometimes share some experiences. But therapy is therapy; it is a personal and private space, and it requires a different kind of trust. It's where I work out my problems so I can open the door to my garden.

References

American Psychiatric Association (APA) (1980). *Diagnostic and Statistical Manual of Mental Disorders (3rd edition)*. Washington, DC: American Psychiatric Association.

Erskine RG, Trautmann RL (1996). Methods of an integrative psychotherapy. *Transactional Analysis Journal* 26(4): 316–328. www.integrativetherapy.com/en/articles.php?id=63 (accessed July 2017).

Fassin D, Rechtman R (2009). *The Empire of Trauma: an enquiry into the condition of victimhood*. Princeton, NJ: Princeton University Press.

Herman JL (1992). *Trauma and Recovery: the aftermath of violence – from domestic abuse to political terror*. New York, NY: Basic Books.

Stutheridge J (2006). Inside out: a transactional analysis model of trauma. *Transactional Analysis Journal* 36(4): 270–283.

UNHCR (2016). *Global trends: forced displacement in 2016*. Geneva: UNHCR. www.unhcr.org/globaltrends2016/ (accessed July 2017).

van der Hart O, Brown P, van der Kolk BA (1989). Pierre Janet's treatment of post-traumatic stress. *Journal of Post-Traumatic Stress* 2(4): 379–395.

World Health Organization (1992). *The ICD-10 classification of mental and behavioural disorders*. Geneva: World Health Organization.

3. Recovery and reconnection
Kirsten Lamb

The right to rehabilitation of survivors of torture is contained in Article 14 (1) of the UN Convention Against Torture and Other Cruel, Inhuman or Degrading Treatment or Punishment (UNCAT) (OHCHR, 1984). This states:

> Each state party shall ensure in its legal system that the victim of an act of torture obtains redress and has an enforceable right to fair and adequate compensation, including the means for as full rehabilitation as possible.

A discussion paper produced by the Medical Foundation for the Care of Victims of Torture, now known as Freedom from Torture, describes how practitioners working with survivors of torture have applied the principles of rehabilitation in mental health to torture-related psychological health difficulties (Smith, Patel & MacMillan, 2010). Anthony (1993) describes rehabilitation as what helpers/services do to facilitate recovery. In the torture field, this includes medical and psychological care, as well as legal support in seeking asylum, and social/educational support.

Recovery is what people do in the face of the catastrophes of life; thus, it is a universal, unifying and unique personal experience (Anthony, 1993). In the mental health field, recovery is the process through which individuals with a mental health condition find ways to live a meaningful life, whether or not they continue to experience symptoms of the condition. Recovery is described as a deeply personal process of changing one's attitudes, values, feelings, goals, skills, and/or roles. It is a way of living a satisfying, hopeful, and contributing life, even with limitations caused by illness (Anthony, 1993). Recovery involves a personal journey of discovery and development of new meaning and purpose in one's life. It also requires a supportive environment, to maximise the person's opportunities and functioning, alongside actively challenging stigma and discrimination.

In my work with survivors of torture, I use Herman's three-stage model of recovery from trauma (1992). Her model applies to the aftermath of prolonged, repeated trauma, where there has been a sustained threat to life, whether perceived or actual, in an interpersonal context. In addition to developing symptoms of post-traumatic stress disorder (PTSD), depression, anxiety and loss, 'enduring personality change' can result from catastrophic experiences (World Health Organization, 1992). Herman names her stages of recovery safety, remembrance and mourning, and reconnection. Here I will describe practice-based evidence and guidelines covering her third stage of recovery, drawing from my work and that of other practitioners in the trauma and refugee field.

From safety to reconnection

Recovery from trauma is about working through the following key processes:

- establishing a level of safety and security
- stabilisation of trauma symptoms
- facing traumatic memories
- the integration of the trauma into a new narrative of self and personality, and
- moving forward to living an ordinary life.

Rehabilitation following torture may also include the opportunity for the survivor to give testimony, to seek access to restorative justice and to pursue survivor activism.

Papadopoulos's concept of the Trauma Grid (2007) has expanded our understanding of the effects of trauma beyond the purely negative. He categorises the effects of trauma under three headings: negative (psychiatric symptoms, psychological distress and ordinary human suffering), neutral (resilience), and positive (adversity-activated development (AAD)). Also positive is the concept of post-traumatic growth, first described by Calhoun and Tedeschi (2006) in the mid-1990s.

Post-traumatic growth describes a post-trauma transformation that exceeds pre-trauma levels of functioning in three broad domains: sense of self, life philosophy and interpersonal relationships. It develops from the resolution of a dissonance between pre- and post-trauma worldviews, where a significant challenge to a person's assumptive world has occurred and their worldview then changes for the better. The negative, neutral and positive categories of the effects of trauma are not mutually exclusive and, according to Papadopoulos (2007), depend on a range of factors other than the actual traumatic experience itself: personal (eg. personality characteristics, history, coping mechanisms), relational (eg. supporting systems), gender, power position, meaning (political, religious, ideological), and presence or absence of hope.

Therapeutic interventions developed from an understanding of post-traumatic growth and AAD can facilitate recovery for survivors of torture. For example, interventions that foster a sense of personal agency have been shown to be important facilitators for growth (Joseph & Linley, 2005). Tedeschi and Calhoun (2006: 292) emphasise the importance of the therapist adopting an open stance with the survivor, and valuing their experiences as 'potential sources for learning rather than approaching the survivor merely as a collection of symptoms to be altered'.

The Trauma Grid describes the impact of trauma at four levels: individual, family, community, and society/culture. This serves to remind us that recovery from torture involves more than one-to-one therapeutic work. Kira's Wraparound Approach (2002) is also multi-systemic and community-based. It distinguishes between the remits of the therapy team and the rehabilitation team. The focus of the rehabilitation team is on body therapy, including physical, dance movement, respiratory, art and music, activity and recreational and biofeedback. Kira describes the body as 'the site of the initial wound in torture', and, therefore, suggests that somatic rehabilitation can be the 'instrument through which the survivor can heal' (2002: 75). He argues that, where psychological therapists have no access to a body therapy team, it is helpful if they hold these aspects of the recovery process in mind and try 'to provide interventions that address both the body and the mind' (2002: 75).

Omeri and colleagues contend that moving from post-traumatic stress to post-traumatic growth is 'not only a function of the therapeutic relationship but a matter of social policy' (2004: 28). In achieving reconnection and integration into living an ordinary life, the torture survivor moves from 'responding to their trauma to responding to the meaning of the traumatic events', and 'that meaning is provided by their surrounding culture' (2004: 28).

I am not going to explore in depth here the various socio-political-cultural contexts in which recovery takes place and how the recovery process is influenced by them. However, it is important to recognise these influences and, where appropriate, acknowledge the political context of seeking asylum and the universal struggle for human rights. Seeking asylum may cause additional traumatic experiences, both in terms of the journey to safety and the legal process. My clients have described waiting for decisions that are beyond their control as another form of 'mental torture'. Survivors describe being detained in the UK as a terrifying and dehumanising experience; many compare it with the experience of imprisonment in their home countries, in that they are powerless and under threat. Minimising the potential for retraumatisation is an important part of the recovery journey.

Herman's three stages of recovery from trauma are not distinct and separate, and it is important to recognise that some processes will be common to all the stages. Joseph distinguishes between avoidance-coping and approach-oriented coping. He argues that, while the latter facilitates recovery, sometimes some avoidance can be helpful (2011: 128–129). The survivor needs to develop flexible and adaptive ways of coping, moving from an avoidant stance to an approach stance. I would suggest this ability is also necessary for the therapist.

Finally, it is important to be mindful of the links between recovery and ending formal individual psychological therapy. Survivors often seek therapy while they are going through the asylum process. There is the risk that ending psychological therapy could become mixed up in their minds with securing international protection. It is important to hold in mind that the goal of therapy is not being granted asylum, but psychological recovery.

The clients' stories in this chapter are fictional and based on amalgamated examples from my practice.

Reconnecting and integrating

From the start of therapy, it is important to have a clear, shared understanding with the client about the purpose of therapy and the route to reaching the therapy goal. Recovery is not simply about dealing with trauma symptoms. The goal is to help survivors connect with this changed person they have become, with the trauma more or less integrated into their autobiographical identity, and to help them live in the present, with a sense of hope about the future and a life to be lived as fully as possible. The therapist is aiming to connect with the client as an individual and help them to understand how their experience of torture has affected them. The survivor also needs support to explore their wider experiences of oppression, both in the UK and in their own country. Finding meaning (personal, social and political) is important in recovery (Bracken & Petty, 1998).

Reconnection starts at the beginning of therapy, and may occur at any point during the therapy. The Den Bosch five-phase treatment model of group therapy, developed in the Netherlands and described by Drožđek and Wilson in their book *Broken Spirits* (2004: 250), defines phase four as covering 'reconnecting the present with the past and the future, damaged core beliefs, roles and identity, coping strategies, current worries and future outlooks' (2004: 255).

Broadly, the reconnection process involves:

- connecting with the therapist
- identifying pre-trauma personality, interests, strengths and resilience
- recognising significant role relationships
- facilitating post-traumatic growth through 'expert companionship' (Calhoun & Tedeschi, 2006: 292)
- reclaiming a physical self
- creating opportunities for new interests to develop
- creating opportunities to reduce social isolation (therapeutic activity groups and/or community activities)
- connecting with a transformed sense of self
- connecting with family, community and culture.

When working in a specialist rehabilitation service for survivors of torture, I am mindful of the need to document the details of my clients' torture experience, as this may be important for the success of their claim for asylum. Survivors may be able to recall and disclose more details about their torture as the psychological therapy progresses. Psychological therapists working in any setting should be aware that they may be asked to document a client's account of torture and its psychological impact in the form of a report or clinical letter. If a report is required by a client's legal representative, therapists should refer for guidance to the *Istanbul Protocol* (OHCHR, 1999).

An important element of reconnection is the ability to establish new, positive relationships with other people. By establishing a therapeutic relationship of trust and safety, the therapist is modelling a template for the client from the very first meeting. If the therapist is working with an interpreter, this offers the client another opportunity for building a positive relationship.

Survivors of torture may need help to reconnect with their own past. Sometimes the therapist can create the barrier to looking back, if they are experiencing vicarious traumatisation and also avoiding the past. Alternatively, if a client's torture experiences occurred in the context of a political conflict that has been widely reported in the western media, the therapist may identify with a client as a fellow human-rights activist. Factors such as these may mask the therapist's ability to access who the client was before they became a survivor of torture. Some survivors may have had other traumatic experiences, including childhood sexual abuse, prolonged exposure to war, domestic violence or sexual exploitation, before the actual torture. For them, it may not be helpful to draw a distinct line between 'before' and 'after' torture. A recovery-oriented assessment needs to be holistic, focus on the whole person, and include a narrative of the client's pre-torture life and any previous trauma experiences, as well as information about their talents, interests, abilities, natural strengths and resources.

For some clients, their identity and their torture are closely linked: for example, if they have been persecuted for being a political activist, a writer, a lawyer, an artist, or because of their sexual orientation. There is some evidence that survivors who were persecuted for their political activism and were prepared for the consequences of their actions are less damaged by the experience, or better able to recover (Başoğlu et al, 1997).

Survivors who were not aware of the risks they were taking may blame their subsequent torture on their interests or work role, and want nothing more to do with them. Clients whose interests have no obvious connection with the torture, such as sports or nature, may be less likely to avoid them. However, they may be unable, for other reasons, to pursue their favourite activities or hobbies, and will still experience loss and disconnection. This can happen if the torture caused lasting physical injury, impairment or pain that prevents the activity being enjoyed again.

For example, a client who was a competitive wrestler in his home country tried joining a football group in the UK. He enjoyed the distraction and physicality of the football, but the pain in his joints afterwards was too great for him to continue.

A family history will have been taken as part of a full assessment. Before the torture, the survivor will have occupied certain social and family roles, such as wife, husband, mother, father, daughter, son, breadwinner – roles that they regarded as positive and valued. Torture and flight will have disrupted these relationships, to varying degrees. The therapist will need to explore these issues with the client, where appropriate, as part of facilitating their reconnection. For example, a client who has left behind a spouse and/or children may be under pressure to send money back to their family, to ensure their survival, but this may not be possible if they are not allowed to work, or are too ill to do so. They may only just be managing to survive themselves, and may have no spare resources or capacity to think about the needs of others. Survivors may protect themselves by deliberately avoiding contact with their family. Thus, their role as a spouse or parent will have changed from a positive aspect of their identity to one that is negative and that they seek to avoid.

Where torture involves sexual violence, this is likely to impact on the survivor's sexual functioning, with implications for the person, and for their relationship with their partner if they have fled with their spouse. Women who have been raped may find it very hard to allow any physical contact or intimacy from their partners. Male African survivors with whom I have worked have described their experience of sexual torture as 'being made to become wives'. This phrase vividly describes an experience of complete emasculation. Trauma-processing work will address the memories and the emotional pain, but the recovery process will need to explore ways for them to regain their sense of masculinity and positive male identity. They may need specialist psychosexual counselling to follow up psychological therapy.

A survivor's marriage or partnership may end while they are in therapy. Perhaps the spouse or partner left behind has had to move on with their life. In some countries, they may need to find someone else to provide for them financially. Clients have said that the news that a relationship has ended or their spouse has found a new partner can be a relief – a release from responsibility for their partner or from feelings of guilt – and also a devastating loss. Therapy may be the only place where survivors can express these conflicting emotions.

Survivors who have left behind elderly or sick parents live with the knowledge that they cannot provide the support that would be expected of them in most cultures. They are in limbo, waiting for possible bad news and living with the likelihood that they may not see their parents again. In addition to managing all the associated emotions, there is the challenge of dealing with role transgression – the son or daughter who is not taking care of their parents when they are in need.

Some survivors in exile have lost all contact with family members. They may have been killed during political conflict, either randomly or in response to the survivor's activities. It may take time for the details to emerge in therapy, due to the guilt and shame. I worked with a client who found it very hard to talk about his children until he was able to face his fears that they had probably been killed in retaliation for his escape. A turning point occurred when he told me about an incident in a shopping centre, when he had run after a young boy who looked like his son, calling out his son's name. He was distraught with shame that he had frightened the boy and the boy's mother by his seemingly bizarre behaviour.

I have also worked with a visual artist whose art had violated culturally acceptable norms in her country of origin. I tried encouraging her to use art materials to express her emotions, but this triggered her traumatic memories and blocked, rather than facilitated, her emotional expression, as she transferred her anger at being tortured to her art and away from the torturers. When I recognised this, and understood that art was just one pathway for her creativity, I explored other ways of connecting her with her creative side: for example, through songwriting and singing. She joined a choir and found a new sense of purpose and a creative outlet while she was still in the second stage of recovery. Thus, although she was unable to use her creative skills for trauma processing, they played an important part in helping her develop a new sense of identity.

The reconnecting process requires the therapist to offer more than the core components of a good therapeutic relationship, which is of course central to all therapy models. Given that many survivors of torture have lost their sense of who they are, and often feel irreparably damaged, the relationship with the therapist may be their only meaningful human connection in the present. Their significant relationships will all be in the past, and either lost or continuing only as abusive voices (of their torturers) in their heads. The therapist needs not only to form a therapeutic relationship with the client but also to become the vehicle for connecting the survivor with their present life. The therapist has to find ways to get to know their client as a person, and help the client to get to know themselves again. An important aspect of therapy will be to help clients find new or different roles for themselves, or change how they view an existing role: for example, as a parent, they may not be able to be a financial provider for their children, but they can still be a provider of unconditional love.

Some clients may be so stuck or lost in the trauma that they become disconnected not only from who they are but also from their asylum application or grant of refugee status. Both the risk of removal from the UK and the benefit of protection in the UK may lose their meaning for or impact on some survivors, so consumed are they by the trauma of their torture and their need to avoid re-experiencing it.

Survivors may present with suicidal thoughts, intentions and plans, or with inertia and little motivation to do anything. Through forming a relationship with the therapist, a client can be helped to re-engage with and actively pursue their asylum application. When survivors of torture first apply for asylum, they are often not well placed to present all the available evidence. Survivors may need to be helped to locate a sense of agency so they can pursue the task of obtaining evidence to support their claim, such as asking people to provide witness statements, getting relevant documents sent from their country of origin and sharing information with their legal representative.

In a human rights-based therapy approach, it is a legitimate aspect of the therapeutic work to help the client to pursue their asylum application, while acknowledging the actual outcome is outside the therapist's control and may not be a just or fair decision.

The therapist can encourage conversations about the therapy room itself. When therapists are working in temporary or shared therapy rooms, bringing in small plants, decorative objects, cushions or pictures can help make the room less anonymous. Discussing the room and/or its contents can provide an opportunity for survivors to make observations about the environment, like the noise levels, the comfort of the chairs, and, more importantly, which chair they prefer to sit on. In this way, therapists can help the survivor value the small choices they are able to make as a gradual step to being able to develop more agency.

The conversation can also be a starting point for the survivor to identify their likes and dislikes. This simple enquiry can indicate how much sense of self they have retained, lost or dismissed. One of my clients commented on how much he liked the plant in the therapy room, as he had always had an interest in nature. I encouraged him to buy one for his bedroom. Psychologically, the plant might function as a transitional object, representing the safety of the therapeutic relationship and carrying that sense of safety into the outside world. Looking after the plant may both rekindle past interests and help the client connect with the caring or responsible part of his past self. Reconnecting work can take place at a metaphorical level and through parallel processing: taking the plant as an example, the therapist could explore the conditions needed for its healthy growth in order to help the client connect with their own daily living needs.

As with the other stages of recovery, the reconnecting process can include psychoeducation, where appropriate, and depending on the survivor's psychological-mindedness. For some clients, a brief description of Maslow's hierarchy of needs can be validating (Maslow, 1943) and may provide a stepwise approach to the tasks of recovery. The therapist needs to be aware of and acknowledge the cultural differences between individualistic and collectivistic societies, while recognising that these are broad generalisations (Takano & Osaka, 1999). Splevins and colleagues (2010) cite the work of Markus and Kitayama, who propose that a critical difference between individualistic and collectivistic cultures is how the person defines their identity in relation to others. In individualistic cultures, identity refers to how a person sees themselves, while in more collectivistic cultures, people tend to define the self in relation to their social (family and community) context.

In individualistic societies, 'priority is given to the actualization of individual potential' (Splevins et al, 2010: 260). The therapist should consider with their client how comfortable they feel about the more individualistic culture here in the UK. I worked with a client who seized an opportunity he would not have had in his own country to enrol on an interior design course; he was the only man in a class of 20 women.

A human-rights approach

For survivors in the UK, it might be helpful to explain that here we have the right to freedom of expression in terms of religious beliefs, sexuality and speech. An exploration of both the client's and therapist's assumptive worldviews can be useful, even at a very simple level. A survivor from an African country where male life expectancy is less than 50 years told me he felt that his life was nearly over. I told him what the average life expectancy was in the UK, as a way of challenging his negative beliefs. With this longer life trajectory before him, he became more optimistic that he had a worthwhile future. Drožđek and Wilson give a similar example from their groupwork, where clients from Africa in their late 30s and early 40s said, 'In our country, many people die in their late 40s, and it does not make much sense to make plans for the future' (2004: 270).

An educational component in the therapy may help a survivor engage more with their legal representative. Many clients do not know what they can expect from a legal representative, and believe they have to wait to be contacted, rather than get in touch when they need information. Survivors may come from cultures where lawyers are seen as elite or authority figures, and clients may not understand that their legal representative is working for them. A relational focus in therapy can help survivors engage more productively with their legal representative, as well as with their GP. For clients who already have the right to settle, the same approach can be applied to their encounters with the various professionals they come into contact with when seeking work, welfare benefits and housing. Survivors may need to be told what they can expect in terms of professional standards and services, such as the right to have copies of all letters written about them.

The police, members of the armed forces, or anyone in formal uniform may present particular challenges, as they can trigger survivors' memories of their torture and, possibly, of their detention in this country. In a human-rights approach, the therapist will be working from the belief that the survivor is entitled to be treated with equality and respect. The trauma-focused aspects of therapy will work on reducing the trigger/PTSD response, and the reconnecting phase will address the client's ability to establish present-day working relationships based on a sense of empowerment and rights. This may include helping a client challenge discrimination based on their race, faith or sexual orientation.

I supported a client after he was struck on the head by a large stone that was thrown at the bus on which he was travelling. He was taken to hospital for treatment and the incident was given a crime number, but he was not interviewed by the police. Upset and angry, he focused on wanting compensation, and I arranged an appointment with Victim Support, an independent charity that supports victims of crime in England and Wales. Then my client began to realise the impact of the attack on how he behaved: he was avoiding taking the bus and he was troubled when he saw groups of young, white men. He felt that the stone was directed at him, as a black person, and now wanted to report it as a racist attack. Two months after the incident, the police interviewed him to establish whether the incident should be reclassified as a hate crime. Thus, recovery involves the survivor being able to shed their victim identity as opportunities to develop other, more psychologically helpful identities arise. One client told me that, after taking part in a group musical performance, he took the event programme listing his name to his next reporting date at the Home Office reporting centre, and announced that he was a musician. He wanted to be recognised as having another identity: he was not just an 'asylum seeker'.

Fostering curiosity and challenging fears

It can be helpful to find out about social, creative and educational opportunities for clients, and encourage them to try out and take part in activities. Even if a survivor says they do not feel well enough to go, or declines the offer, they will now know there are opportunities available at a future date. The therapist is also demonstrating a belief that the survivor is able to undertake and manage a particular activity. Sometimes, in the latter phases of therapy, I have explicitly told clients that the activity itself is not the important thing; it is the vehicle for making social connections or fostering curiosity or challenging fears.

Herman describes how, in the reconnection phase, survivors come to understand that 'their post-traumatic symptoms represent a pathological exaggeration of normal responses to danger' (1992: 197). She suggests this is a time for clients to experiment and take on new challenges. For example, they might learn to ride a bike or swim, if they haven't tried them before. Initially they may be afraid – that they will drown or fall off the bike – and experience a physical reaction through the autonomic arousal response. In this way, in addition to the practical benefits, such activities have a more therapeutic aim of helping the survivor learn to accept a normal experience of fear. Thus, recovery work should include opportunities to retune physiological and psychological responses to fear, as well as focus on restructuring maladaptive social responses such as avoidance of people or seeing oneself only as a victim.

Therapists may need to reflect on whether they are taking on the role of rescuer, as this can maintain the client in a victim position. Having occupied the central role in a client's recovery, the therapist will need to move away from this as the reconnecting phase develops. Survivors will have regained some capacity for appropriate trust through the therapeutic relationship, and they will benefit from experimenting with developing trust in other relationships. This may involve referring clients to other professional colleagues, to other therapeutic or creative activities, to group therapy, or just taking a back seat in relation to their contact with other professionals – for example, no longer making phone calls on a survivor's behalf.

As the trauma-processing work progresses and the survivor becomes less troubled by clinical symptoms, reconnection work may focus on re-establishing a survivor's role within their family. For example, if the survivor is a parent who has left behind children in their country of origin, telephone contact can be painful. The children may ask questions that the survivor can't answer: where are you? when are you coming back? why aren't you here? One client was so troubled by her inability to answer these questions that she avoided speaking to her children for months at a time. She tried not to think of herself as their mother and, at times, the children were so present in their absence that they became an elephant in the therapy room. To work on this, I started with a psychoeducational focus, looking at what being a mother is like and helping her acknowledge her love for her children, even if she couldn't provide for them or be with them. We were able to have gentle conversations about their birthdays and what she would like to tell them about her life in the UK. She wanted to tell them about the first time she saw snow. Then we found a way that she could send them some money, and this proved a breakthrough. She was able to open up to her children, as she could demonstrate to them that they were still at the centre of her thoughts, even though they were separated.

As therapy progresses, the therapist should look out for the following changes as signs of recovery:
- building resilience
- forming an autobiographical narrative as a survivor

- developing a sense of knowing oneself in the present
- developing self-confidence and a sense of self-efficacy
- re-integration of role identity
- re-establishing relationships (family and friendships) and making new ones
- empowerment/finding a voice, speaking out (for some survivors)
- facing endings.

When to end therapy

As therapists, we tend to see the assessment phase as crucial. It undoubtedly determines the flow and effectiveness of therapy, but often the ending of therapy can be more difficult and challenging, on several different levels. During the therapy, clients may have come to regard the therapist or the provider organisation as their new family. The therapist may have been the main witness to their daily life and may have felt like their only source of support. As the meaning of family in different cultures varies and is not necessarily defined by blood ties, it can be puzzling for clients from some cultures to understand the concept of ending therapy.

Some therapists may be constrained by service policies and guidelines that specify a maximum number of sessions. Others may be able to work with an open-ended contract that allows them to decide with the client when to end.

Ending therapy inevitably means facing loss, for both the therapist and the client. For the therapist, this can tap into their personal experiences of dealing with loss. Therapy should be ended in a way that allows the normal feelings of loss to be experienced and activates the healing process of grieving. Clients can be prepared for this, if they have made progress in the areas discussed above.

Ideally, the fact that the therapy is time-limited will be introduced in the assessment phase. Ending therapy should not come as a surprise and, once a client is engaged in therapy, every effort should be made to protect their ability to work towards a planned ending. This is psychologically crucial for survivors of torture, because the torture experience will have forced the ending of most aspects of their past, normal life. Survivors will have experienced numerous abrupt, traumatic and unplanned endings, where the adaptive psychological processes for dealing with loss and death will have been overridden.

It is important that the goals of therapy that were agreed during the assessment phase are revisited during the third stage of recovery, in preparation for a 'good' therapy ending. Goals at the beginning of therapy tend to be aspirational and to give a hopeful message about change and recovery. Herman states that: 'The resolution of the trauma is never final; recovery is never complete' (1992: 211). It is important for therapists to accept this and not seek recovery as an endpoint. Herman describes the process of ending therapy as the shift from 'the tasks of recovery to the tasks of ordinary life' (1992: 212). Drožđek and Wilson list 'psychoeducation, relapse prevention, treatment evaluation and farewell ritual' as the components of the final phase of their therapy (2004: 255).

I recall reaching an ending with a survivor when he said he had 'nothing to speak to me about', even though he still had not had a successful outcome to his asylum application and his situation remained precarious. Previously a fisherman in his country of origin, he was now occupied with the chores and difficulties of his daily life, attending various refugee activity groups and teaching himself to play the guitar. Although the ability to live an ordinary life is not determined by one's residency status, one's income/work, housing and access to education/qualifications are likely to define it, and the ordinary life of a person seeking asylum will be more limited, due to their insecure legal status, lack of control and financial difficulties. This can obscure the psychological progress made when a good-enough-for-now daily routine has been achieved.

For some survivors, a successful asylum application can start the process of ending therapy; for others, it may be destabilising. The therapist will need to assess the impact on clients of such a significant event and not make assumptions about what being granted refugee status means to them.

Sometimes it will be important to celebrate the grant of refugee status, particularly as a client can feel validated by finally being believed by the Home Office or judge. This can facilitate the client's ability to reconnect with themselves. Other clients may need to avoid the reality of being granted refugee status. One client took nearly a year to tell his family that he had been granted protection. If a client is using a high level of avoidance, continuing therapy is generally indicated, although further trauma processing will inevitably be delayed until the client has moved through the transition process and re-established a level of stability in their lives. When a client moves readily into managing the challenges involved in the transition to a more ordinary life, this probably indicates that the time is right to begin to work towards ending therapy, thereby reinforcing a positive message about new beginnings. Survivors will have developed an ability to manage the high stress levels inherent in the major life events of moving house, finding work etc.

Ending therapy

How and when to end therapy will be determined to some extent by the therapy contract agreed at the start of therapy. If the therapy contract offered a set number of sessions, there can be a countdown to the last session. More flexible therapy contracts offer the opportunity to explore with clients how they would like to end therapy – for example, by agreeing an end date or having an agreed number of sessions spread out over time. For me, the crucial component of the ending is that it is planned and transparent.

A planned ending is important as it allows the client to experience a sense of control and uncertainty at the same time. I would suggest that this can be arranged if the client has understood the purpose of ending therapy: that recovery itself is not an end point but a starting point for living an ordinary life, without therapy. Clients can feel a sense of control if they can decide the pacing of the final sessions and have a choice about goodbye rituals. There will be continuing uncertainty about the future and unknown eventualities, which for some may be about family reunion; for others, it may be about employment/training and volunteering opportunities.

Towards the end of therapy, some clients may be able to manage sessions without an interpreter. It can be useful to identify a session where the client can say goodbye to the interpreter; this may be the first time that the interpreter can speak directly to the client. I have observed some heartfelt sentiments expressed between clients and interpreters; exchanges of gratitude and respect are a shared experience of validation. Clients can be helped to see that no longer needing an interpreter is both an achievement and a loss. I see it as my responsibility, as the therapist, to manage the balance of emotions and help the client feel the loss of a relationship and celebrate their achievement in speaking English and moving further towards independence.

To me, there are similarities with the work, described earlier, aimed at helping survivors accept a normal experience of fear: that is, the challenge of helping your client manage ambivalent and confusing emotions as 'normal'. There needs to be a balance between facilitating grieving and acknowledging the positive changes made during therapy. An ending inevitably connects with earlier losses and, for a survivor of torture, the sum of their losses may have been too overwhelming to face. Grieving can be complicated when a survivor has to live with the uncertainty of not knowing whether their relatives who have disappeared have been killed by the authorities or if a family member has died after the survivor fled, and they have no family physically nearby with whom to share their loss. Additional difficulties with grieving can arise when survivors are detached from their cultural rituals and/or have lost faith in their religion.

Ending therapy can provide a kind of parallel process because there is no actual death. The aim is that the therapist is held in mind by the client as an internal 'good' object, and as a resource for the client to fall back on if they encounter difficulties in the future. Saying goodbye in therapy can open up a conversation about how the client can hold lost loved ones in mind and remember them, rather than avoid the emotional pain.

A planned ending gives the opportunity to revisit the work done in the earlier stages of therapy, and to acknowledge fears and unmanageable feelings that have been named and worked through. An example from my work is a male survivor who initially was unable to make any eye contact with me. Given his level of distress, I worried that I would make him feel worse if I mentioned it, and so I avoided exploring it for several months. When we did speak, he gradually explained that he could not make eye contact with anyone because of his shame; he felt if he made eye contact, people would see that he had been sexually violated during his torture. During our ending, we revisited his previous lack of eye contact to demonstrate how he had changed; he had accepted that his internal feelings were not visible to others and that it was his lack of eye contact made him appear different, not his torture experiences.

In the ending phase, it is important to revisit previous fears and avoidance behaviour in order to recognise the changes the survivor has achieved. The client may need reminding of this, so they can take the progress forward into the future. It is also important to identify and reinforce how these changes have occurred – these may be behavioural changes using effective coping strategies, or cognitive ones achieved through developing more confidence and self-belief. Some clients may be able to recognise elements of personal growth resulting from the experience of trauma (post-traumatic growth) (Joseph, 2011).

Towards the last few sessions with a client, I will invite survivors to think about what they would like to happen in our final session. A level of physical contact may already have been established in the therapy, such as formal handshakes or touch as a grounding technique. Alternatively, physical touch may have only happened in physiotherapy sessions or medical examinations. No matter what contact has happened previously in the therapeutic relationship, a planned ending allows this to be discussed and explored in terms of the meaning it holds for the client. These discussions also serve as a dress rehearsal for the final session, so you know whether your client wants to share a hug, shake hands or not have any physical contact. I am left with an empty feeling when a goodbye does not involve any physical contact, and feel this preparation is important for both the therapist and the survivor. There may be other culturally specific goodbye rituals that can be shared.

Sometimes it is possible to share food/drink that is associated with either the therapy or a cultural ritual, or to have a conversation about the food, rather than the food itself. Early in therapy, one of my clients described her struggle to decide what food to bring to the end-of-term celebration at her English language class. She felt very disconnected from what she liked, and found it difficult to make any decisions. In the therapy session, I asked about the food that her mother had cooked when she was growing up. Through this process, she decided on a simple dish to take into college. We spoke about this dish in our last session as the time she began to reconnect with her pre-torture self.

I also invite clients to think if they would like to ask any questions about me. Sharing relevant personal information at this stage can serve to put the therapeutic relationship on a more equal footing. I prepare survivors for possible future contact outside the boundary of therapy and explain that I will always let them decide if they want to initiate any contact. This can puzzle them, if they feel I have become a family member. I still think it's important to have the conversation, to demonstrate that they have a choice and that I will respect that choice. If the interpreter is present at the ending session, it is also important to create space for the interpreter and client to say their own goodbyes in the context of this therapy experience.

Ending sessions may evoke the same high levels of anxiety and emotional intensity that the survivor brought to therapy at the start. Some clients may need some adjustments in the ending phase. Some therapists may be able to offer clients the opportunity to return to therapy at a later date, to engage with further emotional processing. Ending therapy may sometimes be more about taking a break or preparing for future psychological therapy. Some clients may not be able to engage in the trauma processing phase of therapy until they have gained a level of safety through a successful asylum application, or until they are no longer living in an environment where their trauma symptoms are continually triggered.

A planned ending may be sabotaged or avoided. A client may start missing sessions or cancelling them with apparently plausible reasons. This, of course, can happen at any stage of therapy, but it is especially important to address it when a formal ending is being derailed. There is the temptation for the therapist to view this as the client being already in the process of moving on, and to let this happen and disengage. But it could indicate that the survivor is showing emotional avoidance: they may be struggling to express feelings of anger, rejection or loss. If this is the case, it can more helpful to acknowledge the avoidance and try to share an understanding of it, rather than leave it unsaid. I am suggesting that naming the emotions that need to be processed, even if they are not expressed, is more helpful than leaving them as too dangerous or shameful.

Finally, I would like to acknowledge that sometimes endings happen outside the control of both the therapist and client. This may occur if the client is detained for a long time in the UK for immigration purposes, or if they 'disappear' following a failed asylum claim. Both these scenarios, for differing reasons, leave the therapist with an unresolved ending. It is important for the therapist in this situation to recognise their need to process the loss of the client, and to access clinical supervision.

'I am still on the journey to find out...'

For both therapist and survivor, the therapy journey has been driven by hope and expectation, and ending therapy may also involve being left with disappointment, uncertainty and the prospect of an unknown future. As therapists, we tend not to know what happens to our clients – their achievements and the hurdles they face. I feel privileged that some clients have got back in touch to share good news. I once saw a former client performing in a play in a well-known theatre, without him recognising me.

Perhaps unusually, I have also had the experience of a former client becoming a work colleague. I would like to end with some of his reflections on the impact of therapy. As part of his commitment to survivor activism, he wants to be named. In his late 20s, Jonathan fled conflict and torture in the eastern region of the Democratic Republic of the Congo, where he had worked as a teacher. He had no previous experience of therapy: 'It didn't mean anything culturally. The local priest would pray for you, that would be it.' He described how aspects of the therapy have stayed with him years later: he feels he can 'touch things said during therapy'. They were words then, but now they are solid, real and part of him.

> At the start of therapy, I worried about the loss. I was a teacher; what will I become now? But when I look back, I realise I'm a new, stronger person. I don't need to try to become a teacher. I feel like my voice has been found and amplified. I came from a small, remote place, but here I can see my voice travelling and reaching more people than I was when I was tortured.

> I wanted to erase my past... I didn't understand therapy when I started but now, when I look back, I can see a structure to the journey of therapy: first, being listened to, second, being given techniques that have helped, being able to hear the praise and recognition from the therapist, recognising that the therapist believed in what I was and what I could become... facing up to the challenge of knowing yourself better. I now feel I understand myself better.
>
> I didn't know sitting and being listened to could be that powerful. That's what heals you: having time and space, at your own pace to talk about things.
>
> I am still on the journey to find out... what I know now is that I can be in control of what the future is for me.

This chapter has sought to give an overview of the ending phases of psychological therapy with survivors of torture. Jonathan's words reflect the main themes:

- safety and connection in the therapeutic relationship – *'I didn't know sitting and being listened to could be that powerful'*
- loss of self and identity – *'I was a teacher. What will I become now?'*
- timely use of techniques informed by different therapeutic models – *'being listened to... being given techniques that have helped'*
- finding meaning – *'I now feel I understand myself better'*
- growth through adversity – *'I realise I'm a new, stronger person now'*
- a human-rights approach and survivor activism – *'My voice has been found and amplified.'*

References

Anthony WA (1993). Recovery from mental illness: the guiding vision of the mental health service system in the 1990s. *Psychosocial Rehabilitation Journal* 16(4): 11–23.

Başoğlu M, Mineka S, Paker M, Aker T, Livanou M, Gök S (1997). Psychological preparedness for trauma as a protective factor in survivors of torture. *Psychological Medicine* 27(6): 1421–33

Bracken P, Petty C (1998). *Rethinking the Trauma of War*. London: Free Association Books.

Calhoun LG, Tedeschi, RG (eds) (2006). *Handbook of Posttraumatic Growth: research and practice*. Mahwah, NJ: Lawrence Erlbaum.

Drožđek B, Wilson JP (2004). Uncovering: trauma-focused treatment techniques with asylum seekers In: Wilson JP, Drožđek B (eds). *Broken Spirits: the treatment of traumatized asylum seekers, refugees, war and torture victims*. New York, NY: Brunner-Routledge (pp243–276).

Herman JL (1992). *Trauma and Recovery: the aftermath of violence – from domestic abuse to political terror*. New York, NY: Basic Books.

Joseph S (2011). *What Doesn't Kill Us: the new psychology of posttraumatic growth*. New York, NY: Basic Books.

Joseph S, Linley PA (2005). Positive adjustment to threatening events: an organismic valuing theory of growth through adversity. *Review of General Psychology* 9: 262–280.

Kira IA (2002). Torture assessment and treatment: the Wraparound Approach. *Traumatology* 8(2): 54–86.

Maslow AH (1943). A theory of human motivation. *Psychological Review* 50(4): 370–396

OHCHR (1999). *Istanbul protocol: the UN manual on the principles of the effective investigation and documentation of torture and other cruel, inhuman or degrading treatment or punishment*. Geneva: OHCHR. www.ohchr.org/Documents/Publications/training8Rev1en.pdf (accessed July 2017).

OHCHR (1984) *UN convention against torture and other cruel, inhuman or degrading treatment or punishment*. Geneva: United Nations.

Omeri A, Lennings C, Raymond L (2004). Hardiness and transformational coping in asylum seekers: the Afghan experience. *Diversity in Health and Social Care 1*: 21–30.

Papadopoulos RK (2007). Refugees, trauma and adversity-activated development. *European Journal of Psychotherapy and Counselling* 9(3): 301–312.

Smith E, Patel N, MacMillan L (2010). *A Remedy for Torture Survivors in International Law: interpreting rehabilitation*. Discussion paper. London: Medical Foundation for the Care of Victims of Torture.

Splevins K, Cohen K, Bowley J, Joseph S (2010). Theories of posttraumatic growth: cross-cultural perspectives. *Journal of Loss and Trauma* 15(3): 259–277.

Takano Y, Osaka E (1999). An unsupported common view: comparing Japan and the US on individualism/collectivism. *Asian Journal of Social Psychology*: 311–341.

World Health Organization (1992). *The ICD-10 classification of mental and behavioural disorders: clinical descriptions and diagnostic guidelines*. Geneva: WHO.

4. Talking about racial and ethnic differences with torture survivors

Rajita Rajeshwar

Most therapists working with torture survivors in exile are working with people who have a different racial and ethnic background to their own. As the therapist and client make their way through the difficult terrain of managing diversity, differences and multiple traumatic events, at what point should the topic of race be addressed? Is it even relevant? How could the conversation start? And if racial differences are not raised, how does this impact on the therapeutic relationship and the survivor?

This chapter offers my experiences of working therapeutically when race and ethnicity are intertwined with the trauma experiences with which survivors present.

What follows is a personal account drawn from my practice with survivors and my training as an integrative psychodrama psychotherapist. I will be looking at the initial encounter, when and how to broach race issues and how racial and ethnic differences can impact on the therapeutic process. Using 'personal reflexivity', defined by Dallos as 'a conscious cognitive process whereby knowledge and theory are applied to make sense of remembered reflective episode' (Stedmon & Dallos, 2009: 3), I draw on multiple sources, including theories of identity and counselling approaches. Reflexivity can also be a creative and playful experiential process (Stedmon & Dallos, 2009). Therefore, I have included autobiographical accounts of my subjective perceptions of power and equality and the spontaneous ways I have worked with clients. My work is human rights-based, with a strengths and resilience orientation.

The explorations and ideas described here are not prescriptive, and nor are my conclusions. The examples I use are anonymised descriptions of common situations I have encountered in this work. I hope that, by sharing my wrestling with this topic, I will be of some help to other therapists seeking to explore these themes in their work.

Definitions

Cultural identity is not fixed; it is complex and fluid, seeping into every layer of our thoughts, feelings and relationships (Drožđek & Wilson, 2007). Each of us belongs to several different cultural frames, such as gender, disability, sexual orientation, race, ethnicity, migration status, and religious and political beliefs, and, at any one moment, different combinations intersect (Hays, 2008). The therapist and client each bring their own cultural realities that can alternate between different cultural frames in a single session. Verkuyten supports the notion that identities are present at several levels: 'Theories of hybridity reject the notion of homogenous, uniformly defined identities and subscribe instead to the notion of heterogeneity and multiple identities, where the emphasis is on self-definition and personal meaning' (2004: 53).

My focus here is how trauma and race/ethnicity intersect in order to make visible the often-avoided dynamic that lurks in the room and to visibly reintegrate issues of racism, power, oppression and equality back within the therapy space.

Use and understanding of the terms race and ethnicity can vary. They overlap but are not the same constructs. Historically, race has been defined by physical and biological characteristics (Atkinson, Morten & Sue, 1998). Helms offers a more complete definition: 'Racial identity is a multidimensional construct [including] the feelings, thoughts and behaviours an individual has in relation to his or her own race and to people of other races' (1993: 15).

Ethnicity includes these definitions, but also refers to the historical and cultural patterns and collective identities shared by groups from specific regions of the world (Helms & Cook, 1999).

In this chapter, I use the terms race and ethnicity collectively: sometimes race may be more prominent; at other times, I use ethnicity to describe how individuals conceptualise their identity. Acculturation needs also to be brought into the discussion. Acculturation refers to the physical, biological, cultural and psychological changes that occur when an individual or group from one culture moves to an area dominated by another cultural group and there is pressure on the newcomers to conform and accommodate to the dominant culture's way of life and to abandon or devalue their own cultural roots (Chun, Organista & Marín, 2003).

Remer demonstrates how the development of ethnic identity and acculturation can occur simultaneously. This push and pull creates acculturative stress: 'While trying to locate [him/herself] with reference to the dominant group, [s/he] is simultaneously attempting to locate [him/herself] socially and psychologically with reference to an ethnic group' (1999: 99). 'Acculturation stress' can increase vulnerability to physical health problems and psychological distress (Cuellar, 2000).

In the beginning

I will start my exploration with my own experience of intercultural therapy.

I was in my early 30s. I was a desperately lost, vulnerable, second-generation British Tamil. My GP referred me to a therapist. She appeared to me as a strong, 'knowing' white female. I remember talking in depth about difficult experiences and ways of coping. However, throughout my time with her, she never mentioned the colour of my skin and my Indian heritage. On one level, I wasn't bothered by this. I felt invisible in Britain and my complex cultural/racial identity made me feel very exposed. I was happy for us to focus on her agenda; it made me feel as if I belonged.

However, when she asked about my family, I laughed involuntarily. It came from a place of shame and cultural discomfort. The therapist looked puzzled and interpreted this laughter as me discounting my feelings. We never explored what the laughter meant to me. As a result, something inside me began to shut down. I felt I had become a passive vessel, and eventually I left, after six sessions.

Memories of this therapy encounter and rupture have stayed with me for more than 10 years. Looking back, I now understand that my race and ethnicity were shut out. The therapist's failure to explore my ethnicity colluded with my fears of making race visible. My experiences as a racial being and any issues of acculturation and the power dynamics between us were not named; the traumas inherently experienced through my racial identity were buried and could not heal.

My personal experience accords with studies by Work, Cropper and Dalenberg (2014) and Chang and Berk (2009) of cross-racial therapeutic dyads. They found that therapy with people from ethnic minorities with complex trauma often ruptured because race was not discussed in the therapeutic dialogue. Indeed, in these studies, white therapists never mentioned race at all. However, communication also broke down when the issues of race were raised, because the therapist's discomfort either manifested in excessive interest in cultural detail, or they would expect the client to offer their cultural expertise.

Why are racial /ethnic differences not discussed in the therapy room?

There are many reasons why therapists are missing opportunities to have these conversations.

The survivor is likely to present with multiple needs, such as loss of appetite, poor sleep, flashbacks, physical pain, social dislocation and the effects of enforced exile and cumulative trauma. Silove (2004: 60) writes that 'the asylum seeker is trapped in a continuum of threat, loss of control and intensifying feelings of helplessness'.

The therapist, bombarded with these multiple needs, may prioritise establishing a sense of emotional safety. Racial differences and cultural issues may be placed on the backburner. Arguably, though, racial and ethnic identity is inherently entwined with the torture experience. The psychic self is injured by trauma but aspects of identity linked to race and ethnicity may also be adversely affected.

I would argue that the visible aspects of our identities carry meaning, and exploration of this can offer valuable opportunities to deepen the therapeutic relationship and work therapeutically with trauma.

Working with Sum

> 'When and where I enter, then and there the whole race enters with me' (Cooper, in Giddings, 1996).

Sum was implicated in a Liberation Tigers of Tamil Ealam (LTTE) bombing attack on his village in Sri Lanka. As a result, he was imprisoned by the army and repeatedly tortured. Sum finally escaped to the UK with his family. When Sum came to therapy, I experienced him as a desolate and fragile person: he seemed alone, adrift and removed. However, as we talked, I experienced a subtle shift in the boundaries in the room, a growing sense of closeness. Sum asked where I was from, how long I had lived here. I felt a kind of merging was taking place between me, Sum and the female Tamil interpreter, alongside moments of dissociation and a strong sense of loss seeping through the room.

I immediately felt guilty and worried. Was I losing my role as a therapist by compromising my boundaries and not maintaining emotional distance?

These were confusing transferential reactions, which required further attention. Working with survivors can evoke strong countertransference reactions. Dalenberg describes how transference and countertransference reactions are most heightened in trauma-related work (2000). The therapist's initial response to these projections may offer valuable clues about the impact of trauma on the survivor. For example, Sum's dissociation might reflect his desire to escape to a fantasy world, free of pain. However: 'Trauma is not a disembodied construct, as suggested by *DSM-IV*, it is a cultural and historical reality that must be entered into by the clinician' (Aroche & Coello, 2004: 56).

Widening the lens

In considering this, would the course of therapy be different if the therapist explored the interplay of racial dynamics and its impact on the therapeutic relationship? My work with Sum demonstrates the significance of racial/ethnic difference in the psychotherapy process and how acknowledging this may provide further insight into the client's trauma narrative.

Therapists may be sensitive to issues of race and cultural difference, and may have learnt about a client's cultural group, their country of origin, its history, politics, social systems, and its experience of colonial power. This can be a useful way to gain some insight into the client's experience and establish a starting point for questions. However, it can also lead to an illusion of knowledge about the whole cultural background of the client, and shut down conversations about unique individual meanings. Subconsciously, this approach may also serve to intellectualise the relationship and create distance between the therapist and client. The therapist may be seeking to avoid working with racial difference by controlling the discussion, thereby unwittingly keeping the client in the position of the 'other'. Ortega (2011) argues that a rights-based approach to therapy requires practitioners to be grounded in cultural humility rather than cultural knowing.

Therapists may navigate working with racial and cultural differences by focusing solely on the universal characteristics that connect us. Vontress (1988) argues that counselling offers a universal system that transcends culture. Rogers highlights the importance of empathetic attunement: 'Accurate empathy involves the therapist's sensitivity to current feelings and the verbal facility to communicate this understanding in a language that attunes to the client's feelings' (1961: 76).

Williams argues that, within this, there must be cultural safety in the therapeutic relationship. He describes this as 'an environment that is spiritually, socially and emotionally safe, as well as physically safe for people, where there is no assault or challenge or denial of their identity, of who they are and what they need. It is about shared respect, shared learning, shared knowledge and meaning' (1999: 213).

Overlooking discussions around race may model to the client that some aspects of a person are more important than others. The therapist may focus on what feels 'safe' and comfortable to discuss. This may be a defensive strategy to minimise their anxiety about difference. Ultimately this may serve to distance the therapist from the client and their experiences.

Burman urges therapists to give race the space it needs, and my working experience confirms this (2003). Furthermore, raising the issue of race relieves the client of the confusions, burdens and feelings of detachment that may be experienced when their ethnicity is not acknowledged.

In my work with Sum, I asked myself what I might represent to him. Did my visible identity as an Indian therapist inform the dynamics in the room? Would this exploration help explain my feelings of enmeshment and my desire to be a separate and different individual?

Me: Are you curious as to where I come from?

Sum: You are Tamil. I know this.

Me: Yes, a part of me is. I am also Indian and I have spent a large part of my life in England. I am really interested in how being Tamil makes you feel? Is it important for you to be around Tamils?

Sum: Yes, I feel comfortable here.

Me: How do you feel about working with someone with my background?

Sum: You are like my sister, my aunt, my whole village.

Sum reminisced about his village. He had known everyone there and he could talk freely there. He came from a large family and spent a lot of time in his aunts' and uncles' houses.

Me: I am different to the significant people in your village. It feels really important for me to understand your experience. Tell me more about the people in your village and how you see yourself there.

When the therapist asks the client to describe their experience of their race/identity, it avoids stereotyping them and opens the conversation to more intimate disclosures and insights, for client and therapist alike. Furthermore, a therapist's self-disclosure can create an emotional bridge between the therapist and client. Vontress states how 'thoughtful disclosure' encourages the building of trust and rapport in the therapeutic relationship: 'It is the most direct means by which the individual can be known to the other' (1988: 75).

Explorations of each other's racial identity helped Sum understand what I represented to him. Sum told me: 'I have fond memories of my sister. I could tell her anything.' Accessing these memories led Sum to explore other strengths related to his family and community life: 'Everyone in my community would support me... we would talk about my career choices; they would care for me when my father was ill...'

By accessing some positive memories before his trauma, Sum began to create his own internal safe place, which contributed to the stabilising of his mental health in our early work together (Rothschild, 2000; Herman, 1992).

I have found the following questions useful in eliciting this kind of exchange with a client:

- What words do you use to describe where you are from?
- What does it mean to you?
- What is it like sitting in a room with a therapist from [the therapist's country of origin]?
- I may not fully appreciate your experience as I am [the therapist's nationality or race]. Please tell me more about your experience.
- Is there anything about the differences between us that is affecting you?

Models of racial and ethnic identity

Sue and Sue (1990) have developed an influential racial identity model that shows how people move through stages of psychological adjustment as they become ethnic minorities in a new country.

The stages in Sue and Sue's model are described as follows:

- the conformity stage, when the person enthusiastically espouses the values of the dominant culture, and deprecates their own culture group
- the dissonance stage, when they question and withdraw from the dominant culture
- the resistant-immersion stage, when they develop an awareness of oppression and racism and reject the values of the dominant culture

- the introspection stage, when they reconnect with a deeper sense of their identity as part of their minority group, and finally,
- the integrative awareness stage, when they reach a reconciliation between these conflicts, and gain an appreciation of the unique features of both their own and the dominant culture.

Sue and Sue argue that '[e]xploring stages of identity development influences outlooks on life and behaviour for both therapist and client alike' (1990: 234). I think awareness of this staged model can help the therapist and client discuss issues of race in the therapy room.

Returning to Sum, it can be argued that, at points in the relationship, Sum was at an introspection stage, needing to connect with his cultural group. These projections may be linked to Sum's need to identify with a person of similar ethnicity. In these moments, I focused on western therapeutic notions of separateness and boundaries. I responded to Sum's cultural need to connect by creating distance. I avoided eye contact and swiftly moved on from the topic of our shared ethnicity. I adopted a response likened to those at the conformity stage. On reflection, this may have left Sum feeling unsettled and rejected.

One of the dominant discourses of race is that Caucasians do not have to think about being white as an important aspect of their identity. This failure to acknowledge racial difference is dangerous for therapy as it ignores the possibility of different experiences and unique individuality related to skin colour. It can result in the therapy room mirroring the wider systems of oppression, by silencing individual's experience of racism and discrimination.

Rowe and colleagues (1994) argue that being a culturally competent practitioner means also exploring being white. White identity development has been studied by several multicultural theorists (Helms, 1993; Rowe, Bennett & Atkinson, 1994). Helms' (1993) white racial identity model proposes the following stages.

- The contact stage. The person is oblivious to race. Societal influences and stereotypes are accepted without much thought, thus perpetuating a superior/inferior dichotomy between whites and non-whites. The person does not see themselves as having prejudices or being part of a dominant group. Racial and cultural differences are not part of their awareness.
- The disintegration stage. Here, the person may become conflicted with

unresolvable racial/moral dilemmas. They believe they are not racist, but this is not reflected in their lives. For example, they do not know anyone from a minority ethnic group; they may witness oppression, but not acknowledge their unearned white privilege; they may notice but not question the absence of ethnic minorities in senior positions. During this stage, they may experience confusion, dissonance and conflict.

- The reintegration stage. In order to resolve this dissonance, there is a move towards a dominant ideology associated with their race. This stage may be seen as regression, resulting in a tendency to idealise their own racial group at the expense of other racial groups.
- The pseudo-independence stage. This may occur because of a painful/insightful experience – for example, witnessing police mistreatment of Muslim youths. However, the person may attempt to understand this difference from a distance – from an intellectual understanding rather than a lived exploration – by, for example, reading about oppression and racism, rather than reflecting on their own reactions and feelings.
- The immersion-emersion stage. As a result of continuing personal exploration of their racial being, the person begins to consciously explore what it means to be white. The personal meaning of white privilege is explored. In this stage, individuals begin to confront their own biases and directly combat racism and oppression on a personal and possibly societal level. For example, questioning anti-oppressive practice within their organisation.
- The autonomy stage. The person develops an increased awareness of their whiteness as they accept their own part in perpetuating racism and the guilt associated with this. As a result, they become more open and flexible, and believe they have something to offer and something to learn.

I believe that reflecting on one's own racial identity schema will influence how a therapist engages in racial conversations. It may be postulated that therapists who believe 'we are all the same' may be at the contact stage of Helms' identity development and feel no need to bring up issues of race, or may wait for the client to bring up these issues. Those who feel uncomfortable about their privilege may be at the disintegration stage, where the avoidance of conflict and power imbalance leads to uncomfortable feelings of guilt around talking about race, or wishing not to offend. Those who may have an intellectual sense of race issues are more likely to be at the pseudo-independent stage: 'I know race/racism exists but I don't need to talk about it.' However, those with a growing awareness of issues may be at the immersion-emersion stage, resulting in a wish to take personal responsibility for the discussion and the belief that they have something to offer and something to learn: 'I'm going to talk about race, even if I don't do it correctly.' These therapists will consider how race and racism influences the therapeutic space.

Acculturation

An exploration of acculturation models may shed further light on the dynamics in the room. The survivor who is dislocated from their home country and arrives in the host country experiences huge losses. Eisenbruch (1991) coined the term 'cultural bereavement' to describe the loss of a home, possessions, networks, social/spiritual belonging and connection to one's cultural symbols and people.

Berry's model of acculturation (1997) describes how people in minority ethnic groups negotiate the pressures to integrate in their own, unique ways. Berry identifies four models of acculturation:

- integration (the person values their own culture and the dominant culture)
- assimilation (the person values the dominant culture and denigrates their own culture)
- separation (the person values their own culture and denigrates the dominant culture), and
- marginalisation (the person rejects both their own culture and the dominant culture).

According to this model, Sum's survival strategy at this stage in therapy might be described as separation, which Berry defines as the person's need to belong exclusively to their own ethnic group. As an immigrant, I reflected on my own response to migration. I noticed that I had adopted what Berry calls an 'assimilation stance'. When I moved from India to England as a child, I rejected the values of my cultural heritage for those of the dominant white culture. This realisation prompted me to question whether my countertransferential response to Sum, of maintaining an emotional boundary, was a defensive manoeuvre to avoid my own feelings of pain and loss.

Issues of acculturation may be acknowledged in the therapeutic relationship through questions such as: 'How do you see/describe yourself?' 'How do you describe your ethnicity?' 'Has this always been the same or has it changed?' 'How has this affected you and your relationships?'

Moreno's (1947) cultural/social atom is a mapping exercise that looks at the social and cultural aspects of a client's life. It is a visual, projective tool that can help the client focus on their strengths and connections in the present and integrate aspects of their pre- and post-trauma identity, to feel more safely held and less isolated.

The client is asked to find a place on the floor or table and pick an object to represent themselves. Objects can be anything – pebbles, shells, old toys, keys, trinket boxes, scarves. I have collected items that may have a cultural significance for clients, including sari material, a small Buddha, a bell, djembe drums and prayer flags.

The client is then asked to pick objects to represent significant people in their life (living, dead, fictional), major life events, and difficult/happy moments that are important to them in the here and now. To acknowledge their own resources, the client may be asked to explore interpersonal strengths, such as personal qualities, and transpersonal strengths, such as their spirituality or a set of beliefs. The client is then asked to place each of these objects at the distance from the object that represents them to reflect how close they feel to these other people and resources.

In this way, the client is mapping out influences that inform their sense of belonging in the world and the reference points that give meaning to their life and nurture their identity. Where the objects are placed reflects clearly how the client feels about each of these potential resources. Fox states: 'It is from the social/cultural atom that we get our picture of one's inner world' (1987: 72).

Moreno (1969) argues that this is a process of concretisation: the act of choosing an object to give internal experiences a form. The presence of this visual display opens individuals to new ways of thinking. It brings to life relationships, ideas, feelings and concepts in a richer way. Therefore, this approach offers an opportunity for deeper explorations about identity without getting lost in vague intellectual discussion.

Furthermore, the therapist and client may work together to map out several atoms: for example, one before exile, one after, and a future, wished-for atom (Garcia, 2010). The therapist encourages the client to notice any similarities and differences between the atoms, such as the support the client had before exile and now. This could lead to discussions about what the client can change in a future atom and/or new roles the client would like to develop.

Using this exercise, Sum created a social atom of his life in England. He used objects to depict his role as a father, 'asylum seeker', and devout Muslim. Sum remarked on how small it looked. He then commented on the loss of his role as student and being part of a community. He had little contact with the

Tamil community in England. This led to an exploration of a new 'wished-for atom' and aspects of his identity he could develop here. 'I like learning. Maybe I could do a mathematics course here'; 'I want to engage with the Tamil community but I am scared of telling them I am an asylum seeker.' Together we began to explore his fears about connecting with others from his community in the UK.

I-self, we-self

The dynamics in the room may also be affected by different ways cultures see the self in relation to family and community (Sue & Sue, 1990). Western culture, and western psychotherapy by extension, is very individualistic. Scheurich writes (1997: 47):

> We (in the West) think that the private conversations we have with ourselves, our 'I's are the most precious thing. We typically assume that this self, our individuality, our subjectivity, our agency, exists outside of the cultural array, that the individual is an autonomous self largely in control of her/his actions, thoughts. Other cultures similarly produce different kinds of 'I's or selves, some of which are more group orientated.

White therapists may believe in western cultural values such as client autonomy, as defined by independence and individualism. Many therapists may believe that their role is to model a separate and benign internal object to contain the client's distressing feelings and help them develop a sense of separateness (Bion, 1961; Winnicott, 1968). However, this ignores the perspectives of more collectivist cultures, and the importance of emotional openness and intimacy in those cultures.

In Indian culture, the child's secure attachment is built on establishing the 'we-self'. It is the group rather than the individual that is the primary player in the child's early psychological growth, resulting in strong bonds of loyalty to the wider family group (Roland, 1988). Roland argues: 'To be culturally credible we need to conceptualize problems in a manner that is consistent to the client's belief system' (1988: 367).

By exploring my own cultural/racial reference points in supervision, I felt more able to safely embrace the collective pull from Sum, thus respecting his cultural reference point. I felt, that in my opening up, I respected Sum's worldview, which was represented by groupness, sameness and communality

(Perkins, 1985). There was also a further subtle shift: my feelings of tension and weariness were replaced by comfort and closeness as I began to fully experience all the emotional and cultural aspects of Sum's cultural experience. I felt we were being present and truly beginning to encounter one another, in line with Moreno's concept of 'encounter'. This is described as the authentic willingness to engage deeply (Moreno, 1914, in Moreno, 1985). Later in the work, we joined together, enabling Sum to experience a communal sense of grief.

I believe that engaging clients in conversations about racial and ethnic differences plays a critical role in the therapeutic process. In my experience, broaching this topic is never easy. For some clients, this may lead to rich discussions with their therapist. However, others may choose to respond superficially, or not at all. Furthermore, the therapist will need to be sensitive around the timing and pace of these questions, which may lead to one conversation, or several over time as the therapeutic relationship deepens and survivors feel safer to explore these issues. However, what is important is to initiate this conversation, as it demonstrates a willingness to explore differences, while also showing respect for the client's boundaries and their right to choose self-disclosure. In this way, it creates the foundation for deeper trust to develop.

Francine

We all represent things to our clients and they to us.

Rape is a humiliating and degrading form of torture. How it is experienced and viewed is influenced by the cultural and socio-political context. The following case story highlights how exploring racial dynamics can open the discussion to an exploration of the shame and power of rape.

When I first met Francine, she was impeccably dressed. She had arrived from the Democratic Republic of the Congo (DRC) with her children, having fled after she was raped by four men from a militia gang. I felt very small and child-like, sitting in the room with her. I wondered if she felt the same: whether her garments were armour, holding her together. Francine had lost all trust in other people, and would make statements like, 'There is nowhere to be safe,' and, 'I am in hell.'

Concealed identity – revealed identity

I was struck by Francine's impeccable dress, how upright and focused she appeared. I wondered if her outward appearance was a sign that she was hiding the vulnerable parts of herself – the parts of her that may have felt shame, horror and disgust. Goffman (1963) describes shame as a 'spoiled identity', and how people seek to hide this.

Rape can result in what Alleyne calls cultural shame (2004). Here, shame stems from an internalised conflict with an external authority (cultural/societal norms). One's private identity becomes public, and one's view of self is punctured, or shattered. This can lead to the destabilising of a person's sense of who they are, and give rise to an identity split. This form of cultural trauma results in depersonalisation. Francine described how everything around her was drained of colour; she was convinced this was a nightmare she would eventually wake up from. Sarup (1996) highlights how this form of cultural trauma also creates identity wounding, self-hate and damage to relationships. Francine thought it was her independence and defiance that singled her out for attack: 'I know this is why I am punished. I speak for myself. I do not let my husband speak for me.' Francine also told me that she wanted her daughters to be strong: 'They too will become strong black women.' She then paused, and in a quiet voice added, 'but I have failed them. They heard what happened to me.'

As I sat there, I felt the unsettling texture of Francine's shame in the room and her feelings of powerlessness and deflation, as if she were in a state of inertia. How could I honour this hiding away in response to her trauma, this silencing and shutting down of herself through shame? I feared that if I said nothing, this might result in a co-construction of avoidance and concealment, and create further distance between us. Raising issues of racial identity felt appropriate here; if I avoided this part of her identity, I might reinforce her feelings of being denigrated and invalidated in the world.

Me: You look strong when you talk about yourself as a black woman.

F: In my country, I am a commander's wife. He is of the highest rank. I am respected.

Thus, Francine brought a different sense of herself into the room. Francine was showcasing her power as a black woman, her status as a military wife, her role as a political activist fighting injustice. It was as if these declarations would guard her from further pain. The room was suffused with an overwhelming thrust of defiance. It felt as if Francine was declaring her identity and activism as the most important aspects of her self. These aspects appeared to make her feel invincible, as if she could not be harmed by the experience of rape.

My raising the issue of Francine's racial identity gave her an opportunity to take control and reclaim those parts of herself that were untouched by violation. In this way, I supported her to keep alive parts of her identity that kept her grounded. This is in keeping with Kohut's (2004) notion of grounding – offering strength and stabilisation in order to survive and come to terms with the atrocities of rape and cultural shame. It is also in line with Grotberg's (1995) universal strengths model, as well as post-traumatic growth, of which resilience is a major part (Tedeschi & Calhoun, 2004).

The dialogue shifted the power dynamic in the room as, together, we explored her strengths. Francine began to see her identity as having many different meanings, not just linked to the polarities of power and powerlessness, damage and shame.

Internal oppressor – external oppressor

Over the next few months our pattern of relating in the room became apparent. Francine used the space exclusively to express her views about the asylum system and outrage at what was happening to her: 'Here I am treated like an animal.' I often felt locked into Francine's speeches, dominated by their force and afraid to express a different view. Intervening felt risky, and she often responded: 'It's alright for you.'

The Karpman drama triangle (1968) helped me understand the dynamics, shedding light on how trauma is destructive to trust and trauma re-enactment can often occur because of this. Francine's way of managing fear may have resulted in her becoming more rigid and positioning herself, at times, in the role of perpetrator, and me as victim, rescuer and/or helpless bystander.

However, incorporating a race narrative into the understanding of these dynamics highlights further issues. Alleyne (2009) argues that, when discrimination is acknowledged, the power re-enactment can be understood; the internal-oppressor attachment style is made visible. This can be described as an unconscious power dynamic occurring between the therapist and client. It is based on historical oppression faced by black people. In this situation, Francine may have perceived me as powerful, due to my role as a professional.

As a result, the client may feel devalued, internalising and acting out the actions of the perceived oppressor. I felt dismissed and disregarded at times. I wondered if this was how Francine felt at the hands of her oppressors. 'The internal oppressor', or inner enemy, can be described as 'absorbing, consciously/unconsciously, the values and beliefs of the oppressor. Alleyne (2005) cites Bach's assertion that 'the self becomes the inner tyrant, allowing external beliefs and value systems to invalidate one's authenticity'.

Alleyne also discusses how the 'internal oppressor' is triggered in situations of identity wounding, stress and trauma. Historical memories are reawakened, re-opening old wounds and rewounding the self and the person's identity: 'Prejudices, projections, intergenerational wounds and the vicissitudes of our historical past are all aspects of this inner tyrant' (2008: 49).

The response to these wounds creates a defensive behaviour pattern. This can include a fear of relating, a silencing of others and a distancing from others to protect raw wounds. Re-enactments based on the internal oppressor attachment style may be apparent when a client adopts a defensive and fixed mindset: 'I don't do deference to you'; 'I cannot be vulnerable;' 'I don't trust anyone but me.' Therapists may reinforce this by maintaining positions of power (Sampson, 1993). If what the therapist might represent for the client is not explored, it will result in a collusion of these power dynamics.

Alleyne explains how the cultural trauma of racism, the 'grinding down' experience of discrimination and exclusion, can be triggered (2009). Here, the psychic structure may be vulnerable to racial differences, resulting in hyper-alertness and hypersensitivity. These responses may be overlooked among the survivor's plethora of trauma symptoms. Alleyne's research highlights how these experiences can cause interruptions to coherency and continuity and are key to understanding both racist oppression and other cultural oppression. Raising the issues of race, racism, power and oppression can minimise this.

As a result of these insights, I noticed how power can manifest in therapy through the construction of privilege. I wondered if exploring issues of privilege would model a commitment to talking about power differentials and repair this empathic breach. McIntosh describes privilege as 'an invisible backpack of safety and positive experiences that is carried by each member. It cannot be taken off and is rarely noticed by the person who carries it' (2001: 164).

Internally, I was aware that acknowledging privilege induced guilt and shame, which I reclaimed as dynamics I brought to the room. My awareness of this freed me to initiate a conversation about it with Francine.

Me: I know I am in a comfortable position as a therapist, listening to you. What is it like for you, sitting in a room with me? I wonder what it means to you, being here together, talking about discrimination and racism. My experiences are going to be different to yours...

F: You are the first person of colour I have talked to. In the UK, I have experiences of all different people... who do I trust? Some people move away when I walk here. I am an asylum seeker. I am no more than a dog.

As a result, Francine began to talk more freely about her feelings of isolation, frustration and helplessness. These discussions no longer felt oppositional. Instead, I could listen to and validate Francine's experiences. This enabled me to step out of any re-enactments and avoid becoming party to any projections.

Mutual explorers

Bringing the dynamics of difference into our shared awareness felt like a step towards repairing Francine's trust. My willingness to tell uncomfortable truths shifted the power in the room. As a result, it was no longer a battleground. Our discussions about privilege led to Francine sharing a deeper experience of her dislocation.

Acknowledging my place helped her to explore her own loss of status and place and redirect her anger towards structures of discrimination and towards the perpetrators. Thus, I noticed she became more able to feel trust, empathy and reciprocity. Waiving the anonymity of one's own race and privilege can enable the therapist to step out of enactments and projections and deepen the therapeutic alliance.

New possibilities – 'I see things differently now'

Ignoring conversations about race and ethnicity means overlooking issues of power and oppression, which can lead to the denial (by therapist or client) of personal heritage and experiences of relating as an ethnic being. This is as harmful as the denial or erasure of a person's trauma history.

Ethnic, white identity development and acculturation models are vital for the cultural understanding of 'self'. Denying the influence of culture and ethnicity on oneself and issues of cultural shame may result in a shutting down of cultural exploration in the therapy setting. This may be experienced by the client as a dismissal or minimising of experiences of racism and how this impacts on the client's identity.

I found that taking up positions of cultural naiveté, mindfully relaxing the boundaries of my self and embracing not-knowing enhanced the effectiveness of my therapeutic practice. Pedersen and colleagues (2001) advocate befriending complexity – that we should see it as a friend, rather than an enemy, when exploring multicultural dynamics.

In this way, engaging in conversations about race and ethnicity can name and make visible the silenced, uncomfortable parts of ourselves: the resistant, heavy and immoveable parts, the aspects of self that avoid words like race. In taking these risks, we are able to look at 'otherness' with more fluidity;

similarities and differences become part of a co-creative act of togetherness. We can reach a transcultural state of consciousness and inclusiveness, leading to deeper, more enriched practice. As a result, clients are truly held in a safe and trusting relationship.

> For which of us extends loving kindness to all parts of the self? Who does not deny the existence of our censored voices? Do we not project the darkness elsewhere, onto our own foreign bodies, our inner outsider, our hidden 'other'?
>
> By having the courage to explore beyond our familiar sense of self, we extend loving kindness to the different parts of our own heritage – persecutor and victim alike. We highlight the importance of identifying ancestral voices, difference and power relations within ourselves, ultimately honouring those in other cultures. This attentive, loving listening to all our voices, this inner democracy, may be the basis for effective multicultural practice. (Boas & Reeve, 2003: 21)

References

Alleyne A (2009). Working therapeutically with hidden dimensions of racism. In: Fernando S, Keating F (eds). *Mental Health in a Multi-ethnic Society: a multidisciplinary handbook*. London: Routledge (pp161–173).

Alleyne A (2008). The Internal Oppressor and Black Identity Wounding. [Online.] Croydon: RSCPP. www.rscpp.co.uk/article/56/black-white-people-oppressor.html (accessed July 2017).

Alleyne A (2005). Invisible injuries and silent witnesses: the shadow of racial oppression in workplace contexts. *Psychodynamic Practice 11*(3): 283–299.

Alleyne A (2004). Black identity and workplace oppression. *Counselling and Psychotherapy Research 4*(1): 4–8.

Aroche J, Coello MJ (2004). Ethnocultural considerations in the treatment of refugees and asylum seekers. In: Wilson JP, Drožđek B (eds). *Broken Spirits: the treatment of traumatized asylum seekers, refugees, war and torture victims*. New York, NY: Routledge (pp53–80).

Atkinson DR, Morten G, Sue DW (1998). *Counselling American Minorities* (5th edition). Boston, MA: McGraw-Hill.

Berry JW (1997). Immigration, acculturation and adaptation. *Applied Psychology 46, Issue 1*: 5–34.

Bion WR (1961). *Experiences in Groups and Other Papers.* London: Tavistock Publications.

Boas S, Reeve S (2003). Cultural embodiment: reflections on an ADMT conference workshop. *e-motion XIV*(4) :1-24

Burman E (2003). From difference to intersectionality: challenges and resources. *European Journal of Psychotherapy & Counselling* 6(4): 293-308.

Chang DF, Berk A (2009). Making cross-racial therapy work: a phenomenological study of clients' experiences of cross-racial therapy. *Journal of Counseling Psychology* 56(4): 521-536.

Chun KM, Organista PB, Marín G (2003). *Acculturation: advances in theory, measurement, and applied research.* Washington, DC: American Psychological Association.

Cuellar I (2000). Acculturation and mental health: ecological transactional relations of adjustment. In: Cuellar I, Paniagua FA (eds). *Handbook of Multicultural Mental Health: assessment and treatment of diverse population.* New York: Academic Press (pp45-62).

Dalenberg CJ (2000). *Countertransference and the Treatment of Trauma.* Washington, DC: American Psychological Association.

Drožđek B, Wilson JP (eds) (2007). *Voices of Trauma: treating survivors across cultures.* New York: Springer Science & Business Media.

Eisenbruch M (1991). From post-traumatic stress disorder to cultural bereavement: diagnosis of Southeast Asian refugees. *Journal of Social Science and Medicine* 33: 673-680.

Fox JL (ed) (1987). *The Essential Moreno: writings on psychodrama, group method, and spontaneity.* New York, NY: Springer.

Garcia A (2010). Healing with action methods on the world stage. In: Leveton A (ed). *Healing Collective Trauma using Sociodrama and Drama Therapy.* New York, NY: Springer Publishing Company (pp3-24).

Giddings P (1996). *When and Where I Enter: the impact of black women on race and sex.* New York, NY: Harper Collins.

Goffman E (1963). *Stigma: notes on the management of a spoiled identity.* New York, NY: Simon & Schuster.

Grotberg EH (1995). *A Guide to Promoting Resilience in Children: strengthening the human spirit.* The Hague: Bernard Van Leer Foundation.

Hays PA (2008). *Addressing Cultural Complexities in Practice: assessment, diagnosis and therapy* (2nd ed). Washington, DC: American Psychological Association.

Helms JE (1993). *Black and White Racial Identity: theory, research and practice.* Westport, CT: Praeger.

Helms JE, Cook DA (1999). *Using Race and Culture in Counseling and Psychotherapy: theory and process.* Needham Heights, MA: Allyn & Bacon.

Herman JL (1992). *Trauma and Recovery: the aftermath of violence – from domestic abuse to political terror.* New York, NY: Basic Books.

Karpman S (1968). Fairy tales and script drama analysis. *Transactional Analysis Bulletin* 7(26): 39-43.

Kohut H (2004). The role of empathy in psychoanalytic cure. In: Langs R (ed). *Classics in Psychoanalytic Technique.* New York, NY: Rowman & Littlefield (pp463-474).

McIntosh P (2001). White privilege: unpacking the invisible knapsack. In: Rothenberg PS (ed). *Race, Class, and Gender in the United States: an integrated study.* New York, NY: Worth Publishers (pp163–168).

Moreno JL (1985). *Psychodrama: first volume* (4th ed). Ambler, PA: Beacon House Inc.

Moreno JL (1969). *Psychodrama: vol III. Action therapy and principles of practice.* Beacon, NY: Beacon House.

Moreno JL (1947). Organization of the social atom. *Sociometry 10(3):* 287–293.

Ortega RM (2011). Training child welfare workers from an intersectional cultural humility perspective: a paradigm shift. *Child Welfare 90*(5): 27–49.

Pedersen P (2001). Multiculturalism and the paradigm shift in counseling: controversies and alternative futures. *Canadian Journal of Counselling 35*(1): 15–25.

Perkins UE (1985). *Harvesting New Generations: the positive development of black youth.* Chicago, IL: Third World Press Foundation.

Remer R (1999). *Multicultural Therapy/Psychology and Chaos Theory.* Unpublished manuscript. Lexington, KY: University of Kentucky.

Rothschild B (2000). *The Body Remembers: the psychophysiology of trauma and trauma treatment.* New York, NY: WW Norton & Company.

Rogers CR (1961). *On Becoming a Person: a therapist's view of psychotherapy.* London: Constable.

Roland A (1988). *In Search of Self in India and Japan: towards a cross-cultural perspective.* Princeton, NJ: Princeton University

Rowe W, Bennett SK, Atkinson DR (1994). White racial identity models: a critique and alternative proposal. *The Counselling Psychologist 22*(1): 129–146.

Sampson EE (1993) Identity politics. challenges to psychology's understanding. *American Psychologist 48*(12): 1219–1230.

Sarup M (1996). *Identity, Culture and the Postmodern World.* Edinburgh: Edinburgh University Press.

Scheurich J (1997). *Research Methods in the Postmodern Era.* London: Falmer Press.

Silove D (2004). The global challenge of asylum. In: Wilson JP, Drožđek B (eds). *Broken Spirits: the treatment of traumatized asylum seekers, refugees, war and torture victims.* New York, NY: Brunner-Routledge (pp13–52).

Sue DW, Sue D (1990). *Counselling the Culturally Different: theory and practice* (2nd edition). New York, NY: Wiley & Sons.

Stedmon J, Dallos R (2009). *Reflective Practice in Psychotherapy and Counselling.* Maidenhead: Open University Press.

Tedeschi RG, Calhoun LG (2004). Posttraumatic growth: conceptual foundations and empirical evidence. *Psychological Inquiry 15*(1): 1–18.

Verkuyten M (2004). Everyday ways of thinking about multiculturalism. *Ethnicities 1*(4): 53–74.

Vontress CE (1988). An existential approach to cross-cultural counselling. *Journal of Multicultural Counselling and Development 16*(2): 73–83.

Williams R (1999). Cultural safety: what does it mean for our work practice? *Australian and New Zealand Journal of Public Health 23*(2): 213–214.

Winnicott DW (1968). Playing: its theoretical status in the clinical situation. *The International Journal of Psycho-Analysis* 49(4): 591–599.

Work GB, Cropper R, Dalenberg CJ (2014). *Talking about Race in Trauma Psychotherapy.* [Online.] The Society for Advancement of Psychotherapy. www.societyforpsychotherapy.org/talking-about-race-in-trauma-psychotherapy (accessed July 2017).

5. Treat us like people

Prossy Kakooza, in conversation with Jude Boyles

I'm from Uganda. I've been here nine years. In most aspects, it feels like yesterday, and in any other space it feels like a long time. I'm currently working at the Red Cross, with refugees and people seeking asylum who have just arrived in the UK.

I needed to leave Uganda because it's illegal to be gay there, so I was in prison because of that, and that's where I faced torture, and that's why I left. I came by myself; my partner stayed in Uganda and was in prison for about four and a half years before I found her. She's here now, but we didn't see each other for about seven years. She joined me about two years ago.

I was given refugee status a year after I arrived, so I've had my status about eight years. At the time, it [the year of waiting for status to be granted] felt like the longest time, but now, having worked with refugees and asylum seekers, I know that waiting for a year was nothing. At the time, it just felt like forever. Now I know how lucky I was.

When did you first have therapy?

It was actually taken out of my hands. I don't know if you can call it lucky, but when I arrived, I literally came here about a day after my torture, so I left prison like today, spent a day out and then, the following day, I left Uganda. So, when I arrived here, I pretty much still had all the bruises. It was pretty bad, as I had been burnt. The girl I was sharing the accommodation with told me to go to a healthcare walk-in centre in the town. So I went, and they refused to treat me, and they called the police. Not because they were being mean; they were actually nice, but they said it was protocol for these kinds of injuries.

The police took me to a rape referral centre and I was examined. I got the doctor's reports about my injuries and bruises, and they took forensic photos. There were diagrams and photographs. It was traumatic, dealing with the police, because I had just come from prison in Uganda, where I had been badly assaulted by the police. Then I had to be in a car with two policemen, who took me to the rape referral centre. They were probably not to know, but it was really awful. I was literally a day old in the UK. It was just very scary. Looking back, it was probably good for my asylum case, but it's terrible that you get in a situation where you look at it like that.

The centre was really good and supportive. They told me about therapy, and that I could see the counsellor. I wasn't ready. I had not heard of such a thing as counselling and talking to someone about how you're feeling emotionally. From what they explained, it just sounded to me like I was crazy. We didn't have such things in Uganda, and I wasn't ready to talk about it. I just wanted to forget everything. But then I went to see the lawyer and, when I told them about what had happened, I gave them the doctor's letters, and they said it was beneficial for me to see the counsellor for my asylum case. So the decision was made for me, in a way. I felt I had no control over it and it was like I had to. But it was not because I wanted to, not because I was ready to. So that's how I got to know about therapy and counselling. I didn't choose it and I wasn't into it and I was never committed to it.

I really don't think the first counselling worked for me because I went because I had to. I kept going, but I talked about the bare minimum. She said I didn't have to talk about things I didn't want to, so I just ended up talking about my legal case and the asylum process and how it was for me being in this country and the differences. I didn't really deal with things. I was just doing it, but not actually getting involved. I didn't have a breakdown until a year later, after I got my refugee status.

What did you make of counselling?

At that time, I found it extremely intrusive. I was talking to someone who had really no idea about me and my background and my culture and what was going on in my life. So we just ended up talking about how it's illegal to be gay in Uganda, and she said, 'Oh really, oh my God', and then explaining to her about the asylum system. I didn't see the point of it at the time. It was really strange because, essentially, I was talking to this stranger who I really didn't like that much. That's a terrible thing to say, but she just seemed a little bit distracted and sometimes a little bit condescending. That's how it felt, because I was someone seeking asylum, forced into the situation and so I didn't gel with her, and I went just because I had to.

Did you feel safe coming out to her?

I didn't have a choice because of the context; they already knew that about me because of the police report and because I had to explain how I got the injuries and burns. They knew why I was in prison, so coming out was taken out of my hands.

It felt really intrusive at the time, and I wasn't ready for the probing questions. Probably that's why it felt intrusive. I had never willingly come out to anybody and now I was having to tell every single person I met about my sexuality. It was hard. It was a relief when the counselling was over. I felt like my hands were tied. I had to do a lot of explaining about the asylum system and how it works and about why people seek asylum. Sometimes I didn't even know why I was going, because we just ended up talking about other things, rather than the actual thing, so we just skirted around it almost.

After I saw her, I was done with counselling. I got into my campaign to stay and I was all upbeat. But then I got my status, and then I didn't have a focus. Up until then, I was literally breathing and eating my campaign. Then I got this status and I just wanted to talk to my mum and tell her, 'Oh, I've done this,' but I couldn't, because my family disowned me after my sexuality came out – which is how I ended up in prison. I was forced to think about what had happened and why I was here, and how I had ended up here. That's when I had the breakdown, and everything felt extremely pointless and bleak. I couldn't see a way forward, and so that's when I tried to end my life. I was taken to hospital, where I was for a couple of weeks, and then I was sectioned and in a mental health ward for about seven weeks.

I didn't understand it at the time. I didn't understand what being sectioned meant exactly, or what it entailed. It was only after a couple of weeks that I got to understand it, when I wanted to go to the shops and I couldn't. So then they had to explain it to me and it began to sink in. That was devastating. The wards were horrible. I don't know if they've improved, but at that time they were mixed sex. It was traumatising; you were literally separated by curtains. That was really, really horrible. Then I was moved to a single room, so then I was separated by walls, but I still didn't feel safe, because then I felt that I couldn't come out to the communal areas. Everything was mixed and to be mixed with people who are as unwell as you, well, they don't know the boundaries, or they don't know that this is wrong or this is right, because they are as ill as you. Some of them sometimes would remove their clothes, so it was pretty bad on the wards. It was traumatising, and so finding out that I had been sectioned was hard, because it dawned on me where I was and why I was there. In Uganda, there is stigma attached to mental illness. I was like, 'Oh my God, now I'm crazy after everything else that's happened. On top of that, now I've gone crazy, and I'm never going to recover from this. People are always going to know that I'm this person who this happened to.' I just freaked out.

It never happens in Uganda; you're just chained to a tree until you 'snap out of it' or people get killed so they don't put a burden on their families. So it was difficult to get my head around it.

Were there other African people on the ward?

I was the only one. There was one gentleman who liked to say 'crazy black bitch' when it struck him. I just ended up almost confined to my room as I just didn't feel safe on the ward. I didn't want to eat because that meant going to the communal area where I had to eat with everyone. It was a difficult seven weeks.

I had the most obnoxious psychiatrist. He barely took his eyes off the computer. I think staying on the ward got me to a point of accepting the medication and taking it regularly. It was a horrible experience for me and it was damaging, but it did get me to a point of resigning myself to taking the medication. At first it was just like, 'I don't need the medication, it's not going to help me.' It just made me sleep a lot and do nothing and feel lethargic, and I just didn't want to take it. The time on the ward was traumatic, but it helped me understand that maybe I needed that time to just chill and regroup.

Did you get some therapy on the ward?

I did see that psychiatrist. I think he started analysing me. He was a psychodynamic therapist and we talked about my family. He asked about my growing up and my childhood and I mentioned that my dad beat us. Even now I don't consider myself to have been abused or anything like that; that's just how we grew up, all the children in the school, everywhere. That's how it was. You do something, you get smacked. The psychiatrist just kept asking about my childhood and when I told him that, he just kept saying, 'That's what abuse victims say. They say that they were not abused,' and I was like: 'I had a good childhood.' Yes, I was smacked, but I had a good childhood, I enjoyed my childhood. Sometimes we got naughty to see who would get smacked, so it wasn't like abuse. But he just got fixated on that, and just kept making it like that's what happened to me, and what was happening now had something to do with my childhood. It wasn't about the actual things that were hurting me.

I just hated that he didn't treat me as a person, and he was a man. I know that sounds horrible, but that place was filled with men, too many men. I just wanted to talk to a woman who was going to understand me and talk to me properly. It wasn't that I was being anti-man, but my torture involved being gang-raped, and the last person I wanted to talk to about that was a man. He didn't understand me, full stop. I don't think it had anything to do with him being a white man; he just didn't try to understand me as a person.

When I came out of hospital, he referred me to group therapy. So I got a social worker and then I went with this social worker to this group. It was like a rape group session, which I hated because it was just people talking about being raped. I was, like, 'I don't want to be here.' I just stayed a couple of minutes. There were survivors, and some points of it were upbeat, but I hadn't dealt with my own shit, so I wasn't probably in a good space to deal with someone else talking about their own shit.

At that point, I started being helped by a community mental health team. I wasn't allowed to have medication on me then, because that was the way I had tried to kill myself. So they came to the house regularly to give me medication. They were really good. And I had a really, really good social worker. She was the one who explained to me about therapy. She sat me down and explained different types of therapy and what was out there and what I could do and who I could see when I was ready, not because a psychiatrist told me to. She explained to me about CBT, and it sounded like something for me. At that point people were just asking me, 'How do you feel?' But I wanted help to tackle things that had come up.

I wasn't leaving the house. My experience on the ward had increased my fears of being in the presence of men, and it got worse. I didn't have it before but then, when I was there, my fear of being near men increased. It became out of proportion, so I was just stuck in the house. The one time I went to the bank, I literally felt like I was going to pass out, just because a man was asking how they could help me. That's when I knew that I had to find something that was going to challenge the way my brain was thinking. So that's when I started CBT.

I asked if it was possible to get a counsellor who was a black woman from an African country, who would hopefully understand my culture. When I eventually got an appointment, she was from Nigeria. She was lovely, very friendly. But twice she left me in the room to ask her line manager about things, so she didn't instil trust that she knew what she was doing, lovely as she was. She just didn't know what she was doing, I think. Maybe she was a student. But the agency was good, because they understood, and they asked if I wanted to change counsellor. The social worker asked, 'How did it go? Did you like her, because if you don't like her and you don't trust her, it will not work.' I was honest with her. I said she was lovely enough, but this happened and this happened. Then they assigned me to a different lady, J, and that's when my therapy started properly.

She was really nice, very understanding, and she was a little bit aware of problems facing LGBT people in the world. So she wasn't totally clueless, like the people that I had seen before. I think that was a decider for me: that she got that bit, because it was such an integral part of why I left and how I was feeling. To find someone who understood a bit made me more connected, if that makes sense. That started a good rapport, so that's when I started my therapy.

CBT is what worked for me. I'm not quite sure even today if it worked because it worked or if it worked because I connected with the person who was giving me the therapy. Probably both.

I actually worked with her on and off for a couple of years. The counselling service was good because, when I finished my sessions with her, they said, 'The door is open. If you are referred, you can come back.' I did go back for two more periods of therapy – in total, I had 16 sessions. Both times I saw J. It was really good. I didn't have to start again. The last time I had to wait a bit longer, because she didn't have space, but I thought it would be worth it to see the same person who had the back story, rather than starting from scratch.

She didn't presume anything, and she didn't assume that, just because she knew about some of the issues that LGBT people feel, she knew everything I felt. She personalised my problems; she didn't generalise them. When I was nervous about Christmas or birthdays or important things coming up, the counselling was more practical. She was so flexible with my fears of going out; she went places with me and waited outside. She was so nice, because I had that massive fear of going out for such a long time, and she came to the library with me and she waited outside when I went in. She was hands on. I didn't feel like I was a client; I felt like I was a person, you know, for the first time. With the psychiatrist, I felt like he was doing his job, sat behind a computer: it was his job to talk to me. She made it so personal; like almost a friend. It felt like a relationship, and that the label almost went away. It just felt like I was working with someone to get better, so that helped a lot.

Did she do anything that was unhelpful?

I find it difficult to find anything unhelpful – probably, the times that she cancelled on me. It was only twice, but I just started relying on those appointments and then, when they were cancelled, it wasn't great. I panicked, like 'How am I going to cope?' Everything is out of your hands.

At first, I did dread the sessions. Sometimes I would leave feeling like I'd been in a boxing match, but then, as time went on, I was like, 'OK, it's going to feel dreadful to start with, but it feels better afterwards.' So I started looking forward to them, because then it would help me plan out things, and I liked having a plan and something to rely on. When we started setting targets of things to do, I become like a child, and I looked forward to telling her about the little things that I had achieved, to show that we were moving forward. So when the sessions were cancelled, it wasn't great, but it was only twice.

What was it like having a limited time frame?

When the sessions were coming to an end, I got proper anxious – really, really anxious. The first time the sessions ended, I was referred again after about three months. I did try to do the things we set in place and practised, but I was actually quite anxious because I had become reliant on the sessions and they were helping me. It took me some time to proper open up and get to trust her and know her and talk to her. Then, just as we were getting somewhere, we had used up my sessions. I felt I was more confident, but it felt like, because I was more confident, people thought I was OK, but I was just getting there. Then we had to end, and I became proper anxious again. I felt like I needed more.

Were there things that you didn't talk to her about?

That first time, we didn't really go into much detail about what actually happened. I think that I would have trusted her to go there deeply, but our sessions were coming to an end, so we actually didn't talk about that until almost in the middle of the second period of therapy sessions, when I went back. Then we did talk about that, but it took the first cycle of counselling and the next one before I could talk to her about stuff. Even then, we didn't talk about everything.

It helped that she knew about LGBT issues in the world, and also about the asylum process. With the first lady I saw, she had absolutely no clue. I just felt I couldn't really relate. I mean, can you imagine starting from scratch, telling someone about the asylum system? I just felt like, 'Gosh, what do you know? Where do I start with you? How do I tell you about myself, explain what happened, why I'm here and the asylum process, and what I've gone through?' That's why I spent most of the time with that first counsellor talking about the asylum process. She knew nothing. But J knew about the asylum process. I think she had already seen some clients who were seeking asylum, so she was aware, and for me it was important. She didn't know about my back story, about the torture, but at least she had an idea of the asylum system. It's a different type of torture, but at least I didn't have to explain about that.

You originally asked to see an African therapist. Would you have wanted to work with a lesbian counsellor if you were given a choice?

If I had the choice, absolutely one hundred per cent. I feel like I would have related more. They probably would have understood more about how I felt with the sort of torture that happened to me. I felt that they probably would have related more and empathised more. If I had a choice, then one hundred per cent.

I would never have seen a male therapist, but that decision at the start was taken out of my hands. I couldn't do anything about it.

What advice would you give therapists seeing torture survivors in the asylum process for the first time?

Learn at least about the basics of the asylum process. That's the first thing. If you know where your client is from, learn a little bit of the basics of the culture of that country and where their country stands on therapy. It just instils trust if you know a little bit of that country's stance on therapy and also about torture.

With torture, don't dive in too quickly. Don't expect people to open up straight away. And also explain to people about therapy. Make sure that they understand what therapy is and what it entails, what to expect and how they might benefit from it. We don't know.

With the first counsellor, I didn't ask too much. I was just told she was someone to talk to about what's happened; that's it. She probably did say what we were going to do, but it wasn't something that clicked in my brain.

Did your experience in the asylum process affect you when you went to counselling?

I think it affected the way I approached my first counsellor. Because my lawyer said it would be helpful, so it just felt like it was for my case, not about me. I felt I had to convince the counsellor that these things had really happened. In the end, she couldn't even write me a report in support of my asylum case, apart from saying that I went for counselling.

It felt like the counselling was an immigration thing, like I had to be proper and not speak out of line, and I had to talk about what happened, as if our sessions were to do with claiming asylum rather than to support me. I think people need to know what you do with the information they tell you. I thought counselling had something to do with the Home Office. It wasn't explained to me, so that did affect the relationship and the way I came into it. So I felt that this person was going to reveal things about me to the Home Office. I was more wary and more reserved.

I think I got this vibe off this first counsellor. It felt like she was saying that I was only going because of the asylum claim, not because I needed therapy.

You seem good at asserting your rights now, but what was it like at the beginning, when you were up against all this officialdom?
Yes, that's just developed. I got fed up to a point where I said, 'OK, that's enough.' But it hasn't always been like that, especially when I was vulnerable. I wasn't aware who was official, who I could say no to and who was going to affect my case. I wasn't as vocal as I am now; it's just developed over the years. At the time, there were so many things that happened.

When I went to the rape referral centre, they sent a man to do forensic photos of the burns I had suffered, and the other wounds and bruises. I refused at that point; there was no way I was going to remove my clothes for a man, because the injuries were all over my body, including my upper thighs. Then they sent a lady, and she really apologised for that, as normally a woman would be sent, but that was overlooked.

When I asked for asylum at the Home Office in Croydon where my interview was held, I said my English was OK, but they brought in an interpreter for my screening interview. They said, 'We have to confirm that you're from Uganda,' and they brought this Ugandan woman. She said, 'It's people like you who give Uganda a bad name. We don't have lesbians in Uganda,' in my language. I didn't say anything because she was saying it in my language and then repeating what I said in English. But when she was talking to me in Luganda, she said things like, 'You're such an embarrassment, people think that we are crazy, we don't have these things in Uganda.'

Now I look back and I'm, like, 'Why didn't I say something?' Why? Because of where she was. It felt like she was an official and she was with the Home Office. I couldn't say anything, but it's disheartening to think about it. Her name wasn't on the interview documents. Later on, I wanted to report her, but her name wasn't there, so I couldn't.

It was difficult, when I started getting therapy and counselling, to understand accents, to understand what people were saying and what certain words meant. I really have no idea how people feel when they have to use an interpreter; that must be horrendous. It was bad for me, but not as bad as it must be for people who can't really speak English. You're not talking to one person; you're talking to two people. I can't really compare my experience with that. I think this affects many people, not just at the screening interview but in court, where the interpreter may be a person from their community. They just don't want to reveal certain stuff, and then later on the Home Office will say, 'But you didn't say that then,' so it backfires, and that must be hard. That was the only time that I had an interpreter. She was awful, really awful.

Have you seen a therapist since you stopped seeing J?

My partner and I are having some couples counselling. We were separated for so long and we are very different now. I think it's inevitable, because we were separated for seven years, so we deal with things not as we used to before. I'm more assertive than I was back then; I'm more vocal. I think the positions have changed – before, she was the protector and the stronger one of the two of us. She was more out than I was at the time, and now I'm more out. The positions have reversed, because she was in prison for so long, and she's not as comfortable or confident as she used to be. So, we are having some couples counselling, and this time we have found someone for ourselves, who works privately and who is a lesbian and understands.

It's different because I know what I want now. It makes such a difference, but at the same time, it's not as easy because you're not just thinking about you; you have to think about the needs of another person. L hasn't had the therapy that I have had. She's been here two years, but she is still not comfortable with therapy, and she hasn't had as much as I've had. For her, it's almost a new setting, talking to someone. I am still trying to convince her to get therapy for the other things, but she's not ready, and I know from my experience that, when you're not ready, it's not going to be helpful. So, hopefully, at some point, she will be ready, but for now she's not.

There have been quite a few times you have wanted to kill yourself – did you explore this with your counsellor?

Mostly that was when I was still on the ward. They would ask if I still felt that way, and, most times, I did. They would ask things like, 'How would you do it?', and I wasn't going to divulge that because I felt, if I did, then they'd take my means away. When I got out and I started seeing J, I still went through periods where I thought about it. During that time, I still had the community mental health team, and I got calls from them and visits as well. So I probably was more protected in those times when I felt vulnerable.

When I started seeing J, I was more aware of wanting help and I actually wanted the help, so if I had weak moments and I felt like this, there was the community mental health team. It wasn't perfect, because sometimes you would call and nobody was there. They would say to leave a message. I tried the Samaritans, but that didn't work for me, because for me it just felt like calling a stranger who was just going to start from scratch. So I did that once and I didn't do it again.

I found it difficult when I was in those moments to find someone to call who was going to help. I started trusting the friends I had made in that time. I was quite blessed in having two people who were so amazing. I could pick up the phone and call them anytime; they were always there, which was awesome. I was lucky. I know some people don't have that and don't get the help that I got at the time. It could have ended totally differently. I tried to kill myself twice, so I am lucky that I'm here.

What helps people in your situation, do you think?

It is just probably wrong to assume that every type of therapy suits everyone, because it doesn't. I know that if I was to get therapy again, just being asked how I feel wouldn't work for me. It does work when you find the right fit and there's a lot of factors there.

It's not just the therapy; it's not just the person receiving the therapy. It's the setting, it's where you sit, how the person sits when they talk to you. The psychiatrist was sat behind a desk and I was sat across from him. That was off-putting, to say the least. It's so weird how the small things at the time make it not OK. I was so fixated on certain things: on how the person sat when they were talking to me, how they said good morning in a certain tone. I hated it when I went into therapy and the counsellor started straight away getting into things. I would like them at least to ask how my journey was. The counsellor was the only person I was going to talk to that day, so it was important for me for someone to say, 'How are you? How did you get here? How was your trip? How was your week?' Or even the weather! Anything that started the appointment off as a conversation, and didn't make it too clinical.

Don't assume that people are not coming because they don't want to. There's a lot of things like transport that happen – how many buses it takes to get there. If someone is anxious about getting to an appointment and they have to get three or four buses, sometimes just thinking about that journey is hard. You think about how many buses you're going to take, and how many things you're going to go through to get to that appointment, and you think, 'Can I do that today?'

When I missed a session with J, I was worried they were going to say that, because I missed a session, my counselling was cancelled, and they couldn't give me any more. I was worried she was going to think I wasn't taking it seriously, that I was messing her about. Then I worried that I was taking up time that they could have given to someone else. Mostly, I worried that she was going to think that I didn't want to get better. I felt like she wanted me to get better and she was one of the very few people who was in my corner. I felt, if I don't go, she's going to lose interest in helping me to get better, and it really played on my mind quite a lot at that time.

It can be so difficult to get to sessions for so many reasons, and especially when I started. What stopped me going was fear. I would have a sleepless night gearing myself up for this appointment, and then I couldn't go; I just couldn't. Sometimes I would just take a few steps out of the house and then I would just see something or see a man somewhere and just go back in. I just could not bring myself to go, however much I tried. My social worker started helping me to go to the appointments, and she took me to the first couple because I couldn't bring myself to go.

The counsellor leaving the room without explaining why, that really peeved me. It was like, 'Well, you haven't really read my notes and you're not prepared. So you have probably forgot what we talked about last time because you haven't really gone back to it.' That's the feeling I got. I want the counsellor to be prepared and to know. It was important because it shows I'm important. That's probably egotistical, but it was important that they remembered me. I felt so insignificant at the time, totally insignificant, like nobody really cared that much about what I was or where I was or what was going on in my life. So, for me, it was really significant and important that people remembered certain things or they remembered what I told them last week.

The most important thing is that they treat you as a person. Don't treat the person as a client or service user or whatever people choose to call us. Treat them like a person, and when they come to see you, be personable. Pay attention to the little things that are important to them.

6. Working with women survivors of torture and gender-based abuse: a woman-focused approach

Katie Whitehouse

I am a psychotherapist working in a women's counselling service in the UK. The service offers low-cost, often free, long-term psychotherapy of up to two years to women in the city where it is based. We offer a service to women, many of whom would not otherwise choose to access therapy, by providing a space that is physically and psychologically safe. In line with feminist counselling theory, we recognise explicitly the barriers and disadvantages women face in society and the impact of oppression (Chaplin, 1988). We aim to support and empower women to make changes in their lives, and to recognise and sometimes challenge some of the discrimination they encounter.

I have worked in this context for the past three years, as the co-ordinator and psychotherapist in a project that supports asylum-seeking and refugee women, most of whom have experienced gender-based abuse and/or torture.

I have worked as a psychotherapist for 15 years. My academic background is in languages, and I am a qualified social worker. My first encounter with people seeking asylum was in the context of a crisis counselling agency, where I was on placement as a social work student. I worked with a young, pregnant Cameroonian woman, who had been trafficked. I remember my outrage and shock at the complexity of her life, the multiple layers of disadvantage that she encountered, the day-to-day practical difficulties of her life in the UK, in addition to the trauma that she had experienced in her home country. This profound initial experience, alongside my social work background, with its attention to dynamics of power and oppression, laid the foundations for my conviction that psychotherapeutic work with women seeking asylum must attend to a challenging level of complexity.

In our work with refugees, psychotherapy cannot be undertaken without attention to the social, cultural and political context of women's lives, and an understanding of the discrimination women have lived with and continue to live with in their home and host country.

The case studies in this chapter are based on women I have worked with. Names have been changed.

Women's experience of torture and gender-based violence

Grace grew up in a refugee camp run by humanitarian organisations, after her family were driven from their village by civil war. She watched their village burn and her parents and siblings killed as they tried to flee. In the camp, she was raped when she was 13 and gave birth to a son. She later found out that she was HIV positive and that she had passed the virus on to her child. Unable to afford the medication to keep her child well, Grace accepted an offer from a man she met outside the camp to find her work abroad, but had to leave her son behind to be cared for by a friend. When she came to the UK, she was imprisoned in a house with several other women and forced into prostitution.

The UNHCR estimates that there are 59.5 million forcibly displaced people in the world, of whom women and girls make up 50%.[1] Contrary to UK media headlines about the current 'refugee crisis' in the west, around 84% of all refugees live in developing countries, not in wealthy, industrialised countries like the UK (UNHCR, 2016).

While the proportion of women and girls who are likely to be able to access psychotherapeutic support will be small in comparison to these large figures, it is important to understand how their experiences of torture and abuse and of seeking safety and asylum differ significantly to those of men. Berkowitz (2000) notes how, under the Refugee Convention 1951, the 'dominant view of what constitutes a "real refugee" has been of a man'. Girma and colleagues emphasise how, for women, 'the persecution that she experiences is more likely to take place in the private sphere, such as from pimps and family members, in a situation where she feels that she cannot seek protection from her own state... Even if a woman has been persecuted by the state, say for her politics or her ethnic background, the persecution may be more likely to take the form of sexual violence' (2014: 11).

Pettitt (2014) reminds us that, while rape has now been classified as a war crime and a crime against humanity, international law still does not adequately protect women from the range of gender-specific abuses that they flee – such

---

1. www.unhcr.org.uk/about-us/key-facts-and-figures.html

as rape, forced marriage, child marriage, domestic violence, trafficking, female genital mutilation, 'honour' killings, childhood sexual abuse, physical abuse, neglect and/or domestic servitude – or recognise that women may also be fleeing abuse due to the activities or views of their husbands or other male family or community leaders.

Gender inequalities in their countries of origin are often at the root of the particular kinds of abuse women experience. The absence of women's rights and education in countries of origin facilitates an environment in which women are powerless to seek justice or reparation for their experiences. 'Many states exhibit a societal acceptance of widespread and systematic violence perpetrated against women, where abuse forms part of women's daily lives' (Smith & Boyles, 2009: 8).

Fewer women claim asylum than men (Refugee Council, 2012). For example, in the UK, in the fourth quarter of 2016, only 14% of people applying for asylum were women (Refugee Council, 2017). This may be because women do not have the same economic resources as men, and are therefore unable to access the same help to flee their home countries. It may also reflect women's restricted access to education, lack of awareness of their human rights and restriction of freedom of movement in many countries (Smith & Boyles, 2009).

I am frequently told by women that they had never heard about the concept of asylum before coming to the UK. Their stories of flight often include numerous attempts to relocate in their country of origin, which have been thwarted either by state or family members. A common theme is the difficulty women face, when they try to escape, because a single woman, unaccompanied by a man, is so conspicuous.

While the number of women making the journey to the west is increasing (Grandi, 2016), it is hard for a woman to relocate with children or other dependents. The alternative is the heart-wrenching decision to leave family members behind, either to save themselves or as a temporary measure while they establish a 'better life' elsewhere and can reunite the family. Research by UNHCR found that women are particularly at risk when they try to flee. Once they have escaped, they may be stranded for years in refugee camps, where they are less likely than men and boys to have access to even the most fundamental of their rights, such as food, sanitary items, shelter and health care (UNHCR, 2011).

Women who access our service come from all over the world, yet their experiences are notably similar in that the abuses they describe are almost always sexual, sometimes perpetrated by numerous men, and often on many occasions.

How gender-based abuse relates to torture

My experience of working with women concords with Amnesty International's view that 'the experience or threat of violence affects the lives of women everywhere, cutting across boundaries of wealth, race and culture. In the home and in the community, in times of war and peace, women are beaten, raped, mutilated and killed with impunity' (Smith & Boyles, 2009: 5).

For the purposes of this book, I am using the United Nations Convention Against Torture (UNCAT) definition of 'torture' as:

> ... any act by which severe pain or suffering, whether physical or mental, is intentionally inflicted on a person for such purposes as obtaining from him, or a third person, information or a confession, punishing him for an act he or a third person has committed or is suspected of having committed, or intimidating or coercing him or a third person, or for any reason based on discrimination of any kind, when such pain or suffering is inflicted by or at the instigation of or with the consent or acquiescence of a public official or other person acting in an official capacity. It does not include pain or suffering arising only from, inherent in or incidental to, lawful sanctions. (OHCHR, 1984)

More than 94% of women referred to our service have experienced gender-based violence, according to our three-year service statistics. However, the percentage of women who, at first glance, fit the UNCAT definition of 'torture' is far lower. This is because their abuse typically takes place in the private sphere and is perpetrated by people who are not state agents: they may have been trafficked, or forced into abusive marriages, for example.

The women I work with regularly refer to their experiences as 'torture', and they would be dismayed to think that their suffering would not be immediately recognised as such.

The inadequacy of the Refugee Convention (UNHCR, 1951) to protect the rights of persecuted women is recognised. Amnesty International and REDRESS talk of a new 'imperative to provide a remedy and reparation to victims of torture at the hands of both state and non-state actors... a state is implicated in acts carried out by non-state actors by its failures to prevent and respond to such acts' (2011: 7).

Key to understanding how gender-based abuse fits the international definition of torture is to recognise how a state may either fail to offer a person protection from abuse, or systematically collude with and facilitate the abuse committed in the domestic sphere, as illustrated by the case below.

Mariame was told that she was to be married to a rich and significantly older man at the age of 13. She ran away before the wedding ceremony, but the marriage still took place in her absence. She was caught by the police as she tried to cross the border to a neighbouring country, and was returned to her family. Mariame experienced daily violence and abuse from her husband and her in-laws. She reported her abuse and showed her injuries to the police, but was told to return to her husband. Her only respite was when her husband travelled away on business trips. She remained in the marriage for seven years, unsuccessfully trying to escape whenever she was allowed to visit her own family. Each time Mariame fled, she was returned by the police to her husband.

A woman-focused approach: holistic, responsive and flexible

The complexity of working therapeutically with refugee populations is well documented, and it is now recognised that psychotherapists should be aware of the impact of gender and appreciate fully the experiences and needs of refugee women (Kastrup & Tata Arcel, 2004). When working with women, the impact of gender and disadvantage is always in the forefront of my mind. A woman-focused approach has the dual aim of recognising and naming the disadvantage and discrimination a person may face because she is a woman, while seeing women as individuals and as equals. Such an approach accords with the human rights-based approach that is fundamental to my work with asylum-seeking and refugee women. In Sands' words: 'The... idea of human rights is that they are available to all human beings, an expression of common humanity, of the bare minimum that should be available to all' (cited in Girma et al, 2014: 3). Furthermore, as Brown notes (2012: 3), women's therapy is 'a politically informed model that observes human experience within the framework of societal and cultural realities, and the dynamics of power informing those realities... Therapy is not construed as happening solely during the session or in the consulting room; it is linked to the events of daily life and to the politics of power, privilege, and disempowerment that are inherent, overtly and subtly, in all of the cultures'. In this way, a woman-focused approach directly addresses the dynamics of power and difference in the therapy room.

The importance of a holistic assessment that recognises the range of factors impacting on a woman's wellbeing is a vital start to therapeutic work. Women survivors of torture and gender-based abuse often struggle to access and engage with psychotherapeutic support in statutory mental health services. Waiting lists for these services can be long, and the pathways to support from statutory settings can often be too inflexible to accommodate the chaotic patterns of engagement that are characteristic of traumatised clients. Services can rarely guarantee a woman the right to see a female practitioner and/or interpreter, and may require her to sit in waiting rooms with men or use mixed-gender facilities that may feel unsafe. Specialist women's services and organisations that work therapeutically with survivors of sexual violence can provide a safe, responsive and flexible service.

A holistic assessment allows a psychotherapist to understand the client in the context of her life in the UK, but also enables the therapist to pick up any factors that may potentially present barriers to the therapeutic process.

Farideh had been referred for psychotherapy in the NHS. She was assessed, but deemed too unstable to engage with psychotherapy. She was referred to our service, and we were asked to undertake preliminary therapeutic work to stabilise her so that she was 'ready' for therapy. After a thorough assessment, it became apparent that difficulties with Farideh's housing were constantly retriggering her post-traumatic stress disorder (PTSD) symptoms. Her psychotherapist made a referral to another voluntary sector organisation to help her get rehoused and to another organisation to provide a mental health support worker to help her with day-to-day practicalities. As well as addressing the social difficulties that were causing such distress, Farideh's psychotherapist supported her to begin to tell her story and understand her mental health symptoms as resulting from the trauma she had experienced.

Knowledge of the asylum system and refugee life is vital to understand the complex interplay of factors impacting on a woman. Critically important is a compassionate understanding of the way in which symptoms of PTSD, the requirements of the asylum system, financial hardship and language barriers combine to make it hard for women to engage in therapy.

Hibo struggled to attend therapy sessions regularly, although, when she attended, she used the sessions well and clearly valued them highly. Hibo's psychotherapist realised that, although Hibo's travel costs were reimbursed, she had no cash to pay for the bus fare in the first place. Hibo had a significant mobility difficulty, and walking was not an option. The psychotherapist started providing her with her weekly bus fare in advance, and downloaded the application for a disabled person's bus pass from the internet, which Hibo got her GP to sign. Hibo was granted a free bus pass, which enabled her not only to attend therapy regularly but also to access other health appointments that she had been missing for the same reason, which had further benefits for her health and wellbeing.

Working holistically with torture survivors is especially important, as they are some of the most vulnerable and disenfranchised people in our society. Kastrup and Tata Arcel talk about 'the complex interrelationship between the health of women and their social, political, cultural and economic situations... we cannot consider the treatment of traumatized women without grasping the complexity of the social context in which they live' (2004: 549). The scarcity of services to meet women's particular needs means that a woman often presents with a bewildering array of practical and psychological difficulties that require consideration. At assessment, exploration of her immediate practical difficulties might have to take precedence over her traumatic experiences. A psychotherapist might have to set up an appointment with an advocacy worker or contact a client's legal representative. This human rights-based approach might add to a psychotherapist's workload, but it contributes greatly to the client's trust and the building of the therapeutic relationship. Women are often disorientated and confused about the services available to them, and may turn to their psychotherapist for advice and guidance. It may not feel immediately comfortable for a psychotherapist to be in this advice-giving or signposting role, but, given the circumstances of a newly arrived refugee, it is humane and therapeutically appropriate that they should provide such information when they can.

It is important for a psychotherapist to be aware of the particular vulnerability of women seeking asylum who are destitute. Women may be relying on friends to provide shelter and food. I have known women who, in return, have had to provide free childcare, domestic work, care for elderly family members or sexual services. In such circumstances, it is difficult for a woman to prioritise her own therapy session, as she is entirely reliant on the good will of whoever is providing her with shelter. In such circumstances, it's essential for the psychotherapist to be flexible, when necessary, around session times. A bus pass and access to free childcare and interpreters can also make all the difference to whether a woman can access therapy or not.

Traditionally, psychotherapy is undertaken with clients whose basic needs for shelter and nourishment have been met. However, this may not be possible with this client group. A woman may be homeless at the start of therapy, or become homeless during therapy. In these situations, a psychotherapist needs to be responsive to the immediate needs of the client. The psychotherapist may need to accept that she may sometimes have to step outside her formal role and advocate on behalf of the client, if the therapy is to proceed. It is not unusual for a client to arrive at a session and present her therapist with a letter that needs careful explanation, and for reassurance to be offered, before they can move on to other material. It is important to be mindful that a psychotherapist's role can become diluted by the overwhelming practical difficulties of clients' lives. At the same time, I can think of occasions when I have made a telephone call in session time (perhaps because a client has no credit or could not make the call themselves), and witnessed the client's relief, and this has enabled them to make better use of the therapy session.

In some settings, this kind of work might be done by an advocacy worker, but many services do not have on-site advocacy workers. While it is important to reflect on and understand how these activities can impact on therapy, it is also the case that practical responses can communicate compassion and understanding, and sometimes be necessary – for example, supporting a client to find a safe place to stay that night. Undertaking practical tasks, when appropriate, can strengthen the client's trust and so enhance the quality of the work. However, it is also important that the therapist is aware when they are being drawn into practical responses because they cannot bear the client's pain, and because of the impotency they feel about the client's situation. Wherever possible, I try to direct the client to an appropriate organisation that can support them to resolve their difficulty, so that we can concentrate as much as possible on the task of therapy. Sometimes this is not possible, because increasingly such resources do not exist.

Gender and disadvantage

Many women who have experienced torture and gender-based violence will also be seeking asylum. Understandably, their experiences of seeking asylum and the strain of the asylum process becomes a significant part of the therapeutic work. It is, therefore, important that a psychotherapist understands the context of a woman's life within the asylum system, the way in which the discrimination she may have experienced as woman in her home country continues to affect her in the UK, and how it is also compounded by the failure of the UK asylum system to adequately consider issues of gender.

Women's experiences of discrimination before coming to the UK often make the process of claiming asylum even more difficult. 'Many women come from cultures which condone gender inequality and systemic violence against women' (Smith & Boyles, 2009: 3).

Women may have had very little education, and may not be literate in their own language. They may have little experience of speaking up for themselves, and may be used to relying on their husband or other male family members. They may be afraid to speak out in front their husband/male family members, or concerned that their experiences of abuse could bring dishonour to the family. The bureaucracy and paperwork of the asylum system can be overwhelming, and it may be difficult for women to articulate their own experiences and make sense of the complicated information provided by legal representatives.

The unfair treatment of women in the asylum system in the UK has been recognised for some time. In 2000, the Immigration Appellate Authority published its Asylum Gender Guidelines, to help decision-makers assess more fairly applications for asylum by women, especially where a woman claimed to have experienced gender-based persecution. In 2004, the Home Office issued its own Gender Issues in Asylum Claims (UK Visas and Immigration, 2004), after significant lobbying from non-governmental organisations and refugee support groups. Yet, in 2006, the Refugee Women's Resource Project still found that 'Home Office Gender Guidance is far from being systematically implemented... the impact of the Guidance not being followed will include unnecessary distress... late or lack of disclosure leading to poor quality decision making... and when women's experiences are not recognised, bias against women's claims' (Ceneda & Palmer, 2006: 3). This discrimination persists in the UK. In January 2016, Asylum Aid issued a briefing paper still asking that 'women seeking asylum are provided with relevant information; female interviewers, decision-makers and interpreters trained on issues relating to sexual violence and trauma; childcare and counselling' (2016: 1).

A psychotherapist should be aware that a woman may not know that she can ask for a female legal representative, if one is available. Women can request a female interviewing officer from the Home Office for their substantive interview, and can record a request for a female interpreter. The Asylum Policy Instruction on asylum interviews (Home Office, 2015) does state that people should not be interviewed about their claims in the presence of family members, because it is inappropriate. It also says that interviews should be scheduled when childcare can be arranged, and if none is available, that childcare should be provided on or near the Home Office premises where the interview is to take place. However, children must attend the initial screening interview if they are to be included as dependants on their mother's asylum application.

While a psychotherapist might not traditionally position themselves in the role of advocate, she might be the only person with whom the client has contact who is able to provide this information. Similarly, a psychotherapist might be the most likely person to liaise with a legal representative about information emerging in the therapy that might make the difference between a successful and unsuccessful asylum claim. It is important to understand that women may have been threatened with terrifying consequences if they disclose their experiences, and this will influence the extent to which they can open up in therapy and to their legal representatives. Often, women only disclose the full extent of their experiences as their sense of safety of the therapeutic relationship grows.

Marie was distraught when her initial asylum claim was refused. She had a private legal representative, but, because he was a man, she had only felt able to talk to him about certain aspects of her multi-layered asylum claim. Marie told her psychotherapist how she did not feel able to speak openly to a man. Gradually, Marie began to talk to her psychotherapist about her experiences of female genital mutilation (FGM), how she had been forcibly 'circumcised' after she was raped, in order to be quickly married. Marie described how her mother was a 'cutter' and she was expected to take on this role after her mother. When Marie's mother died, she sought asylum in the UK to avoid this. However, Marie had been too frightened to tell her legal representative her real reason for coming to the UK, having been told that she would be cursed if she ever spoke about FGM and that she would die a horrible death. It was only when Marie's asylum claim failed and her fear of being returned was greater than her fear of speaking about FGM that she tentatively began to confide in her psychotherapist. Her psychotherapist understood the enormous barrier Marie faced in having a male legal representative and contacted a local firm that could access legal aid for her appeal and offer a female legal representative. Finally, Marie felt comfortable to talk about her experiences, although she was still frightened. In the light of this, legal aid was obtained for an expert country report focusing on FGM. It was largely on the basis of this information and new evidence that Marie was given leave to remain in the UK.

A psychotherapist must also be aware that many asylum-seeking and refugee women will have been detained during the process of seeking asylum, and recognise that this is likely to have had an impact on their mental health and their feelings about their host country.

Despite the Home Office's guidance that survivors of torture should only be detained in exceptional circumstances, and the UNHCR guidelines

(1999) stipulating against the detention of survivors of rape, sexual violence and gender-based persecution, women with such experiences are regularly detained in the UK for long periods of time (Girma et al, 2014). The negative impact of detention is well documented (Girma et al, 2014). Indeed, many women I work with link significant and long-lasting deterioration in their mental wellbeing with their experiences of detention: 'For me being locked up reminded me so much of being put in prison back home, it brought back all the memories of torture... I hear the banging of the doors and the sound of their keys. Even though I'm out of detention, I'm not really out' (Besong, quoted in Girma et al, 2014: 2).

This treatment by their host country impacts significantly on women's feelings of trust and safety, especially when they have experienced further abuse in detention: 'When I was in Yarlswood [Removal Centre], I found it hard to believe that I was in the UK. It seemed to be a place where human rights don't exist... I am still so shocked and traumatised about the way I was treated there' (quoted in Girma et al, 2014: 27).

The prevalence of sexual violence

Statistics indicate that 80% of torture perpetrated against women is sexual (Smith & Boyles, 2009). Women may have been trafficked and forced into prostitution; they may have been imprisoned and repeatedly raped; they may have been forced into marriage and raped by their husbands. Women may also have experienced sexual violence in the country in which they have sought asylum, or during their journey there. In any society, it can be hard for a woman to speak about experiences of sexual violence. Moreover, many women will come from cultures that actively blame and shun a woman who has been subjected to sexual violence. In many cultures, a woman carries the honour of the whole community, or her whole family. A woman's worth may depend on her virginity and chastity; if they are lost, she is then considered worthless, a burden, and bringing shame to the family or community.

It is unusual for a woman who has experienced sexual violence to seek any form of redress, and even if she does – by, for example, reporting a rape to the police – it is unusual for her allegations to be taken seriously or for any form of rehabilitation or redress to be available (Pettitt, 2014). Sometimes a community solution is found: a woman might be forced to marry the man who raped her, or be rushed into a forced marriage. A woman may be so frightened of the reactions of her family that she is forced to flee.

Agna lived with her aunt; she was treated like a slave, and was required to do all her aunt's domestic chores. Isolated and lonely, Agna was befriended by an older man in the village, whom she saw as a friend. On one occasion, when Agna visited him, she was taken ill and fainted. A month later, she found out that she was pregnant, and that he had drugged and raped her. Living in a country where sex outside marriage was a crime for women, Agna felt she had no choice but to flee to a neighbouring country, where another friend helped her get a flight to the UK. Agna has now been living in the UK with her son for several years, and is still waiting for an outcome from her asylum claim. She fears she will be killed if she returns home, and her son, if he was not also killed, would be sent to an orphanage.

The severity of the psychological consequences of rape and sexual violence cannot be underestimated. The United Nations Security Council (2008) explicitly recognises rape as a tactic of war. Croatian author Slavenka Drakulic, who has documented war crimes in the Balkan conflicts, has called rape 'a kind of slow murder'.[2] The fact that many refugee women come from countries that stigmatise women who have experienced sexual violence only compounds and increases the feelings of shame that are a common reaction to such violations.

Furthermore, while the experience of sexual violation may be just the beginning of a woman's trauma history; it may also leave her vulnerable to further exploitation, sexual or otherwise, as was the case for Marie (already discussed above).

Marie was captured and held hostage for three days by rebel forces. She was tied up and repeatedly raped by different men. Marie was fortunate to escape alive, but her family blamed her for the abuse. A husband was quickly found and Marie was married at the age of 13. Her husband was in his 40s and had several other wives. He beat and raped her regularly. The ex-rebel forces who had kidnapped her were granted immunity and Marie would continually see her abusers in the community.

Often women's history of sexual violence may have begun in childhood. When women are trying to escape an initial experience of abuse, they are often extremely vulnerable to further abuse.

Mercy came from a poor background. She was unable to finish her education as she had to help her mother sell produce from their small plot of land at the

---

2. www.ohchr.org/en/newsevents/pages/rapeweaponwar.aspx (accessed July 2017).

market. Mercy was sexually abused by her stepfather from the age of 13, and at the age of 16 she ran away, to escape. She survived by sleeping on the streets and undertaking domestic work. One day, Mercy met a man who promised her a job abroad. He was kind at first and paid for Mercy's flight and passport, but once she arrived in the UK, he changed. He took Mercy to a family, who, he explained, had paid for her to come to the UK. Mercy had to work for them from early in the morning until she went to bed at night, doing domestic work and looking after the children. She was not allowed out of the house and she would sometimes be forced to sleep with men who were brought to the house. One day, when buying milk from the local shop, Mercy fled. She sought help from the local church, who helped her relocate and found her a family to live with. This family was kind to her, so, when they introduced her to a man from the community and suggested that they move in together, she trusted them. Mercy was shocked by his violent temper and mood swings; however, she was pregnant, and dependent on him and his family. It was not until he kicked her in the stomach when she was six months pregnant that she sought help and was advised that she could get support to leave the relationship.

For many women I have worked with, it is the experience of rape and sexual violence that has been the most devastating. Due to profound feelings of shame, many women have never talked about their experiences to anyone, let alone sought professional help or reparation. In the words of a survivor: 'Women suffer many things that it is hard to... speak about. It is very hard for a woman to say that she has been raped' (Besong, quoted in Girma et al, 2014: 2).

Hinshelwood emphasises 'the silence in which women suffer' (1997: 10): often a woman has been keeping her experience of sexual violence a secret for years, hiding her distress and trauma symptoms from those closest to her. This can create many difficulties, as family members struggle to understand a woman's continuing distress. If a woman is keeping these secrets from her immediate family, she may not feel comfortable using an interpreter, despite the confidentiality agreement; interpreters may have close connections with members of the same community.

Azar was held in prison and tortured for several months. Her family managed to secure her escape, and she sought asylum in the UK. After a year of therapy, Azar asked to speak to the psychotherapist without the interpreter, and said that she wanted to have sessions just with the therapist. The psychotherapist was not entirely surprised, as she had felt that there was something Azar was not talking about. Without the interpreter present, Azar could disclose that, while in prison, she had been held in solitary confinement and every night the guard would rape her violently. Azar's family did not know and she feared that disclosure would bring too much shame and distress to her family and that she would also be blamed.

Understanding sexual violence in this context explains the immense power of rape and sexual violence as a method of abuse and torture. It also highlights the enormous potential of the therapeutic relationship, where a woman may feel able to speak about sexual violence for the first time in her life. This may be the first and only place that a woman can speak about her experiences and feelings. Sometimes the overwhelming emotional impact of talking about her trauma may prevent a woman disclosing, or fully disclosing, her experiences. The traumatic memories may also make it hard for her to give consistent testimony about the abuses she has experienced: 'Women have difficulty in recalling aspects of their abuse... fragmented memories can both lead women to doubt themselves... and affect the apparent credibility of their account' (Smith & Boyles, 2009: 11).

A psychotherapist is in a unique position to help a client process the trauma they have experienced. This will not only improve their mental health but also help them feel better able to describe their experiences to their legal representatives or in the asylum system, where necessary. Psychotherapists need to be aware that the barriers women face in disclosing sexual violence may have a significant impact on the success of their asylum claim. The 'key problem women seeking asylum encounter in the refugee determination system [is] negative credibility assessment' (Asylum Aid, 2016: 5). A woman may feel unable to disclose sexual violence in her screening interview or substantive interview, and shame and trauma often lead to late disclosures and inconsistencies in testimony. If later, out of desperation and fear of being returned, a woman does disclose sexual violence, she is at risk of being seen by the Home Office or the Asylum Tribunal as lacking credibility, and this will often further weaken her claim.

Despite demands for Home Office interviewers and decision-makers in the asylum system to be given better training in the impact of sexual violence and trauma on memory (Asylum Aid, 2016), in my experience, the asylum system in the UK still fails to consider the impact of trauma on a women's ability to recount her experiences, as was the case for Marie.

Marie contacted her psychotherapist in a panic after her appeal hearing. She had been cross-examined by the Home Office Presenting Officer at her appeal hearing and had found herself unable to remember the date of her mother's death. The Home Office had repeatedly drawn the judge's attention to a discrepancy between her substantive interview and her written statement about the date when she was raped and held hostage. Marie was terrified that the judge would think that she was lying, despite the extensive supporting evidence of her PTSD symptoms and the impact on her memory.

Working with trauma

The typical stages of trauma recovery, as detailed by Herman, remain largely undisputed (1992). It is well accepted that, for an individual to recover from trauma, control and safety must be first be established, and that remembrance and mourning follow, 'which starts the process of recalling and retelling', and then reconnection and reintegration (Elsass, 1997: 89).

Most of the women I work with have experienced multiple traumas. In addition, the harsh and prolonged process of seeking asylum in the UK keeps women in a state of ongoing instability, in which the threat of being returned to their home country adds to the original trauma that caused them to seek sanctuary in the first place. Rothschild (2010) feels that the essential instability in the situation of a person seeking asylum means that it is unlikely they will move beyond the stage of stabilisation, and warns against the over-zealous practitioner who may push a client to confront their trauma before they are ready.

Most trauma psychotherapists accept the primary importance of stabilisation work: 'Helping the client to feel safe must be the first step' (Rothschild, 2000: 87). Stabilisation work can take different forms: psychoeducation, grounding techniques, and resource building. As Fisher emphasises, 'a trauma survivor can have a meaningful, productive life without... processing the trauma, but she cannot have such a life without doing the work of stabilization... the psychotherapist's job is not just to be a witness... but to teach the patient how' (1999: 2).

Indeed, it is important to recognise the level of trauma women may experience in telling their story, and it should not be assumed that narrating the trauma story is a therapeutic necessity. In Rothschild's words: 'I question the regular practice of investigating and revisiting trauma memories over and over... it is significant to note that a good proportion of trauma victims suffer a worsening of symptoms when encouraged or forced to remember their traumas' (2010: x).

Elsass emphasises 'the importance of proceeding cautiously and accepting a tempo the client can tolerate and accept' (1997: 38). Some of my clients have never told me their story in detail, yet significant therapeutic change has still taken place.

For others, initially it can be an enormous relief to find a confidential space in which they can talk openly about their experiences. Women often present at assessment with an overwhelming array of psychological symptoms. They may arrive at the service in an extremely distressed state. Some may have actively sought talking therapy; others have little idea why they have been referred, or what for.

Often women come from cultures in which mental distress is perceived as a sign of mental illness, and deeply stigmatised. Elsass underlines how 'many cultures take no interest in the introspection that psychotherapy takes for granted and are ashamed of talking about psychological problems' (1997: 110). Some women will, for this reason, struggle to talk about their experiences with people from their own country. The opportunity to explore their experience in a safe and non-judgmental space, while welcome, can be a bewildering new experience at first.

A psychotherapist should appreciate the enormous cultural leap that may be required of such a woman to begin to participate in weekly therapy sessions, where her thoughts and feelings are given precedence. It is also important to remember that many women are coming from cultures where talking about emotions, feelings and mental health symptoms is uncommon. Overwhelming emotion may be perceived as scary and threatening, and may cause clients to become avoidant and reclusive. Psychoeducation should not be overlooked: 'Sometimes teaching theory itself to the client will be just what is needed' (Rothschild, 2000: 96). A simple explanation of traumatic memory can give a new level of understanding to a client who is plagued by flashbacks and nightmares. Likewise, a client who is barely leaving the house because of symptoms of panic can find a simple explanation of the physiological symptoms of anxiety allows them to begin to confront their anxiety. While symptoms of PTSD can be broadly similar across cultures, an understanding of the cultural significance of their symptoms is also important. For example, in some cultures, dreams may be perceived as premonitions; the client not only suffers the terror of the dream itself but is also deeply troubled as to its meaning for days afterwards.

Mariame, who is mentioned earlier in the chapter, had been in a long and abusive forced marriage, and would often hear the voice of her husband when she was under stress. Mariame saw this as concrete evidence of his ability to continue to terrorise her psychologically across continents, via his dealings in 'black magic'. In this instance, her psychotherapist was able to help her see her experience differently, by gently offering an alternative perspective on her suffering, based on the psychotherapist's understanding of trauma, while acknowledging and understanding her experience from her cultural perspective. Mariame felt heard and empowered to challenge the destructive belief that her husband could still control her, despite the thousands of miles between them, and this was a turning point in her recovery.

Women who come from cultures where male violence against women is condoned may struggle to connect their symptoms of distress with the severity of abuse that they have experienced. Again, simple explanations about trauma can be very helpful.

Women often present with physical symptoms that they find overwhelming. These symptoms may be trauma-related, and it can be useful to help the client understand that 'emotions are inseparable from the body' (Ogden, Minton & Pain, 2006: 12): 'Clients often find themselves struggling with the effects of overwhelming emotion with little awareness of how the body participates in creating and sustaining these emotions' (p13).

Levine notes a polarity whereby 'traumatized individuals... are either overwhelmed by their bodily sensations or massively shut down against them' (2010: 282). Supporting the client to develop body awareness through meditation and mindfulness techniques can help her manage these troubling trauma symptoms. Sometimes a woman may communicate her suffering by describing her physical pain. What she needs is to be heard. She may find it easier to talk about physical pain and symptoms in the initial stages of the therapeutic relationship. The psychotherapist may have to be patient and gain the client's trust before she (the client) feels able to voice her psychological suffering.

Healing from trauma

In all psychotherapy, 'the work with relationship and attachment bonds between client and psychotherapist is of the greatest therapeutic importance' (Elsass, 1997: 87). However, given the extreme violations of relational bonds experienced by women survivors of torture, this focus is especially restorative. Through demonstrating attentive responsiveness, the psychotherapist communicates her esteem for the client, and this creates a sense of safety and being cared for. In the words of one of my clients, 'You are not like other counsellors. I know that, when I leave the session, you do not forget about me.'

Most women I have worked with have had very low self-esteem; hence the psychotherapist showing an interest in and attention to a client's resilience and strength is restorative, as is an emphasis on empowerment in the present – the fact that the client survived (Rothschild, 2010).

Women and violence

> Torture... is a display of force... it breaks down parts of the victim's personality. The greatest challenge to the torture survivor is therefore to remain a human being under these inhumane conditions. (Elsass, 1997: 1)

It is important to remember that, as well as having experienced abuse, women may have also abused and/or harmed others. While a woman may have had no choice over her involvement, especially if she was a child when forcibly recruited, she may still hold significant feelings of guilt and self-hatred.

Favor was abducted from her village by rebel forces when she was eight years old. As a young girl and a virgin, she was highly prized by the rebel forces, and seen to bring good fortune to their cause.

Brutalised and repeatedly raped, she joined an army of child soldiers, both boys and girls, who were used by the rebel forces as a first line of attack against government strongholds during the civil war. The children were immediately given guns and taught how to fire repeated rounds of bullets as they approached their targets. If Favor had not obeyed orders, she would have been killed, but she now lives with the memory of the lives she has taken. Favor escaped from the rebel forces several years later and returned to live with her family. She was pregnant when she returned and was taken to have an abortion. Her community was aware of her involvement with the rebels, and she was ostracised and lived in hiding. After Favor escaped to the UK, she was finally able to talk in therapy about the violence she had perpetrated and the feelings of horror and shame she still experienced.

As well as bearing witness to the atrocities a woman may herself have experienced, a psychotherapist needs to facilitate an environment where her client can talk about abuses that she has committed. Most media reports of forced involvement in armed combat typically focus on boys and young men, and ignore the fact that, in many parts of the world, girls and women are also forced to take part in fighting. That they are used as 'troops' and also to satisfy the sexual needs of male soldiers adds to their traumatisation.

Sexuality

In my experience, many women who identify as lesbian, bisexual or transgender are forced to seek asylum. The abuses they are fleeing are due to their sexuality, and are usually gender specific, such as rape or forced marriage. These women have not only experienced significant discrimination as women, but are also likely to have lived in fear that they would be killed if their sexuality were ever known.

Nadia comes from a country in which it is illegal to be a lesbian. Nadia realised as a teenager that she was attracted to women, but knew she had to keep it a secret. When she was 20, she found out that her father had set a date for her to be married. Having witnessed the abuse of her mother and her aunts by their husbands, Nadia felt that she had no choice but to flee the country. Nadia's parents, angered by her disobedience, had also heard rumours about her sexuality, and disowned her and made threats against her life. Nadia is now seeking asylum in the UK.

Although these women may be living in the relative safety of the country where they are seeking asylum, they are often still in hiding, still fearful of telling anyone in their community about their sexuality, or the sexual violence that they experienced as a result. The relief a woman feels when she can talk openly in therapy about her sexuality and experiences is significant.

Women-only service and specialised women's services

In my experience, women who have experienced torture and gender-based abuse almost always feel more comfortable working with a woman. To be met by another woman creates a sense of safety and, to a degree, a sense of shared experience. Women generally feel safer with other women, and the sense of safety aids disclosure of traumatic material (Women's Resource Centre, 2007). More often than not, but not exclusively, a woman's abuse has been perpetrated by a man. In addition, women often come from cultures where they are subordinate to men; therefore, to speak openly to a man would feel very difficult. The sexual nature of the abuse means that details are often intimate and a woman may feel less ashamed to talk about them with another woman.

Offering psychotherapy to women who are fleeing persecution means appreciating the specific circumstances women refugees encounter as women.

They will be daughters, sisters, wives and mothers, and often they may have been forced to flee, leaving their loved ones behind. It is not unusual to encounter women who have had to leave their children as babies and are still seeking asylum in the UK, years later. Kastrup and Tata Arcel emphasise how many refugee women come from societies where 'women's role is primarily centred around the home' (2004: 547).

A women's loss may also be conceptualised in terms of women's traditional roles within the family and home, and how this loss could be different to that of a male partner. It is heart-wrenching to sit alongside a mother's grief as she talks about having missed her son/daughter's childhood or how she has no idea where her children are, or about their safety. Sometimes a woman may have had to seek asylum because of her partner/husband's activities, not her own, and as a result may have ambivalent feelings towards him that she may struggle to voice.

When Fatima's husband decided to convert from Islam to Christianity, it became more and more dangerous for the family to continue living in the country. They left their four children with her sister temporarily, and claimed asylum in the UK. Fatima had been led to believe that claiming asylum would be a straightforward process, and that she would quickly be able to reunite her family in the UK. Seven years later, the couple were still struggling with their asylum claim. Fatima was desperately concerned about the wellbeing of her children and their safety in a largely Muslim country where Christians are a persecuted minority. While her husband was sympathetic, there was often conflict between them. Fatima felt that she could not express her feelings fully to her husband and that he could not understand the extent of her suffering. She felt that she had been forced to choose between her children and her husband, in a society where women cannot survive without the support of their menfolk. In her own words: 'I ask myself, am I a mum? I have left my children but I cannot live without my husband... I feel so much guilt, for the last seven years there has not been a night that my pillow has not been wet from tears.'

As her therapist, it has been particularly hard for me to witness a mother's extreme distress at being separated from her young children, knowing that, at the end of the day, I can go home to my own. However, I continue to be amazed by the power of empathy and connection to override feelings of envy and anger, even in these distressing circumstances, and to sustain both client and psychotherapist.

Many of the women that we work with are single mothers. Often, they have been raped or trafficked, or have fled abusive marriages. Their children may be the result of the abuses they have experienced. Despite the traumatic circumstances in which their children have been conceived, they may be the woman's reason for living. Yet, with this, a woman may also feel some ambivalent feelings towards her child.

Mercy, mentioned earlier in the chapter, is seeking asylum and is a single mother. She suffers ongoing mental distress as a result of the violence that she experienced at the hands of her ex-partner. At times, her son's behaviour is challenging and reminds her of his abusive father. Mercy feels frozen, and finds it hard to manage her son's behaviour.

Women also talk about their difficulty adjusting to childrearing in a western culture. They may struggle in particular with boundaries and behaviour, having come from cultures where physical punishment is accepted, and often having been physically abused themselves. It can be hard for women to reconcile the privilege and freedom that their children enjoy in comparison with their own childhoods. I have worked with some women whose children have had social services involvement. In our experience, it has been important to liaise closely with social workers and police to help them understand the particular difficulties that such women encounter in the UK, and how this affects the wellbeing of both the women and their children. It has also sometimes been necessary to challenge the racism and homophobia that women have encountered from social services and the police.

Issues of culture, difference and power

When I'm asked how I address issues of race, culture, power and difference in the therapeutic relationship, I can sometimes struggle to come up with an articulate and polished response. Although I am a psychotherapist who works every day across the 'ethnocultural divide', putting into words the subtleties of forging a strong therapeutic relationship across the cultural chasm between me and my client is difficult (Aroche & Coello, 2004: 69).

Aroche and Coello ask: 'Is any of what Western psychology has to offer relevant and acceptable, not to mention appropriate, when working with clients from such different cultures and world views?' They conclude that 'there are no definitive answers, yet the questions remain valid for every client we see' (2004: 69–70).

For me, a position of genuine interest and caring is crucial. Aroche and Coello also state that 'acknowledging and being prepared to address... diversity and its complexity is crucial to connecting with the individual' (2004: 55). In my experience, clients who have had their trust broken can easily see if a psychotherapist's interest is not genuine and heartfelt. Genuine respect for a client and their culture helps mitigate against inequalities in power. Before meeting a woman for the first time, I always make sure that I have some understanding of her country/community of origin, and, I think, this is appreciated.

Yet, being prepared to admit to the limits of one's own knowledge of a client's culture and one's own cultural position is also important. As Glenn says: 'It is of enormous value in all interactions to adopt a "not-knowing" position... and to be curious about the narratives of others. However, simultaneously, I hold beliefs and values that inform... a view of the world I live in' (2002: 187). Boyles writes: 'A commitment to working within a human rights framework also means naming and exploring such issues of power and privilege, such as my power as a UK citizen, as a white person and other structural powers I may have' (2006: 163).

When I take a summer break, my clients often remark that I have been away. While my privilege and freedom (including the freedom to cross national boundaries) makes me feel uncomfortable, it is far better than I openly acknowledge my position to my clients and give them the opportunity to express their feelings about it, rather than avoid the inequality.

A proportion of clients referred to the service express a preference for working with a white woman. This preference surprised me at first, until I began to understand the fear of these women that people in their community here will get to know about their experiences. Some women have expressed a fear of being 'shamed' in communities here, as they would have been at home. Although I always explain the counselling service's confidentiality policy, it seems that it can be hard for a woman to feel comfortable with someone who she thinks may have a link to her community.

Unfortunately, many women cannot choose to see a female psychotherapist: in our under-resourced counselling services, a male psychotherapist might be the only one available. In these circumstances, the male psychotherapist needs to understand how this might impact on the client. He can help a woman feel more comfortable by telling her that he understands this might be difficult for her, and trying where possible to give her the power to make choices in the therapy room – where she sits, and how long she stays, for example. If the therapist is a man, it is very important that the interpreter is a woman.

It may raise complications when a woman is working with a psychotherapist or interpreter who is from a refugee background themselves, and/or speaks the same language as the client. It is always important to explore how a client feels about working therapeutically with someone they may perceive as coming from the same culture. Sometimes, it can be a relief to work with a 'sister' who comes from the same culture and has had similar experiences of racism in the UK. However, it can feel threatening: for example, it may be hard for a client to truly trust the service's confidentiality policy if the therapist or interpreter is from the same community. Numerous factors can influence the dynamics between therapist, client and interpreter when working transculturally. It is impossible to predict them, which is why it is so important to see every client as an individual, each bringing their own dynamic. As far as possible, a client should be offered a choice of therapist and interpreter in terms of race, gender and sexuality. However, this is not always possible, given that many services are predominantly staffed by white people.

'I know that when I leave the session, you do not forget about me'

With the increasing numbers of people fleeing their home countries, experience of working with refugees and people seeking asylum is becoming more and more necessary for psychotherapists. Yet, for many psychotherapists, it can be a daunting prospect. Many times, I have heard comments such as, 'That sounds challenging,' or, 'How do you cope with the trauma?' or even, 'I wouldn't want your job,' or, 'I couldn't do your job.' These understandable feelings may come from a fear of vicarious trauma, and an awareness of the chaotic nature of the work and the impact on therapeutic boundaries. They are justified, and that is why it is so important for the psychotherapist to look after herself. It is vital to recognise the impact of countertransference – to understand that it is normal in this work to experience powerful feelings of hopelessness, stuckness, frustration, and anger, and that these are important communications of the client's experience.

Undoubtedly, this field presents significant challenges to any psychotherapist. A therapist needs flexible yet firm boundaries, the resilience to sit with and witness the most harrowing human suffering, and the ability to bear and work with the most overwhelming feelings of powerlessness.

The impotence the client feels in the face of the asylum system in the UK can feel paralysing, and can also impact on the psychotherapist. In the face of such adversity, I often find myself wondering how psychotherapy can possibly help, but I am presented with plenty of evidence that it does. Women attend regularly and eagerly, despite their chaotic lives, and express great appreciation of the service they receive. They make significant psychological improvements and give consistently positive feedback.

Trying to understand and articulate how the therapeutic experience heals, I fall back on Herman:

> The core experiences of psychological trauma are disempowerment and disconnection from others. Recovery, therefore, is based upon the empowerment of the survivor and the creation of new connections. Recovery can take place only in the context of relationships; it cannot occur in isolation. (1992: 133)

The experience of torture and abuse destroys a woman's sense of safety in the world, and their faith in the safety and reliability of others. The security of the therapeutic relationship allows a woman to dare to trust and hope again for a world in which she might be safe and respected.

References

Amnesty International/ REDRESS (2011). *Gender and Torture: conference report.* London: Amnesty International/REDRESS. www.amnesty.org/en/documents/IOR50/001/2011/en/ (accessed July 2017).

Aroche J, Coello MJ (2004). Ethnocultural considerations in the treatment of refugees and asylum seekers. In: Wilson JP, Drožđek B (eds). *Broken Spirits: the treatment of traumatised asylum seekers, refugees, war and torture victims.* Hove: Brunner-Routledge (pp53–80).

Asylum Aid (2016). *Double Standards Facing Women Seeking Asylum in Europe: Asylum Aid briefing paper.* [Online.] London: Asylum Aid. www.asylumaid.org.uk/wp-content/uploads/2016/01/Double-standards-briefing.pdf (accessed June 2016).

Berkowitz N (2000). Gender guidelines for the UK. *Forced Migration Review* 9 December. [Online.] www.fmreview.org/sites/fmr/files/textOnlyContent/FMR/09/06.htm (accessed July 2017).

Boyles J (2006). Not just naming the injustice: counselling asylum seekers and refugees. In: Proctor G, Cooper M, Sanders P, Malcolm B (eds). *Politicizing the Person-Centred Approach: an agenda for social change.* Ross-on-Wye: PCCS Books (pp156–166).

Brown L (2012). *Feminist Therapy.* Washington, DC: American Psychological Association.

Ceneda S, Palmer C (2006). *'Lip Service' or Implementation? The Home Office Gender Guidance and Women's Asylum Claims in the UK.* London: Asylum Aid.

Chaplin J (1988). *Feminist Counselling in Action.* London: Sage Publications.

Elsass P (1997). *Treating Victims of Torture and Violence: theoretical, cross-cultural and clinical implications.* New York, NY: New York University Press.

Fisher J (1999). *The Work of Stabilisation in Trauma Treatment.* Unpublished paper presented at The Trauma Center Lecture Series 1999. [Online.] http://janinafisher.com/resources.php (accessed September 2016).

Girma M, Radice S, Tsangarides N, Walter N (2014). *Detained: women asylum seekers locked up in the UK.* London: Women for Refugee Women. www.refugeewomen.co.uk/2016/wp-content/uploads/2016/07/WRWDetained.pdf (accessed September 2016).

Glenn C (2002). 'We have to blame ourselves': refugees and the politics of systemic practice. In: Papadopoulos R (ed). *Therapeutic Care for Refugees: no place like home.* London: Karnac (pp167–188).

Grandi F (2016). *Women Refugees and Asylum Seekers in the European Union.* Address to the Chamber of the European Parliament to mark International Women's Day, Strasbourg, 8 March 2016. [Online.] www.unhcr.org/uk/admin/hcspeeches/56dec2e99/women-refugees-asylum-seekers-european-union-ceremony-mark-international.html (accessed July 2017).

Herman JL (1992). *Trauma and Recovery: the aftermath of violence – from domestic violence to political terror.* New York, NY: Basic Books.

Hinshelwood G (1997). *Gender-Based Persecution.* United Nations Expert Group meeting on gender-based persecution. Toronto, Canada, 9-12 November, 1997. www.un.org/documents/ecosoc/cn6/1998/armedcon/egmgbp1997-rep.htm (aAccessed July 2017).

Home Office (2015). *Asylum Policy Instruction: asylum interviews.* Version 6.0. London: Home Office.

Immigration Appellate Authority (2000). *Asylum Gender Guidelines.* [Online.] http://doubleviolence.free.fr/spip/IMG/pdf/GB_gender_-_copie.pdf (accessed May 2016).

Kastrup MC, Tata Arcel L (2004). Gender-specific treatment. In: Wilson JP, Drožđek B (eds). *Broken Spirits: the treatment of traumatised asylum seekers, refugees, war and torture victims.* Hove: Brunner-Routledge (pp547–571).

Levine PA (2010). *In an Unspoken Voice: how the body releases trauma and restores goodness.* Berkeley, CA: North Atlantic Books.

OHCHR (1984). *Convention against torture and other cruel, inhuman or degrading treatment or punishment.* Geneva: OHCHR. www.ohchr.org/EN/ProfessionalInterest/Pages/CAT.aspx (accessed July 2017).

Ogden P, Minton K, Pain C (2006). *Trauma and the Body: a sensorimotor approach to psychotherapy.* London: WW Norton & Co.

Pettitt J (2014). *Rape as Torture in the DRC: sexual violence beyond the conflict zone.* London: Freedom from Torture.

Refugee Council (2017). *Quarterly Asylum Statistics: May 2017.* [Online.] London: Refugee Council. www.refugeecouncil.org.uk/assets/0004/0488/Asylum_Statistics_May_2017.pdf (accessed July 2017).

Refugee Council (2012). *The Experiences of Refugee Women in the UK.* [Online.] London: Refugee Council. www.refugeecouncil.org.uk/assets/0001/5837/Briefing_-_experiences_of_refugee_women_in_the_UK.pdf (accessed June 2016).

Rothschild B (2010). *8 Keys to Safe Trauma Recovery: take-charge strategies to empower your healing.* London: WW Norton & Co.

Rothschild B (2000). *The Body Remembers: the psychophysiology of trauma and trauma treatment.*

London: WW Norton & Co.

Smith E, Boyles J (2009). *Justice Denied: the experience of 100 torture surviving women of seeking justice and rehabilitation*. London: Medical Foundation for the Care of Victims of Torture.

UK Visas and Immigration (2004). *Gender Issues in Asylum Claims*. London: UK Visas and Immigration. www.gov.uk/government/uploads/system/uploads/attachment_data/file/257386/gender-issue-in-the-asylum.pdf (accessed July 2017).

UNHCR (2016). *Global Trends: forced displacement in 2016*. Geneva: UNHCR. www.unhcr.org/uk/statistics/unhcrstats/5943e8a34/global-trends-forced-displacement-2016.html (accessed July 2017).

UNHCR (2011). *Survivors, Protectors, Providers: refugee women speak out: summary report*. Geneva: UNHCR. www.unhcr.org/uk/protection/women/4ec5337d9/protectors-providers-survivors-refugee-women-speak-summary-report.html (accessed July 2017).

UNHCR (1999). *Revised Guidelines on Applicable Criteria and Standards Relating to the Detention of Asylum Seekers*. Geneva: UNHCR. www.unhcr.org/uk/protection/globalconsult/3bd036a74/unhcr-revised-guidelines-applicable-criteria-standards-relating-detention.html (accessed July 2017).

UNHCR (1951). *Convention and Protocol Relating to the Status of Refugees*. Geneva: UNHCR. www.unhcr.org/uk/protection/basic/3b66c2aa10/convention-protocol-relating-status-refugees.html (accessed July 2017).

United Nations Security Council (2008). *Resolution 1820: adopted by the Security Council at its 5916th meeting, 19 June 2008*. New York, NY: United Nations. www.un.org/en/ga/search/view_doc.asp?symbol=S/RES/1820(2008) (accessed July 2017).

Women's Resource Centre (2007). *Why Women Only? The value and benefit of by-women for-women services*. London: Women's Resource Centre. http://thewomensresourcecentre.org.uk/wp-content/uploads/whywomenonly.pdf (accessed July 2017).

7. Alone in the world: therapy with separated young people
Ann Salter

Separated young people are a unique group in the UK. Their experiences are almost beyond imagination for most of their peers: forced separation, at a young age, from families, communities and homes; journeys across the world that are filled with terror and involve life-threatening danger, and arrivals at destinations where they are often met with suspicion and hostility.

The separated young people I see for therapy have all been tortured, most of them when they were still children. No country admits to the torture of children under its jurisdiction, yet, as was noted by the United Nations High Commissioner for Human Rights:

> The torture of children and adolescents is still a shocking reality. Even young children are... subjected to various forms of torture, including through the use of specific machinery to administer pain, mock executions, sexual abuse and assault, and being forced to witness pain, abuse, violence or humiliation being inflicted on other children or family members. Children are frequently targeted because they are children, as a way to intimidate entire communities or to force their parents or other relatives to endure additional torture. (OHCHR, 2016)

The use of sexual violence and rape as a means of torture of children and young people is widespread, and affects both genders, but predominately girls. This is used as a means of control and subjection:

> Girls are generally one of the least powerful members of society and least able to protect their rights or gain redress if their rights have been violated. If the law regards a woman

> as a second-class citizen, and a child as a non-person, there is
> little chance of respect for the human rights of girls. Girls from
> minority or marginalised groups are victims of even further
> prejudice. (Mann, 2000: 29)

The vulnerability of children and young people who have been tortured is greatly increased when they are separated from their family and community. Separated young people have no one to turn to for protection, nurture or comfort.

Young people may be left at a motorway service station or in a city centre by a people smuggler, with no food or money and nowhere to go. They may have little or no English, and they certainly do not know how to navigate the local systems to find help.

I have been working as a psychotherapist with separated young people for more than 10 years. I work in a human-rights non-governmental agency in the UK that provides rehabilitation to survivors of torture. Before this, I worked for a number of third-sector organisations as a therapist, with a variety of client groups, including separated young people, young people with mental health difficulties, adult refugees and people seeking asylum. I take a human-rights approach in my work. I believe that we, as the host country, have a duty to welcome and provide rehabilitation and redress to people who have been at the receiving end of global injustice and human rights abuses, including torture. I demonstrate this in my work by actively engaging with young people about their rights. I am not neutral as a therapist: I believe that separated young people have a right to be in the UK and to receive support and care, and that this right is not dependent on their asylum status. This will sometimes mean that, in my practice, I will advocate on behalf of young people – for example, in interactions with a social worker or teacher. I may also liaise with their legal representative.

In this chapter, I aim to share my rights-based approach to working with young survivors of torture and describe how I incorporate advocacy into therapy with separated young people who have been tortured. It is becoming increasingly common for therapists in settings such as schools, further education colleges and child and adolescent and mental health services (CAMHS) to come into contact with this client group. I hope to highlight some of the challenges in the work and illustrate approaches that I have found effective in my therapeutic work with young people.

This chapter will include the voices of separated young people. The case studies are fictional and based on amalgamated examples from my practice.

Part of a human rights approach is to bear witness, and I hope to bear witness to the children and young people with whom I have worked in the past 10 years who have experienced human rights abuses through torture and conflict. These young people have not only managed to survive, but, in many cases, have built a new life and found a way of living with profound losses. In writing this chapter for therapists, I also hope to pay testament to the many young people who have shared their experiences with me.

Who do we mean by separated young people?

The consequences of torture on the individual who survives are profoundly personal, isolating and shameful. Torture has a physical, emotional, psychological and spiritual impact on children and young people. Rehabilitation for adult survivors of torture often works from the principle of helping the individual to reconnect with the person they once were. Children and adolescents, who are still on the path to adulthood, do not have a fully-formed self to which they can return. In addition, children and young people who have been separated from their family are deprived of the close emotional bonds from which they might have derived some comfort and emotional holding during the rehabilitation process.

Who do we mean by separated young people? At the simplest, we are referring to those children and young people who have entered the UK having been separated from their usual caregiver, and are thus denied their protection (emotional and physical). The Immigration Law Practitioners' Association (ILPA), in their guidelines for working with children and young people subject to immigration control, uses the following definition:

> 'Separated children' is the term used in most countries to describe those children who are outside their country of origin and separated from their parents or legal or customary primary carer... In each case, separated children are, by definition, children who have been deprived of their family environment. (Crawley, 2012: 10)

Adam and van Essen point to the vulnerability caused by separation from family and community, combined with loss of country: 'For adolescents, the forced separation from family and friends coincides with the loss of parental country and culture... these processes... involve double losses and double mourning' (2004: 524).

This describes both the vulnerability faced by children who are 'deprived of their family environment', as well as the lack of choice available to them – the choice is usually made for them by adults and dictated by life or death situations. But the term 'separated children' also points to strength and resilience: despite everything, this young person has survived, and with survival comes the potential for thriving.

Another term in common use, particularly in statutory children's services in the UK, is 'unaccompanied asylum-seeking children' (UASC). This is often used to refer to children under 18 who have applied for asylum in the UK and for whom the local authority has a duty of care. As separation is such a key part of the asylum experience for children and young people, I will be using the term 'separated young people' in this chapter.

I use the term 'young people' to refer to anyone between the ages of 14 and the early 20s. This is an approach commonly taken by young people's services in the UK, and reflects the fact that development continues up to the age of 25, as confirmed by recent neurobiological research (Montgomery, 2013). Any reference to child/children means a person deemed to be under 18 years.

Most of the separated young people that I have worked with in my clinical practice have been male, and this is reflected in the examples explored in the chapter. This is also evident in the statistics of separated young people who arrive in the UK. In 2015, more than 90% of applications were made by males and nine per cent by females (Refugee Council, 2015). This statistic is striking and it is important to consider some of the reasons behind it. Men still hold most power globally, and in many societies and cultures (including in the west), the life of a boy is deemed more important than that of a girl. We can be certain that girls and young women suffer at the hands of repressive regimes and as a result of conflict. A session of the UN Commission on the Status of Women on 12 March 2015, held to discuss how rape and displacement affect women in war zones, reported that: 'Women and children were disproportionately affected by conflict, accounting for a large percentage of displaced populations' (United Nations Commission on the Status of Women, 2015).

Girls are more likely to be forced into marriage as children, are victims of gender-based abuses such as female genital mutilation (FGM), and are at risk of domestic violence and 'honour' killing. Why then are so few girls and young women able to flee? Primarily this is because priority is given in many cases to saving the life of the boys in the family. But there are additional risks for a girl travelling across the world unprotected. Girls and young women are more likely to be sexually exploited and abused, and an unprotected girl or young woman travelling alone is likely to become a target for traffickers.

The UK has had an obligation since 2008 under the UN Convention on the Rights of the Child (UNCRC) to consider the best interests of the child in any decisions about them, regardless of immigration status. For many years, children subject to immigration control were denied this right. On signing the treaty in 1992, the UK entered a general reservation on Article 22 of the Convention. This reservation denied the rights contained in the Convention to children seeking asylum, which meant that unaccompanied children seeking asylum in the UK did not have recourse to the full range of rights and protection afforded to other children. Health and education services were uncertain as to their statutory obligations for this group, and separated children were left even more vulnerable. After campaigning by a variety of organisations, including children's charities, the government removed the general reservation in 2008.

In principle, then, any child living in the UK, including unaccompanied children seeking asylum, are entitled to have their best interests considered in any decision affecting them. The application of this principle, however, is not always straightforward.

An age-disputed young person is a child or young person who has given their age on arrival to the UK, and the age they have stated is not believed by the UK authorities. In most instances, the young person is assessed as being older than the age they have given on arrival, and this may result in a child being unable to access support from children's services and being placed in adult services. Only unaccompanied children are entitled to local authority care under the Children Act, so being classified as adult can have devastating consequences for vulnerable children. Instead of being accepted as a child, and being treated as a 'looked-after child' by the local authority, with all the support and entitlements that accompany that status, they are placed in Home Office multiple-occupancy accommodation designed for adults, putting them at immediate risk of abuse and exploitation, and denying them access to appropriate healthcare and education.

There are various reasons why the UK authorities may not believe the given age of a newly arrived child. Home Office guidelines stipulate that the 'benefit of the doubt' should be given, but in my experience this guidance is not usually followed (Home Office, 2011/2015).

The Coram Children's Legal Centre (2017) states that age assessments should follow a protocol that incorporates a holistic assessment, including understanding contributory factors from a child's cultural and ethnic background that may impact on their development

Age assessments frequently conclude that the child is not the age they say, which can leave a child feeling undermined and confused. In 2015, 3,253 unaccompanied children claimed asylum in the UK, of whom 789 had their ages disputed. This represents about a quarter of unaccompanied children seeking asylum (Refugee Council, 2015).

The process of age assessment can be retraumatising to children. One of my clients once said: 'My age is the only thing I have left from my mother – she told me how old I was. Now even that has been taken away.' It can strike at the heart of a child's identity.

Ali was left alone in the centre of a strange city, in a new country, where people spoke an unfamiliar language. He was 17. His journey to the UK had lasted almost a year. He had been forcibly recruited to a Taliban training camp, where he was tortured, forced to participate in the mistreatment and sometimes killing of other children, and expected to become a suicide bomber. A camp guard had helped him escape. He fled Afghanistan with his father, and had seen him killed by a roadside bomb when they were crossing the border into Iran. Ali's mother and younger brothers had remained in Afghanistan, as there had not been enough money for them all to leave.

Ali stayed in Iran with a friend of his father's, where he worked for 10 months in a factory doing manual labour to earn his passage across Europe. An agent (or 'people smuggler') took Ali, along with others, on the long and hazardous overland journey. Ali saw many of his travelling companions die during the journey, particularly when they were crossing the mountain ranges. There was no possibility of stopping to help, and, to ensure his own survival, Ali needed to keep up with the rest of the group.

He was left on a bench in the city in the strange country (which he later learned was the UK) by the people smuggler, whom Ali had come to see as his protector over the last few months. He was told to remain where he was, while the man went away to 'sort something out'. He would return in 20 minutes. Ali never saw him again. He waited for nearly 24 hours before a member of the public approached him and took him to a police station. Ali feared that he would be arrested and beaten.

When I first met Ali, he was silent and withdrawn. I greeted him, and introduced myself and the interpreter. I invited Ali to say a little about himself and his current situation, and explained what I and the organisation could offer. Despite the presence of the interpreter, I was not sure that he understood what I was saying. Whatever statement I made was met with silence, and any questions that I asked were responded to with one-word answers. I started to feel increasingly ungrounded, unsure of what I was doing and of what I should do next. At the end of the session, we made an appointment for the following week, but I suspected that he might not return.

Ali was one of the first separated young people with whom I worked. Reflecting on that initial session, I realise that there was a potent mix of anxiety and uncertainty coming from all three of us in the room: therapist, interpreter and client. I was unsure how to explain psychotherapy to a bemused-looking teenager from Afghanistan. I did not know what I could possibly do that would be helpful to someone so young, who had survived such horrific experiences, and who was yearning for his family. Surely anything I had to offer was a poor imitation of what he actually needed?

Ali did in fact return the following week. We worked together for two years, during which we were able to build a strong therapeutic alliance. Ali had been initially fearful that I was going to report him to the Home Office. His asylum application was in process, and Ali was frightened that I might not believe him, as his age was disputed and he felt that no one believed what he had to say.

During my work with Ali, I developed a deeper understanding of how psychotherapy can benefit separated young people. As a result of the therapy, he started to feel safe in himself and with others. He was able to learn to live with the memory of some of the terrible things that had happened to him. This included being tortured by the Taliban in Afghanistan, undertaking the hazardous journey to the UK, and the memory of seeing his father killed. Ali frequently asked why all these bad things had happened to him. In therapy, he was able to find some kind of meaning that fitted with his worldview and personal faith. He was able to regain a sense of his own future, which had seemed so terribly curtailed. He continued to miss and long for his family, particularly his mother. He had not been able to contact her since leaving Afghanistan, and had no way of knowing whether she was safe, or even still alive.

Ambiguous loss

The loss of family is often the most painful experience for a separated young person, and the most difficult to integrate. In the chaos of fleeing and the journey to the UK, young people might have seen their family members killed, or they might not know whether their family is still safe. It is very easy to lose contact with people in a conflict zone or in transit across countries.

The kind of loss that Ali was facing is very common among separated young people. He was caught in the agonising situation of desperately longing for his mother, and not knowing whether she was safe or even alive. He had no evidence to suggest that she had died, but, at the same time, no proof that she was still living. He would think about all the dangers she might face in Afghanistan, including being targeted by the Taliban because of his actions. His greatest fear, which he was unable to voice but which was enacted in his nightmares, was that she was dead. The tension between the intense longing for his mother and the fear of what might have happened to her became increasingly unbearable for him.

Boss (1999) refers to this as 'ambiguous loss', in her book of the same name. She writes of the simultaneous psychological absence and presence of a loved one whose fate is unknown, and the resulting 'frozen grief'. Ali at first found it impossible to express the fears and complicated emotions of his loss. As he had no contact with his family, community, or anyone who knew his mother, there was nobody to share these feelings or concerns with. This in turn led to intense isolation and loneliness.

The therapist in this situation can encourage the young person to connect with their memories of the missing family member. This relationship, even when there is no contact or knowledge of the current situation, is often experienced as real and ongoing. Children and adolescents often have creative ways of fostering this connection, and I believe that it is the psychotherapist's role to encourage and nurture this creativity.

Klass, Silvermann and Nickman write of a 'new understanding' of grief, which they call 'continuing bonds'. This proposes that an ongoing relationship with the deceased is a normal (and desirable) state for many people:

> Survivors hold the deceased in loving memory for long periods, often forever, and that maintaining an inner representation of the deceased is normal rather than abnormal... these relationships can be described as interactive, even though the other person is physically absent... other relationships characterised by physical absence... can have a similar influence on the lives of the individuals involved. (1996: 349)

For a separated young person who has experienced a relationship from a caregiver that has been in any way nurturing, this relationship can still be felt as supportive, even when they do not know if the person is alive or dead. This may not bring closure or healing, but there can be comfort in being able to turn to the 'inner representation' of the mother, for example.

Marie was 18 years old and pregnant when she arrived in the UK. She had been captured by soldiers in the Democratic Republic of the Congo two years earlier, and had lost contact with her family at this time. Once she was safe from the soldiers, she had tried to get in touch with her family, using her last known contact, and had also tried to trace people from her community who might have been able to provide support. She had not been able to make contact with anyone she knew. A Jesuit priest arranged for her to fly to the UK, using a false passport.

Marie was initially detained for immigration offences when she arrived at the airport, before she was found to be pregnant. She was able to make an asylum claim, and was housed in asylum accommodation and assigned care for her pregnancy.

Marie's midwife referred her for therapy after the birth of her baby, as she was 'struggling to cope'. The baby had been conceived when Marie was raped while she was in captivity, and looking at the baby reminded Marie of what had happened to her. She was also feeling desperately isolated and lonely, and did not know anybody who spoke her language (Lingala). She talked about wanting her mother there to help her look after the baby, and that her mother would 'just know what to do'.

Marie's baby, Eva, was 12 weeks old when I first met them both. I knew that Marie was receiving support from both a midwife and health visitor, and Marie agreed that I could exchange information with them, so that between us we could provide the best help for her and her baby. I could see that Marie had ambivalent feelings about Eva, and she appeared low in mood. I was concerned about Marie's isolation, so we agreed that I would try to help her find groups where she could take Eva and get some social support and contact with other women with babies and young children.

In our sessions together, I became aware that Marie was emotionally remote from her child and sometimes responded to Eva's cries with annoyance. Marie talked about her mother, who had had seven children and would often be called on for advice and help with other children in the community. I asked Marie if she could imagine her mother giving her any advice now. Marie's response was that her mother would take the baby so that she could have a rest. I asked what it felt like for Marie to imagine being looked after like that. 'It feels like my Mum giving me a hug.' Marie appeared to soften towards Eva after thinking about her own mother, but she would also sometimes become distressed. She seemed to move between feeling some comfort and intensely missing her mother.

Some young people make drawings of their absent family, or arrange dolls in a doll's house to show the family group. Some describe dreams, talk about childhood memories, and even express remorse and guilt for misbehaving as a young child. This can connect with a range of other losses, such as friends and a lifestyle that will never return.

Ali told me about his memories of standing on the roof of his house, flying kites with his father. He also recalled children and adults being hurt or killed by falling off the roofs, but this did not lessen his grief that he would never again see or experience flying kites with his father.

Working with complex trauma

Therapists new to work with this client group may feel overwhelmed by the degree of loss and trauma experienced by separated young people. It is helpful to think and formulate in terms of 'complex trauma'. Herman proposed what was then a new diagnosis of complex post-traumatic stress disorder (PTSD) to describe a syndrome shown by survivors of 'prolonged, repeated trauma' that includes torture, repeated childhood abuse and captivity, where escape is not possible (1992: 119).

This diagnosis, and the three-phase approach of recovery that Herman proposed, is widely recognised by therapists, psychologists and trauma specialists, including the Complex Trauma Task Force (CTTF) of the International Society for Traumatic Stress Studies (ISTSS) (2012).

The ISTSS task force definition of complex PTSD includes the core symptoms of PTSD, such as re-experiencing of the traumatic event, avoidance/numbing and hyper-arousal, in conjunction with a range of other disturbances related to an individual's capacity for self-regulation. This includes the ability to relate to others, emotional regulation, dissociation and somatic symptoms. This diagnosis can be a helpful way of understanding children and young people's responses to extreme events.

When working with separated young people, we need to remember that they are not yet on stable ground. They are experiencing often intense cultural displacement and are trying to adjust to life in exile, without the key family and community figures who would normally be there to guide and protect them. They are frequently in the asylum process, with all the fear and uncertainty that brings, and may be age disputed and at risk of exploitation, including sexual exploitation. The therapist may feel overwhelmed by the multiple layers of trauma, loss and current risk. It is therefore important that therapists give sufficient time for a thorough assessment process.

The process of initial assessment should aim to be collaborative. It is important to find out how the young person understands their situation, and to explore together how therapy might be helpful. The assessment should aim to be holistic, in that it includes both psychological and physical health, educational and welfare needs, housing, social functioning and the young person's legal situation. While the therapist is unlikely to be an expert in all these areas, it is important that they can ascertain where there is a problem, and signpost to or approach organisations that can help with any specialist area of need.

Risk assessment

Risk assessment forms part of any therapeutic assessment; in work with separated young people, the monitoring and management of risk is ongoing. It is always important to ask the young person directly about whether they have had thoughts or feelings about wanting to end their life or to hurt themselves. The answer to this question has almost always been 'yes', in my experience. Asking this question clearly and 'normally' can help reduce the shame, stigma and, in some cases, taboo that can be associated with suicide and self-harm in many cultures.

Risk assessment with separated young people presents additional challenges for the therapist. Separated young people are often isolated, may not speak English and may have limited access to health and support services. This is particularly the case if they are age disputed or over 18, as they would not then be able to access mental health services available to children. This may leave the therapist holding more responsibility for a young person's safety than would normally be the case.

Young people may hold cultural beliefs about suicide and self-harm that make it difficult for them to talk openly about suicidal thoughts or plans. The young person might also feel too ashamed to talk about these feelings in front of an interpreter from the same culture or religion, for fear of being judged. These challenges mean that the therapist needs to be able to carry out risk assessments with the young person on an ongoing basis, involving the young person in the process.

For some young people, risky behaviour is an expression of distress, rather than a clear desire to die. Ali would have nightmares in which he repeatedly saw his mother attacked by snakes, while he looked on, powerless to help. At these times, he could not bear to stay in the house and would sometimes wander through the streets in the early hours of the morning, and spend the night sitting in his local park. When I explored the risks of this with him, he responded by saying, 'It is all Allah's will.' This was a complex situation, in which what might appear to be a strategy to manage his distress (going out of the house to walk around) was in fact risky and potentially harmful behaviour. By making this explicit, we could explore other ways for Ali to manage his distress during the night. Ali was able to admit to himself that there were times when he felt that life was 'too much' and that he 'had enough of living'.

Trafficking and sexual exploitation

The term 'trafficking', as used in the UK, refers to the movement of people both from overseas and within the UK for the purpose of exploitation. Children are trafficked into the UK for various purposes, including sexual exploitation and exploitative labour.

ECPAT UK, formerly known as End Child Prostitution, Child Pornography and the Trafficking of Children for Sexual Purposes, is a third-sector organisation in the UK that campaigns to end trafficking. It refers to 'myriad complex factors that make children particularly vulnerable to trafficking', which include poverty, gender inequality and exploitation of children: 'Once trafficked, these children are often controlled through violence, being deprived of their freedom of movement... and a deep-seated fear of authority instilled by their trafficker' (ECPAT UK, 2015).

Farhad, a 17-year-old young man from Afghanistan, had been coming to therapy for several weeks when he started talking about 'the man in the restaurant'. I was unsure at first who this man was and what role he had played in Farhad's life. Was he someone from Kabul who had also been part of the Taliban who had tortured him? It became clear as the sessions progressed that Farhad had been brought to a restaurant on arrival in the UK, and had been told that he needed to stay with the man who worked there, who would look after him. The man repeatedly sexually abused him, and told Farhad that the police would beat him and send him back to Afghanistan if he reported what was happening. Farhad was terrified that he would be found, not only by the Taliban, but by the man in the restaurant.

With Farhad's agreement, I told his legal representative about this, who was able to refer his case to the National Referral Mechanism (NRM), a process set up by the government to identify and support victims of trafficking in the UK. There was also a police investigation to ascertain if there was enough evidence for a prosecution.

Therapists working with young people may find it helpful to have some training with a local organisation working with trafficked young people, so they know the signs that may indicate that a young person is at risk of or being exploited.

If there are concerns about the possibility of trafficking, then it is vital to contact the local authority safeguarding team, (the local government agency in the UK that has a duty to protect children and young people) and specialist agencies working with trafficked young people.

Detention and destitution in the UK

One of the risks inherent in the asylum process for separated young people is destitution when they become 'appeal rights exhausted' (ARE). At this point, a young person may also be detained in an immigration removal centre (IRC), in preparation for return to their country of origin. They should not be detained unless removal is imminent.

A young person who no longer has an active claim for asylum will be evicted from their accommodation and will lose all financial support. At this stage, many young people become destitute – that is, homeless, with no source of income. In addition, there is the constant fear of detention and return to the country where they originally fled from torture. The threat of this happening can cause a great deal of distress and anxiety.

Children under the age of 18 are no longer subject to immigration detention (under the Immigration Act, 2014), but can be held with their family in 'pre-departure removal accommodation'. However, if a child is age disputed and being treated as an adult in the system, there is the possibility of detention, both on arrival in the UK and as a prelude to removal once they become ARE.

A human-rights approach involves being active in supporting a client in the asylum process to work towards being granted some form of asylum in the UK. This may mean that the therapist will engage with a young person's legal representative to ensure the young person is kept informed of the progress of his or her asylum case. If a young person does not have an effective legal representative, they may need support to access one. The people involved in the care of the young person would normally aim to ensure that they are represented for free by lawyers specialising in immigration, under a Legal Aid Agency (LAA) contract.

The importance of active engagement with a legal representative becomes clear in times of crisis. Serge was an 18-year-old young man from Cameroon who had fled torture when he was a child, but he had been denied asylum in the UK. He was ARE; he was also age disputed. He had been assessed as being aged 19 on arrival in the UK, when he was in fact 16.

Serge was detained by the Home Office, and transferred to an IRC close to an airport. He was informed that he would be returned to his home country, where he had no known family and was still a target for the authorities, due to his father's previous political activities. This removal was prevented, as the legal representative was able to submit a letter from his therapist to the Home Office, confirming that he was in therapy and detailing the impact of torture on Serge's mental health.

Therapists may sometimes be required to write a letter or report describing their clinical work with the young person. Clinical letters should be written with the principles and guidance of the *Istanbul Protocol* in mind. The Istanbul Protocol is the internationally accepted guideline on the investigation and documentation of torture and its consequences, produced by the Office of the United Nations High Commissioner for Human Rights (OHCHR, 1999).

Young people who become destitute often show considerable resilience and may be able to rely on networks of friends or acquaintances to provide a temporary sofa or room. Young people can be referred to night shelters or hostels, and make use of services such as soup kitchens provided for homeless people. Sometimes these systems break down, however, and a young person may become street homeless. This clearly renders them highly vulnerable; they may become at risk of exploitation, physical attack, health problems, and drug and alcohol use.

It is useful for therapists to make links with agencies that provide destitution support to refugees and people seeking asylum. There is a network of such agencies in most cities where people seeking asylum are accommodated. Having access to this support might prevent a young person from street homelessness.

Asylum process

It is useful for therapists to have some understanding of the asylum process and the support arrangements available to young people. Unless a separated young person has already been granted some form of protection, they will be going through the asylum process. This is often a major source of distress and confusion.

Children who arrive in the UK without either of their parents are required to make an independent claim for asylum. They should always be advised and represented by a legal representative, through legal aid, and they are entitled to 'the benefit of the doubt' from the Home Office, which processes the claim. In asylum law, it is understood that children are usually less able to recount logically and sequentially what has happened to them, due to various factors, including the child's stage of development, and the fact that children might not be aware of all the factors that put them at risk. Children may also have seen things that they do not understand or do not have the words to articulate. For example, a child who has witnessed or been subject to a sexual assault might find it impossible to describe what has happened. This can depend in part on the child's age and how much they know about sex. It is also due to children and young people's feelings of fear and shame after being subject to or witnessing sexual assault. This can make disclosure difficult in any context; in the context of a formal asylum interview, the potential for fear and shame in disclosure can be overwhelming.

A child or young person over the age of 12 must usually be interviewed by the Home Office about their asylum claim. Anyone under 18 has the right to have an independent adult with them at the interview, and this is usually a social worker. Legal aid is available for their legal representative to represent them at the interview too. If the child's asylum claim is accepted, then they will be granted protection in the UK. However, unlike adults, children do not have the right to family reunion under the immigration rules, which means that they cannot automatically apply for their parents and siblings to join them in the UK, even when they know their whereabouts.

A refusal of a claim for asylum can be devastating for a child or young person. They face return to a place where there is nobody left to protect them, and where they can expect torture and death. On refusal, a child will be granted limited leave to remain for 30 months, or until they are 17½ years old (whichever is sooner). This uncertain future can make it very difficult for a young person to start adjusting to a new life in the UK.

It can be difficult for therapists to hold this uncertainty with the young person. The feelings associated with this lack of safety and continued threat can begin to dominate the therapy. The focus of the work at this point will often be on finding some degree of safety, located internally and in relationship to others (including the therapist), as well as practical work, such as liaison with the legal representative and other agencies.

The young person has told their story in the asylum process and has not been believed, and so it is important for the therapist to remember their role of bearing witness to the human rights abuses the young person has experienced. This can be profoundly important for a young person and can contribute to their recovery and rehabilitation.

Building safety and the therapeutic relationship

In the early stages of therapy, my aim is to provide a sense of containment and to work with a young person to develop a sense of stability and safety. Central to this phase is acknowledging and building on a young person's resilience in the face of loss and trauma.

Ahmed was 20 when he came for his first session of therapy. He had been in the UK for six months, after fleeing detention by the government in Syria, where he had been tortured, due to his family's political activism. Ahmed appeared angry as we entered the room together. While we were still standing, he asked me if I was a doctor. I said no, and started to introduce myself. Ahmed sat down, opened his rucksack and started to pull medications and prescriptions out of his bag and throw them on the floor. 'What can you do for me? I need a doctor. See how much pain I am in; I need someone who can help me.'

Ahmed was in a hyper-aroused state and was so anxious that he took little notice of me or the interpreter. He was angry, and his anger was directed initially at me and the organisation. I felt that his anger was in fact linked to his experiences of torture in Syria, his journey to the UK, and his current situation. He had no expectation that anybody would be able to help him, and he appeared to have lost hope in any future. I knew that I needed to help him move from this state in order for him to be able to experience me, the interpreter and the setting of the organisation as safe and containing. As Ahmed seemed unable at that time to find any stability in himself or in the environment, I used my voice and my physical presence to try to help him become calmer. I spoke clearly and slowly, realising that it was the tone and rhythm of how I was speaking that was important. The interpreter spoke with the same intonation as I did. By the end of the session, Ahmed was able to hear what I was saying a little bit more, and to agree to another appointment.

This initial phase of therapy with Ahmed helped him to develop some understanding of his feelings of intense distress and to develop ways of coping with his symptoms of trauma. We did this through careful use of psychoeducation, where I explained the impact of traumatic events on the brain and body, and we explored ways of managing distress that he found useful. These included distracting himself by listening to music when he experienced flashbacks, and getting out of bed and drinking water when he woke from nightmares. Ahmed was not at this stage ready to connect with physical sensations. When I suggested that he pay attention to his breathing as a way of becoming calmer, for example, he became agitated and distressed.

As the therapeutic relationship is built, a sense of safety can be developed, from which it is possible to start addressing and processing trauma. It can be useful to think of the therapeutic alliance in terms of an attachment relationship, particularly for separated young people, who have been deprived of their key attachment figures at such a critical time in their development. They will have lost these people at a point when they are most in need of the comfort that person (very often the mother) would have provided. Holmes makes an explicit link between the therapeutic relationship and attachment:

> The basic interpersonal architecture of therapy is (a) a person in distress seeking a safe haven, in search of a secure base; (b) a care-giver with the capacity to offer security, soothing and exploratory relationship; and (c) the resulting relationship, with its own unique qualities. This process applies to the initiation of therapy itself, to the start of ongoing sessions, and to moments of emotional arousal as they occur within the session. (2013: 17)

Thus, a separated young person needs to be able to find a safe haven in the therapist, in order to have a sufficient sense of safety and security, both internal and external, to be able to explore the multiple layers of losses and trauma. However, the therapeutic relationship brings with it its own particular complexities for separated young people. While forming a bond with the therapist, the young person is usually longing for his or her lost family.

Trauma processing

It is inevitable that such loss and trauma will have a profound impact on the mental health of a child or young person. For a separated young person who has been tortured, a significant part of their distress is the separation from family and community. It is important to remember that, in processing the trauma of the experiences of torture, or of the journey to the UK, the loss of the family will form a significant part of the picture. Therefore, it is particularly important that young people have developed a sense of safety if they are to be able to undertake deeper exploration and processing of past events.

Van der Kolk stresses the importance of breathing as a way to self-regulate: 'Learning how to breathe calmly and remaining in a state of relative physical relaxation, even while accessing painful and horrifying memories, is an essential tool for recovery' (2014: 207).

Helping a young person to develop this ability is important if they are to be able to start processing trauma. Being able to revisit the memories of traumatic events, while staying present, embodied and in psychological contact with the therapist, is an important step to recovery.

This does not have to be spoken, however. Children and young people may struggle to find words to describe an overwhelming memory. Creative materials and use of a sand tray can be very helpful. Ali used a sand tray throughout our work together. He would regularly put objects into the sand to build a narrative of the past, and to express his feelings about his current life in the UK. During one of our sessions, he used miniature figures and objects to make a representation of the Taliban training camp where he had been detained and tortured. He did this in concentrated silence, with me watching. While Ali was concentrating and absorbed in what he was doing, he was also clearly aware of my presence. When he had finished placing the objects and buildings in the sand, and having moved and altered some of the small wooden buildings and the trees, he looked up at me. 'They made me do horrible things. They said they would kill me and my family if I didn't do what they said.' Ali was then able to tell me, over the course of the next few sessions, about the beatings he had endured and the executions he had witnessed and been forced to participate in. He was able to share how terrified he had been.

The sensory experience of using a sand tray can be soothing, and can help towards a reconnection with physical sensation, which can be helpful in trauma reprocessing. Van der Kolk writes of the disconnection many traumatised people feel from their bodily sensations: 'Traumatized people chronically feel unsafe inside their bodies. The past is alive in the form of gnawing interior discomfort... People who cannot comfortably notice what is going on inside become vulnerable to responding to any sensory shift either by shutting down or by going into a panic' (2014: 96 – 97). The sensation of the sand is soothing, and can bridge the gap between a dissociative 'shut down', and a hyper-aroused panic.

Working with the sand tray in therapy has enabled young people to express anger and outrage. One young person from Cameroon buried figures that represented his torturers in the sand, then took them out one by one and beat them against the side of the table. This was done carefully and deliberately. Although he was clearly angry, the young person was not reliving his distress and was connected to me as he shared his story and expressed his outrage and anger as it affected him in the present.

Reconnection

A major dilemma in the lives of separated young people is how to move into early adulthood in a very different situation to their previous expectations. Any notion of what their adult lives would become has to be radically changed. In addition, they do not have the family and community that they could have expected to support them through this transition into adulthood.

The therapist needs to enable a reconnection between the child or adolescent they once were and the adult that they are becoming in the UK. This might involve an acknowledgement of what they once had hoped for and planned, in comparison with the possibilities open to them now. There are new possibilities to explore and new relationships to be formed. This is only possible if enough time has been given to mourning what has been lost, and enough attention paid to the family whose whereabouts and fate remains unknown.

Once a young person has been able to revisit and process some of their traumatic experiences, they are usually able to then find a way of reconnecting with their past self. Ali began talking to me about his place in the world. His asylum claim was still ongoing, so he did not know whether he would be granted protection in the UK. 'The world is a big place, but there is no place in it for me.' I found this difficult to bear – almost more difficult than some of the details of his torture. I needed to stay with the existential loneliness of this young adult, still a teenager, who in a very literal sense had no place to call home. Papadopoulos writes of the central place that 'home' has in the refugee experience: 'Homecoming is... about the re-establishment of all meaningful connections within one's own family and own self' (2002:14). This may be a lifelong journey for Ali.

Ali and I started to explore what he might like to happen in his future. He had been successful in learning English, which can be a struggle for some traumatised young people. Ali talked about becoming a car mechanic, as he had learned about engines from his father and uncles while still in Afghanistan. We were able to talk about what his family would think if they knew that he would pursue the same work as his father: 'My father would be very proud.'

Ali was granted refugee status at his second appeal hearing at the Asylum Tribunal. He had been in therapy with me for two years, and was 19 when he was finally safe. He was attending a further education college, and had applied to do a car mechanics course.

When I first met Ali, he appeared fearful and traumatised. He was now at times happy and confident, and looked forward to his future. He still encountered difficulties, and he still had occasional nightmares where he relived aspects of his experiences in the Taliban camp. And, of course, he still desperately missed his family. However, I started to recognise that the therapy was approaching the end of its course, and Ali did too.

During our last session together, Ali told me how coming to see me in therapy had helped him: 'There was a stone in my heart. Now my heart is lighter.' This is the best description of the therapeutic process that I have heard, from anyone.

'I can think of my future now'

Separated young people who have been tortured show a remarkable ability to survive. They have been separated from their family, having endured torture; they may have witnessed the killing and deaths of others, and they have survived the gruelling and long journey to the UK. They may also be disbelieved about their history, about where they have come from, and their age. Separated young people are trying to make a new life in the UK, while still not knowing whether their claim for asylum will be accepted and whether they will be allowed to stay. Young people often come for therapy feeling overwhelmed, confused and disorientated. It is therefore understandable that therapists may feel the same when they start therapeutic work with them.

In writing about therapy with refugees, Papadopoulos emphasises the need for the therapist to understand that:

> ... what is 'traumatic' for refugees is not only the 'devastating events'... but the totality of their situation... An exclusive focus on the devastating events tends to suppress the totality of their experience and creates a skewed perception of them, of their history and of their stories. (2002: 157)

I find this to be particularly true in my work with separated young people. They are living with trauma, and they are also living with so much more. This includes trying to make sense of what has happened to them, trying to find some meaning in their lives now, and trying to find some hope for the future.

I occasionally see former clients around the city where I live and work. I was recently walking through a public square when I saw Ali with two other young men. Ali came up to me and shook my hand. He told me that he was on his way to college with his friends. He looked relaxed and happy; I felt delighted to see him.

This is part of the reason that I continue to do this work. I am constantly touched by young people sharing their experiences of loss, despair, life and hope. Separated young people can and do manage to recover sufficiently to make a new life, with a new future. It is a privilege for the therapist to be part of this.

References

Adam H, van Essen J (2004). In-between: adolescent refugees in exile. In: Wilson JP, Drožděk B (eds). *Broken spirits: the treatment of traumatized asylum seekers, refugees, war and torture victims*. Hove: Brunner-Routledge (pp521–546).

Boss P (1999). *Ambiguous loss: learning to live with unresolved grief*. Cambridge, MA: Harvard University Press.

Coram Children's Legal Centre (2017). *The Age Assessment Process*. Migrant Children's Project fact sheet. London: Coram CLC. www.childrenslegalcentre.com/wp-content/uploads/2017/03/Age-assessment-process.march_.2017.pdf (accessed July 2017).

Crawley H (2012). *Working with Children and Young People Subject to Immigration Control: guidelines for best practice*. London: Immigration Law Practitioners' Association.

ECPAT UK (2015). *Working Against Child Trafficking*. [Online.] London: ECPAT. http://new.ecpat.org.uk/content/working-against-child-trafficking (accessed July 2017)

Herman JL (1992). *Trauma and Recovery: the aftermath of violence – from domestic abuse to political terror*. New York, NY: Basic Books.

Holmes J (2013). Attachment theory in therapeutic practice. In: Danquah A, Berry K (eds). *Attachment Theory in Adult Mental Health*. London: Routledge (pp16–34).

Home Office (2011/2015). *Assessing Age for Asylum Applicants*. [Online.] London: Home Office. www.gov.uk/government/publications/assessing-age-instruction (accessed July 2017).

ISTSS Complex Trauma Taskforce (2012). *The ISTSS Expert Consensus Treatment Guidelines for Complex PTSD in Adults*. [Online.] www.istss.org/ISTSS_Main/media/Documents/ISTSS-Expert-Concesnsus-Guidelines-for-Complex-PTSD-Updated-060315.pdf (accessed July 2017).

Klass D, Silvermann P, Nickman S (1996). *Continuing Bonds: new understandings of grief*. Philadelphia, PA: Taylor & Francis.

Mann N (2000). *Children, Torture and Power: the torture of children by states and armed opposition groups*. London: Save the Children.

Montgomery A (2013). *Neurobiology Essentials for Clinicians: what every clinician needs to know*. New York, NY: WW Norton & Co.

Office of the High Commissioner for Human Rights (2016). *How Can Children Survive Torture? Report on the Expert Workshop on Redress and Rehabilitation of Child and Adolescent Victims of Torture and the Intergenerational Transmission of Trauma*. Geneva: United Nations.

Office of the High Commissioner for Human Rights (1999). *Istanbul Protocol: manual on the effective investigation and documentation of torture and other cruel, inhuman or degrading treatment or punishment*. Geneva: United Nations.

Papadopoulos R (2002). *Therapeutic Care for Refugees: no place like home*. London: Karnac Books.

Refugee Council (2015). *Asylum Statistics: annual trends*. London: Refugee Council. www.refugeecouncil.org.uk/assets/0003/6286/Asylum_Statistics_Annual_Trends_Nov_2015.pdf (accessed October 2016).

United Nations Commission on the Status of Women (2015). *Targeted attacks, rape, displacement threaten women in war zones, commission hears as delegates call for swift action, sustainable solutions*. Wom/2028. 59th session, 7th & 8th meetings. [Online.] New York, NY: United Nations. www.un.org/press/en/2015/wom2028.doc.htm (accessed October 2016).

van der Kolk B (2014). *The Body Keeps the Score: mind, brain and body in the transformation of trauma*. London: Penguin Books.

8. Understanding shame with survivors of torture

Colsom Bashir

At a conference, some years ago, I sat in the audience while a highly experienced systemic psychotherapist spoke eloquently about the need for sensitivity when engaging with survivors of torture and their families, because shame was experienced differently in other cultures and had unique effects on victims. This caught my interest; it sounded promising to me, as a practitioner who dealt regularly with the tricky and frustrating aspects of shame. She spoke about how shame required us to be careful, to understand that we could not comprehend how sexual assault, for instance, was experienced by women from other cultures and relationships. I heard how this different kind of 'shame' *particularly* silenced victims and prevented them from seeking help. I heard that, if I was not sensitive to this shame, I would alienate clients by misunderstanding its cultural inevitability.

I was left with the vision of the 'poor refugee woman', crippled by shame, and the 'powerful psychotherapist', who had to be cautious and sensitive when referring to the sexual assault, which is often a part of torture. I am sure it was not the speaker's intention, but she implicitly constructed shame as a particularly unique issue for women from 'other cultures', and perhaps beyond the comprehension of therapists in the host country. The decision to raise the issue of sexual assault must be left to the survivor, we were told, when they were ready to overcome the shame. To be directive about it would reinforce the shame, further silence the victim and charge up the dynamics in this refugee's family, who did not want to deal with the sexual assault because shame prevented them from doing so.

The speaker had spoken from a position of 'whiteness' and 'imperialism', in such a way that constructed the 'victim' as a woeful refugee woman, from some 'backward' country that still viewed raped women as shamed. While she had made a promising start by raising the issue of shame and refugee women's experiences of sexual assault, much of the rest of the presentation had devolved into conceptions of shame presented from a white, imperialistic standpoint, rather than considering the social and political functions of shame in reinforcing gendered and, from my perspective, racialised positions.

The lack of consistency in formulating psychological health from a political perspective was disappointing. I was taken aback by the speaker's lack of political perspective and contextual formulation in constructions of rape in war and as a method of torture. These limited formulations were riddled with the disease model of mental health (or, more accurately, mental illness) and resulted in what I regarded as limited psychotherapeutic interventions. Therapy was aimed at healing people from the pathogenic process of one individual raping another, with no collectivist or systemic position on rape, globally, in society or during war or conflict. The construction of shame was limited to a decontextualised intrapsychic factor, without any ownership of the therapist's standpoint and how it might influence and, in this case, reinforce shameful experiences and identities.

My direct and supervisory work with survivors of torture had led me to understand that what is shameful remains hidden and will not often be purposefully brought into the discussion by survivors themselves. My work has led me to the clinical opinion that practitioners should accept shame's important role in ongoing distress and disengagement. This standpoint then necessitates a sensitive and purposeful exploration, directly with survivors, of shame and its effects. Ultimately, this allows us to therapeutically engage with individual narratives of shame and begin to collectivise embodied experiences of shame by linking them with its wider narratives and social purposes. The aim of this chapter, therefore, is to examine shame and how it is intertwined individually, socially and politically, to help inform psychological formulation and ultimately therapeutic intervention with survivors of torture.

This chapter is not intended to be an exhaustive review of the psychology, sociology or biology of shame, but rather an invitation to take an interdisciplinary perspective on psychological formulation that will drive us towards transformative interventions with survivors.

Shame as a socially constructed phenomenon

Shame has been associated with a range of psychosocial problems, including depression, anxiety, post-traumatic stress disorder (PTSD), substance abuse, eating disorders, violent behaviour and domestic violence, among others (Dearing & Tangney, 2011). Generally, in psychotherapy, and specifically in our work with survivors of torture, we may see shame as one dimension of a complex set of reactions and effects within an individual's life history. Its manifestation is often attributed to the individual's psychic state as a function of pathology.

The tendency for psychological therapists to view shame as a unitary, individual phenomenon is described as attention to the primacy of *dispositional shame*, which is problematic, because it reinforces shame's essence as a 'context-free intrapsychic variable [that serves]... to mask the social constitution of shame' (Leeming & Boyle, 2004: 375). This de-politicisation and de-collectivisation of shame might be seen more broadly as part of the agenda of individualism and the neoliberal ideologies that underpin psychological models, or the result of the prevailing reductionist disease model of human psychology. However, a deeper probe reveals that the causes, functions and effects of shame are much more far-reaching than its embodiment in the individual.

It is easy to drown oneself in the river of writings on the meaning and function of emotion without arriving at an integrated standpoint, and there are good reasons for this, as Misheva summarises (2006: 128): 'Emotions are dealt with in psychology, psychiatry, sociology, philosophy, theology, anthropology, linguistics, history, classical scholarship, as well as primatology and a vast range of neurosciences... The specialized literature clearly indicates that the word 'emotion' simultaneously signifies many disciplinary notions and images that are unrelated to each other.'

I would direct the reader to the array of stimulating writing produced in sociological and cultural studies on the social embeddedness of emotion (see Harré, 1986; Ratner, 1989; Ratner, 2002; Boiger & Mesquita, 2012; Ahmed, 2014). This body of literature is the backdrop to the argument that shame is a socially constructed phenomenon (see Scheff & Retzinger, 1991; Munt, 2007). For example:

> 'Social constructionists maintain that emotions depend on a social consciousness concerning when, where, and what to feel as well as when, where, and how to act.' (Ratner, 1989: 211)

> 'There is evidence for the social construction of emotion in three embedded contexts: in-the-moment interactions, relationships, and cultural contexts. Studies of children–caregiver and adult dyadic interactions provide support for the idea that emotions are constructed in the process of interaction.

> Moreover, these interactions are embedded in the context of relationships, which shape and are shaped by the emotions of the people committed to these relational engagements. This process of construction unfolds within a rich environment of cultural meanings and practices (ie. cultural models) that render certain emotional themes, meanings, or actions salient for the emoting self.' (Boiger & Mesquita, 2012: 227)

Ahmed argues further that psychological or sociological positions are both incomplete because emotions are not polarities that originate internally and move outwards, and nor are they external phenomena that somehow embed themselves in us. Emotions become 'crucial to the very constitution of the psychic and the social as objects, a process which suggests that the "objectivity" of the psychic and social is an effect rather than a cause' (2014: 10). Emotions provide information about how we have come to accept and internalise social norms. The quality of emotion belies how much we have become invested in received norms as rules we adhere to and live by. Expression of such emotion reveals and reiterates norm-based values, thereby reinforcing them. This repetition cyclically strengthens the individual display of an emotion *and* the cultural narratives that it references. How we perform emotions as individuals sets us apart from others, creating boundaries, or, when we choose to link our responses to a social group, we develop a sense of experiencing with others in relation to received ideas. It is between *or among* the embodied expression and the social norms to which it alludes that physical manifestations of emotion therefore have a separating or collectivising role. Ahmed argues that our task in furthering a complete understanding is to establish the connection between emotions, the body and language to uncover this 'circularity of affect'.

Liddell & Jobson (2016) review neural processes in PTSD symptoms across individualistic and collectivistic cultures. While this binary view of culture is limited, their review challenges the assumption that brain processes are universally similar, and argues for the interdependence of culture with neural activation. Their work reveals that the variation in neuro-expression of PTSD symptoms is influenced by culture. For example, they outline the neural evidence suggesting a collectivistic cultural tendency towards focusing on background/contextual details during peri-traumatic exposure, as opposed to the focus on specific and central detail in individualistic cultures. Furthermore, they show how much we focus on the self in relation to others: ie. the interpersonal is dependent on cultural norms, which therefore influences perception and attention bias and ultimately affects recovery pathways.

In particular, they propose five aspects of PTSD experience modulated by cultural variables: '... fear perception and regulation, attentional biases (to threat), emotional and autobiographical memory, self-referential processing and attachment systems (2016: 1).

This review invites us, once again, to critically appraise received ethnocentric, individualistic wisdom influenced by models that disembody emotions from the cultures within which they are produced. In particular, it is important that we reflexively appraise our beliefs about the cultural relevance of what is feared peri- and post-traumatically.

If shame is the foremost threat intra- or inter-personally, then survivors from collectivistic cultural backgrounds may require specific, sensitive interventions to support the processing of central details alongside the contextual and background information that drives their PTSD. As practitioners, this position will enable us to stand alongside survivors of torture as they develop culturally congruent understandings of what constitutes threat stimuli and threat cues, rather than standing above, by, for example, imposing our 'objective knowledge' on their experience. Shame, a pervasive socio-cultural phenomenon, will be enmeshed with survivors' considerations of distress. I would also suggest that individualism and collectivism are viewed dimensionally, rather than as fixed polarities, to ensure nuanced formulations that are sensitive to changing historic-temporal, socio-cultural and migration contexts.

The bottom line for us here is that this literature directs us to learn more about 'the *operations* of culture, and specifically the cultural and discursive practices that articulate emotions and the self' for a comprehensive appreciation of the lived experience of human emotion (Doyle McCarthy, 1994: 267). The multidimensional nature and functions of shame are therefore best revealed using an interdisciplinary approach. I believe it is our task, as practitioners, to familiarise ourselves with an individual's shame by tracing its origins, embodiment, meaning and function within the cultures where it is expressed – to fully appreciate its impact intra-psychically, socio-politically, across borders and interpersonally.

'Culture' is not monolithic but dynamic, subject to changing temporal and social contexts. Differences in cultural norms are apparent in relation to ethnic group, class, sexual identity, gender, familial group, and religious beliefs, among others. Cultural pluralism may also be valued or devalued within nations, which would mean that there exist implicit imperatives driving individuals to adhere to some context-dependent social rules and not others, which has implications for how people experience and understand shame and shaming. Further, Ahmed describes 'national shame', where nations express shame about historical wrongdoings or failings (towards, for example, indigenous cultures), to arrive at a disembodied 'collective shame' (2014: 108). The operationalising of national shame, Ahmed contends, serves to reify a unique national identity, while simultaneously othering the groups towards whom shame is expressed. For example, the way in which social narratives drive views of how the individual shamed woman tarnishes the honour of the nation, which then makes her a target for further abuse. Examples of this proliferate on social media in relation to the current treatment of (particularly lower caste) women in India. Furthermore, in the context of a host country, the contact points between mainstream society and individuals who have been ostracised in their home country results in further marginalisation (for example, survivors in a refugee context) and, in particular, reinforces ideas of unworthiness or otherness that make up social shame (Kinouani, 2015).

For our purposes, here, cultures and national identities might impact on the individual survivor in multi-dimensional ways that shape whether shame is experienced at the level of the self, the body, the group, the nation, or across nations. The notion of intersectionality (Crenshaw, 1991) may be useful in helping practitioners to appreciate how the interconnected nature of social categorisations/cultures/positions (eg. race, ability, sex, gender, sexual orientation, class, caste, religion, ethnicity) create overlapping and interdependent systems of influence over shame for survivors of torture. This idea stems from the post-structuralist position, which views identities as fluid rather than fixed, and specific rather than global (Bhavnani & Phoenix, 1994). Thus, aspects of our identities are created or emerge, depending on the location, who we are in conversation with, the power differential, and other aspects of the context.

For example, an Ahwazi Arab woman may voice difference aspects of her identity depending on her location and if her situation evokes an aspect of her identity. In the south-west of Iran, where her community and family are located and where there is a resistance movement, she may mostly evoke her activist identity as an Arab, as part of a political movement, or perhaps particular aspects of her relationship with the Iranian majority group. Outside of this context, where her ethnicity is less visible, other narratives around identity might predominate: for example, what it is to be a woman, or what it is to be an Arab minority. In the UK context, she may reference a more global Middle Eastern or Persian identity. This is relevant in that emotions may be represented differently within each of these aspects of identity. So, in our hypothetical example, she may be a proud Arab but a shameful Iranian, or a proud mother but shameful woman and so on. Thus, shame experiences that emerge during therapeutic encounters may manifest differently (if they emerge at all), depending on the purpose of the exchange, the context being invoked, the power differentials and whether the person is in the majority or minority in that context.

Intersectional formulations would therefore serve to bring into focus survivors' nuanced understandings of the disparate values and expectations that shape their experience of shame locally, nationally, and within a global context.

Sally Munt considers the cultural politics of shame. Her descriptors of the essence of shame expose how it exceeds the bounds of a unitary emotion. She describes the qualities of shame as:

- an *intense emotion* experienced momentarily in response to acute embarrassment or humiliation which maintains and reinforces the sensory memories it leaves
- a *transitional affect*, passing through which, cumulatively, leaves a psychic trace *embedded in the self*, with a sticky quality that brings with it powerful reactions such as contempt, rage, disgust, humiliation, mortification at the self
- an *embodied experience*, where the body becomes saturated with the cumulative effects and reactions to shame, or is, indeed, the source of such experiences. (2007: 2)

Munt argues: '... shame, working at different levels, performs culturally to mark out certain groups' (2007: 2). As we examine manifestations of shame in our clients, we begin to identify *themes* in its impacts on people, relating to sex, gender, age, culture, caste, class, ethnic group, race and sexuality. These *patterns of impact* are more noticeable as we begin to collectivise our 'data' or client accounts. This process reveals the dynamics of shame and the social and cultural prescripts that contribute to how shame is systematically deployed and how people accept, interact and transact with, and, ultimately, internalise shame. Munt describes these thematic patterns as 'shared shame scripts' (2007: 3) that provide us with the means to analyse the materiality of shame as well as its mentality, and that are operationalised at individual, national, social, and global levels. She argues:

> **Histories of violent domination and occupation are found frequently lurking behind these dynamics of shame, and the**

shame, although directly aimed at the minoritised group also implicates the bestower... Shame is peculiarly intrapsychic: it exceeds the bodily vessel of its containment – groups that are shamed contain individuals who internalise the stigma of shame into the tapestry of their lives, each reproduce discrete, shamed subjectivities, all with their own specific pathologies. (2007: 2)

For instance, particular sociopolitical and cultural prescripts, standards or rules will have informed and consequently shaped the specific form of torture or humiliation used against survivors, for maximum shaming impact. This might include specific methods of degradation and humiliation, including sexual torture and rape, that operationalise shame in particular ways, based on how gender, caste, or class are located culturally. Therefore, it is by collectivising shaming experiences that we begin to understand that shame is a powerful sociopolitical and cultural tool, pervasive in everyday experience, which serves to regulate and shape behaviour. I argue that, at the therapeutic level, we need to pay attention to this global, social, and interpersonal context, alongside the intrapsychic considerations, in order to build integrated interventions that move people away from the alienation inherent in shame to a more participative and self-efficacious position.

Nevertheless, Munt (2007) goes on to suggest that shame has been much maligned in the therapy world, where it is viewed as a toxin that must be excavated, processed and removed from the psyche. She argues that, in fact, shame also has a prosocial function that is helpful in shaping our ethical responsibilities to others, because such a response would indicate that we are aware of a moral transgression. The binary opposition of pride and shame, evident in gay liberation movements, is an example of how shame might be transmuted into pride as part of a strategy for marginalised and excluded groups to overturn the discourse, demonstrating that 'collective emotions do cause social change' (2007: 4).

Liberation is therefore not just about the social freedoms it brings but also the liberation from shaming narratives. Excluded groups begin to collectivise their experience and understand how shame not only alienates and socially positions them but also limits their opportunities. This results in a sense of social, political and cultural agency that activates a demand for human rights.

I would argue that this positioning can be channelled resourcefully in a therapeutic context, by connecting survivors of torture with existing insights (eg. they may have been activists with clear ideas of the impact of sociopolitical narratives on the self), initiatives or new awareness and activism (eg.

challenging the global defamation of refugees or challenging women-blaming rape myths). When survivors begin to shed the responsibility they accept for their torture by regarding shame as an inherent tactic of political repression and torture, they begin to develop a collective appreciation of how they *are and have been* corralled into shamed positions. This collectivised insight may then be used to claim a political presence and reclaim a sense of identity that is based on rights and protection. Herein is perhaps an opportunity for torture rehabilitation services to drive forward a collective position that aims to de-shame survivors and reinforce activist identities at a global level.

It is important to note that human rights discourses have themselves been criticised from a social constructionist standpoint as, for instance, emerging from western democratic ideals based on liberal individualism (Stammer, 1999; Gregg, 2011). It is beyond the aims of this chapter to expound on these important critiques. However, the overarching thrust of my argument is that human-rights discourses have emerged from social justice movements. This has contributed to legislation to protect the rights of people based on specific characteristics (such as age, gender reassignment, sex, disability, sexual orientation and so on), where it is recognised that groups of people exist that experience particular vulnerabilities at a societal level. Inherent in this formulation of rights (and, I would argue, often side-lined) is the standpoint of examining the socio-political and legal circumstances within which rights abuses occur. Therefore, I argue that the therapist who is driven by a human rights position has a responsibility to consider the wider contexts within which psychological harm has occurred, to enable appropriate redress. Within the context of psychological suffering as a result of torture, it is clear that the context of the torture history is vital to holding the state accountable for its actions (OHCHR, 1984). Our natural enquiries, as human rights-driven clinicians, would enable us to integrate an appreciation of the sociocultural context of humiliation and other shame-engendering tactics to widen our focus beyond the dispositional aspects of shame.

An exhaustive formulation of the layers of shaming narratives and the individual's perception and interaction with them will involve uncovering the intersection of multiple identities and positions that survivors occupy within both their home and host contexts. In the example provided at the outset, the psychotherapist's stance as a white, English, upper middle-class female was not acknowledged, and nor was her positioning of the survivor's home culture as implicitly 'backward', or at best conservative. This resulted in several missed opportunities that may have enabled the individual to emerge from the morass of shame.

The remainder of this chapter will consider Fila's experience to consider how shame formulations may be developed to incorporate the ideas presented here. I will also include recommendations for practice at appropriate intervals.

Fila

Fila is a 39-year-old middle class professional, who arrived in the UK from Iran with her seven-year-old daughter. Her husband arrived six months later. In Iran, she had a supportive and extended family network. She was independent, self-sufficient, and known as the 'go-to person' to solve problems and 'get things sorted.' She had always had a supportive relationship with her husband, and often took a lead role in decision-making, within the constraints of an Iranian family.

However, her in-laws did not like her. They denigrated her independence and power, seeing them as inappropriate in a woman. They also criticised her for her inability to become pregnant, and Fila had sought fertility treatment at her husband's request, which had resulted in a precious daughter. She shrugged off her in-laws' criticisms, confident in the knowledge of her unremitting support from her husband and her own family, which acted as a buffer against the tide of negative attitudes over the years.

This reinforced a strong sense of self-worth and entitlement to her basic human rights as a citizen, a woman, a mother, and someone in the workforce. Like many others, Fila participated in post-election peaceful protests in Iran, to demand an undefiled democracy to which she believed citizens were entitled. She was arrested, detained and physically and sexually tortured over a 28-day period. The torture included extreme humiliation and degradation. Methods included multiple and repeated rape by three prison officers, threat of rape/harm to her and her family, verbal insults and humiliation, being handcuffed, blindfolded, interrogated, kicked, punched and slapped 'like a man', kept in isolation, in the dark and naked, physical degradation, being urinated on and having her own faeces thrown over her.

When she was released on bail pending a court hearing, she was treated for sexually transmitted infections. Her in-laws heard she had experienced rape in detention and did not hesitate to highlight how this had tarnished her reputation as a pure and respectable woman. In turn, this brought to bear questions about her position as a mother, wife, daughter-in-law and ultimately her acceptability in their respectable society. They were ashamed that she had been raped, and questioned her ability to parent their granddaughter now that she was a 'contaminated' woman. Her husband indicated that he would continue to accept her, but refused to hear the details of what had happened to her.

Fila was afraid of further detention and torture after her court hearing, knowing she was unlikely to be able to tolerate it and its effects on her family. This, coupled with her in-laws' threats to take her daughter away from her, prompted her to leave the country and seek asylum in the UK. She was housed by the Home Office in a small town on the outskirts of a larger city, pending her claim. She eventually described her double, triple and quadruple shaming in solicitor and asylum interviews (attended by male interpreters and interviewers).

Highly articulate and gently spoken, with a warm and engaging demeanour, she tried to look composed and well at all times. However, it took several assessment sessions before she could tolerate discussing her deeply embedded and multi-dimensional sense of shame. This complex set of responses was elucidated as beliefs that her past self, untarnished by shame, was annihilated; peri-traumatic experiences of shame during her rapes, torture and humiliation; social and personal experiences of post-traumatic shame; and the impact of the dynamic of shame on her relationships with her husband and her in-laws. It took much longer to build the therapeutic relationship to engage in trauma-focused work, in particular due to the block that shame placed in the way of her engaging in recovery both in and out of the therapeutic context.

Recommendations for practice 1

I would argue that we are required to collaboratively develop with the client an understanding of the contextual variables that contribute to shamed identities with survivors of torture. One method of doing this is by embedding our existing therapeutic models within narrative practice to externalise shame and begin to understand the social contexts that thicken shame narratives for ourselves and survivors (White, 2007). Figure 1 identifies the areas discussions might focus on. My richest conversations have emerged from providing a brief psychoeducational overview of my position on shame as a cross-cultural phenomenon; as a normal part of socialisation; as a tactic of social control especially; as having helpful and unhelpful consequences, and as a debilitating intrapsychic and interpersonal experience. Where gender, rape and domestic violence are relevant, I have provided statistics (if available) on the rape of women, domestic violence and the use of rape as a weapon in war and conflict globally. I have found some survivors have idealised views of the position of women in western societies or outside of war and conflict, where they assume rape is not a commonplace occurrence. Therefore, I provide details of its incidence and prevalence in the UK to inform survivors and place their experience within the global context of violence towards women. It is my experience that this helps to connect, normalise, de-stigmatise and collectivise women's experiences across cultures within a rights and justice discourse, in contrast to specifying the peculiarities of individual cultures and labelling them as particularly backward, in isolation of the global narratives that result in violence towards women.

Figure 1: Factors to consider in the social construction of shame

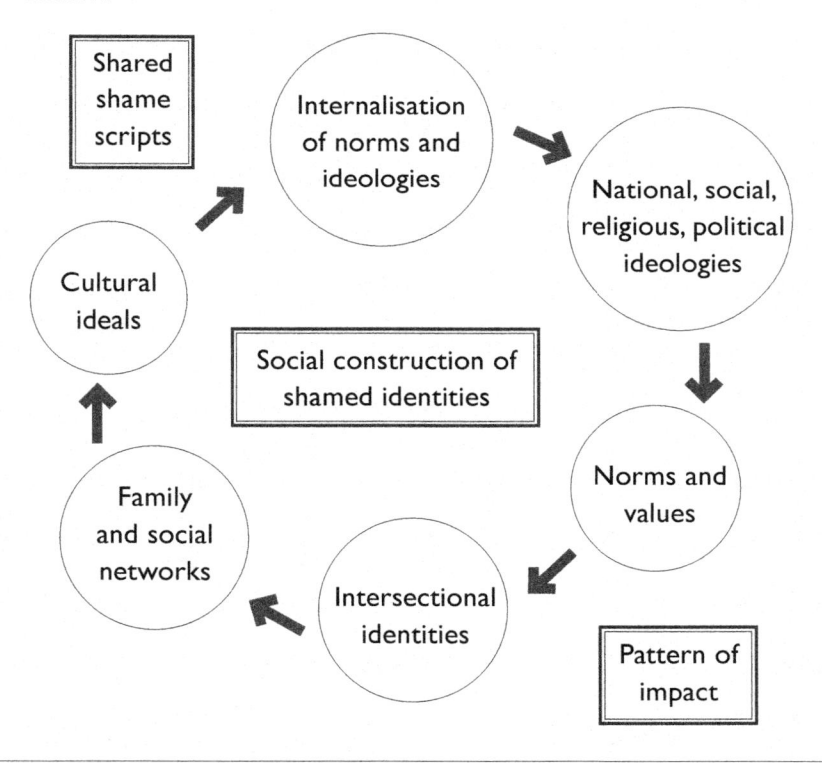

- Shared shame scripts
- Internalisation of norms and ideologies
- National, social, religious, political ideologies
- Cultural ideals
- Social construction of shamed identities
- Family and social networks
- Norms and values
- Intersectional identities
- Pattern of impact

Narratives of shame

In the previous section we established how shame is embedded in the fabric of culture and society, and influences socialisation. These wider sociopolitical 'meta-narratives' shape individual experiences and appraisals of shame and their subsequent actions. A social constructionist framework offers therapists the supplementary opportunity to consider transdisciplinary perspectives as 'narratives' that inform how they construe shame. In what follows, I will provide an overview of some of these perspectives. It is important, however, to start by setting out the differences between shame and guilt.

Shame and guilt: being and doing

Quite often, guilt and shame are used interchangeably to describe overlapping emotional states. In the literature, attempts to find the key cause, effect or mechanism that distinguishes shame and guilt result in a narrative tongue-twisting that risks losing us in the labyrinth of explanations. The social psychological literature conceptualises shame and guilt as part of a range of prosocial 'self-conscious emotions' that include pride, guilt, shame, and embarrassment (Fischer & Tangney, 1995). These aversive emotions function as 'moral barometers'; their emergence indicates that we have transgressed some standard, the consequences of which will differ, depending on the emotion (Tangney, Steuwig & Mashek, 2007: 128).

Fontaine et al (2004: 274) summarise four psychological approaches that describe the specifics of shame and guilt, respectively, as:

a) orienting our attention internally *versus* externally
b) resulting from a violation of norms *versus* a failure to meet our obligations
c) an experience of deficiency in the global self *versus* a behavioural transgression, where guilt is a 'communal oriented emotion leading to a restoration of the balance in interpersonal relationship'
d) the experience of being negatively evaluated by the self *versus* others.

However, there appears to be some theoretical consensus:

> Guilt is generally described as resulting from the feeling that one is *responsible* for harming others, either by omission or by commission... Shame, on the other hand, is assumed to be triggered by situations in which one has the feeling of being negatively evaluated by others or by the self. In shame, the *negative evaluation* would generalize to the whole self. (Fontaine et al, 2004: 143)

Thus, with shame, the individual focuses on an 'unacceptable self', whereas with guilt the focus is on an 'unacceptable behaviour'. The conclusions drawn from the emotional experience result in an evaluative statement that either there is 'something wrong with me', or there is 'something wrong with what I did', respectively.

Fontaine et al (2004) go on to explain that shame results in global feelings of deficiency, inferiority and worthlessness, and positions the self as passive and powerless, which leads to behavioural avoidance and withdrawal. This has an impact on being. Guilt, however, results in feelings of responsibility, and positions the self as in control with a focus on behavioural agency, and therefore doing. Tangney, Steuwig and Mashek (2007) neatly summarise these positions. They suggest that the focus of shame is on the entire self, comprising global self-judgments that are experienced as profoundly wounding and that cause individuals to shrink and retreat from others. Guilt, however, is experienced as less painful, and focuses on specific behaviour that the individual feels regretful about, resulting in an experience of dissonance, which causes them to move towards reparation. Thus, shame and guilt lead to an internal or an external orientation: that is, either a passive versus active self.

Furthermore, some writers argue that guilt is an adaptive emotion, unlike shame, which is destructive and has little adaptive value (Tangney & Dearing, 2002). Others see guilt as linked to anxiety, depression and anger (Ferguson et al, 2007). Ferguson and colleagues (2007) argue that guilt may co-exist with shame and it may be more meaningful to attend to the situations in which these emotions are aroused. In particular, they argue that the perception of control over one's circumstances is associated with the degree of negative impact of shame and guilt.

In the refugee context, where survivors of torture are grappling for anchors to establish control, this might be particularly problematic. In such cases, experiences of guilt, where there are circumstantial, legal, social and individual barriers preventing reparative action, may be one of the routes into experiencing a global sense of deficiency, and so shame. Moreover, Morling et al (2002) argue that shame and guilt are less differentiated in collectivistic versus individualistic cultures. This is ascribed to cultural imperatives in individualistic cultures to pursue self-set goals versus the fulfilling of socially prescribed roles expected in collectivistic cultures.

It is important for us also to consider whether empirical measures to identify shame and guilt are helpful in our formulations. Fontaine et al (2006) provide a critical review of research methods that attempt to measure them. They indicate that measures that seek to label the frequency of shame and guilt using questionnaires, as opposed to those inviting self-labelling of shame and guilt using scenario-based measures, do not yield theoretically consistent results, and that further investigation into the causes of this is necessary. In particular, they show that methods provide convergent evidence about the impact of shame and contradictory evidence about the psycho-pathological consequences of guilt. I would conjecture that the construct validity of such methods is flawed due to the challenges of attempting to reduce and quantify shame and guilt rather than view them from an interdisciplinary position. In my opinion, an integrated theoretical position, combined with individual history taking, is the most appropriate way to identify whether shame and guilt are the key components of a survivor's experience.

It is evident that the psychological literature attempting to delineate shame and guilt lends further credibility to the argument that shame and guilt are culturally contingent, and that emotional construction and perception are socially and interpersonally interdependent. This suggests we need to be mindful of cross-cultural perspectives on the nature of guilt and shame, and ensure we confirm with survivors their culturally ascribed meanings and the impact of transcultural migration. The socio-cultural context of shame and guilt are powerful maintaining forces that push back against any attempts to therapeutically address shame and guilt and therefore must be central to our formulations.

Recommendations for practice 2

Fontaine et al (2006), in a cross-cultural examination of shame and guilt, established two underlying dimensions to categorise the impact of cultural values, which are helpful to our formulations with survivors. These are that:

a) culture has effects at a situational and/or personal level, and
b) this impact is specific and/or generalised.

This is represented diagrammatically in Figure 2 (opposite).

Thus, they summarised that culture:

1. determines specific situations that are relevant for each emotion (situational and specific)

2. impacts on the relevance or threshold for emotional reaction (eg. lowering one's eyes) (personal and specific)
3. determines whether there is an interpersonal (external) versus intrapersonal (internal) orientation roughly mapping onto collectivistic versus individualistic societies (situational and generalised)
4. determines how courses of action are favoured: for example, 'Personal control is more favoured in cultural groups with an independent construction of the self' (personal and generalised) (Fontaine et al, 2006: 290).

Figure 2: Impact of cultural imperatives on experiences of shame and guilt

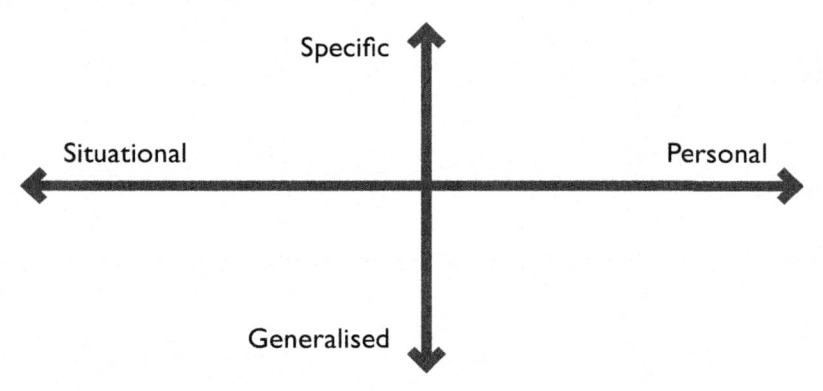

```
                    Specific ↑
                             |
    Situational              |              Personal
    ←────────────────────────┼────────────────────────→
                             |
                             |
                   Generalised ↓
```

This graphic is helpful for practitioners to begin to consider cultural imperatives for both their own social group and the survivor of torture.

Shame as affect and emotion: biological narratives

Affect theorists (eg. Tomkins, 1962; Ekman, 1973; Nathanson, 1992) focus on emotions as internal, individual bodily and sensory experiences, seeing them as hardwired physiological dispositions. In contrast to cultural theories of emotion, these ideas are rooted in essentialism (the viewpoint that the underlying essence of things is biologically universal and unchanging) and originate from Darwinian data and assertions that primary *affects* are universal, and accompanied by the same signals, regardless of nationality or culture, such as 'common facial expressions and postural characteristics' (Taylor, 2015: 2). In this context, there are spectra of primary affects that correspond to experiences of shame, anger, sadness, interest, surprise, fear, joy and disgust.

Tomkins (1962) sees the affects as part of a biological system that controls and regulates how we focus our attention. Thus, affects that operate innately in the nervous system provide information about the internal or external environment. In particular, they provide information about the significance of events in our environment, drive our attention and motivate our behaviour to maximise our chances of survival.

Affect theorists distinguish between affects, feelings and emotions, and note that a range of feelings and emotions correspond to each of the affects. Thus, *feelings* occur because we become aware of *affects*. They break down *emotions* into the components of feelings, cognitions and behaviours linked to memories that then amplify (or perhaps reduce) the intensity of the *affect*.

In affect theory, shame results from the interruption of positive affects and experiences (Tomkins, 1962). Scheff and Retzinger label it the 'master emotion of everyday life', responsible for evoking a range of other emotions (2000: 303). Taylor lists the bodily signifiers of shame, which include 'the breaking of eye contact, the lowering and turning away of the face, upper body slump, and dilation of blood vessels of the face and neck [blushing]' (2015: 2).

Cognitive therapies primarily view attention as the director of patterns of thinking and behaviour following shame affect. That is, *attention* is the central motivator for behaviours such as avoidance, rumination and worry, which (while helpful in the short term) directs and maintains psychological suffering in the long term because it draws us to focus on and perpetuate the problematic aspects of experience that would thicken narratives of self-blame and shame (White, 2007).

Taylor (2015), in line with cognitive models, elaborates on the distinction between *primary* and *secondary* emotion. Using her model, primary experiences of shame are those that are experienced at the moment of torture, peri-traumatically. Clearly, fear must be among these primary experiences but, interestingly, Taylor cites the work of Grey and Young (2005), who found that traumatic memories were mostly related to a severe, negative view of the self – that is, primarily shame. Secondary affects are those that are generated from attributions or appraisals of primary experiences. Thus, Fila undeniably experienced a primary sense of shame peri-traumatically. On recall, however, she viewed her torture solely through this lens of shame, which drove her to notice incidents and experiences that were consistent with this view of self, which thickened her shamed self-narrative. Her post-traumatic fear during flashbacks was a fear of re-experiencing shame and the visibilising of the shamed self. The emotional constellation of secondary affects, emanating from post-traumatic appraisals, result in stronger shame narratives. Taylor (2015) notes that shame is negatively associated with post-traumatic stress disorder (PTSD) recovery rates.

Nathanson (1992) suggested that shame has the effect of reducing our ability to interact with others, because it results in cognitive shock that prevents us from using higher order cognitive processes. Thus, it leads to a plethora of shame-related cognitions, evoking memories of the worst and most damaged aspects of the self. He categorised shame-related responses using a 'compass of shame' (see figure 3), with the *affect* of shame at its centre, emerging from a thwarted desire, or even need. Responses then included an orientation to shame affect along two dimensions: avoidance/withdrawal and attack self/attack other. Here, awareness of the *affect* might lead to *avoidance* of the shame message, or, at the other end of the axis, acceptance of the shame message leads to *withdrawal* from connection. Either way, acceptance

Figure 3: Compass of shame (adapted from Nathanson, 1992)

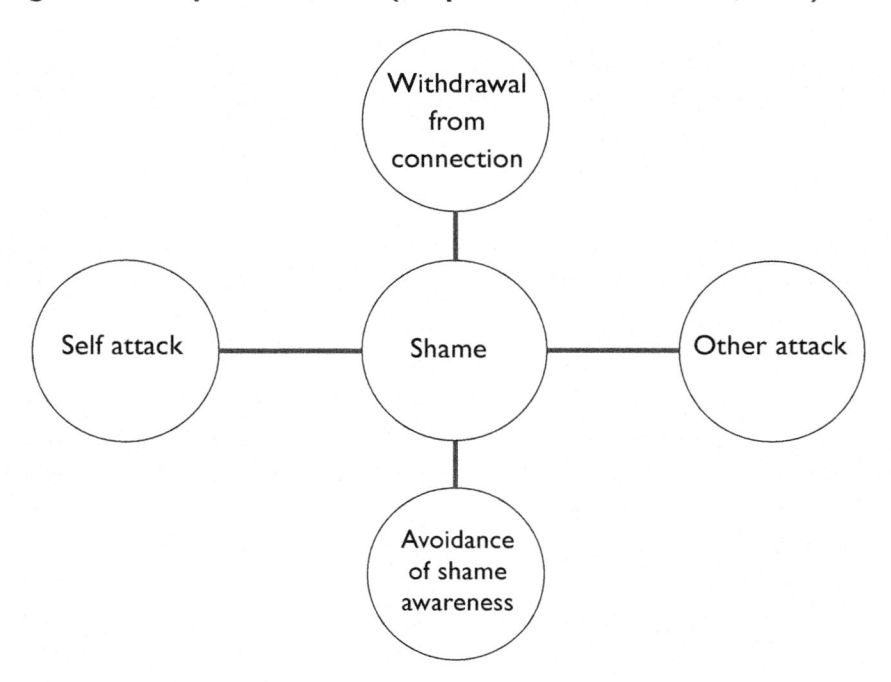

and rejection of shame both result in compensatory responses of *self-attack*, which leads to continued self-abnegation and/or *other-attack* involving over-compensation by asserting one's authority or domination in response to shame.

Fila's responses focused on self-attack, rather than other-attack, and withdrawal from connection. For example, her acceptance of the shamed narrative resulted in an ongoing intrapsychic sense of shame during flashbacks, and simultaneous secondary shame in relation to her belief that others would agree with her view of herself as shamed. This resulted in complex manoeuvres to establish safety by hiding her shame from others and attempting to bypass the experience in order to function in a new country. Her ability to function was also self-judged through this shamed narrative.

I argue that, in order to understand the internal landscape of shame, our formulations should encompass cognition, emotion, and primary and secondary affect, and how these mediate higher order cognitive processes such as attention, judgment and decision-making about behaviour. Moreover, the demarcation of the *feeling* component of emotion is essential to formulations, but is often forgotten. Franks (2010) uses the tricky neuroscientific notion of qualia (or quale, in the singular) to describe the unique subjective experience of affect. Attention to the qualia of shame may result in idiosyncratic formulations that represent the intersection of the biological, psychological and social experience of shame for survivors of torture.

It appears from affect theory that emotions have inter-related components: the biological activity and arousal, the sensations they produce, the feelings and qualia, the understanding and interpretation of these, and the rise of cognitive behaviours and physical actions in response to them. All of these, I argue, are influenced by sociocultural narratives. Therefore, we need to consider this range of possible configurations with survivors in order to offer a multi-dimensional therapeutic approach, in the absence of holistic, inclusive, evidence-based approaches.

For instance, when Fila experienced unexpected touch, it re-ignited peri-traumatic fear and shame sensations, which then directed her attention towards threat. (It could be argued that the immediacy of this response indicated a hypervigilance to threat, signifying the body was already aroused.) The bodily sensations were overpowering because they were intertwined with rape and torture imagery: ie. peri-traumatic affect and event, with their multi-sensory activity, coupled with a perception of the imminence of threat and a 'flight or fight' anxiety response. When her attention was fully directed by trauma sensations and memories, this sometimes led to avoidance of memories/

emotions/affect/sensations, frenetic distraction activity and interpersonal withdrawal, and at other times, rumination about herself as a 'contaminated' woman, and self-recrimination about participating in a public protest and subsequent experiences of shame and loss. When not focused on the past, she worried about her mental state and ongoing post-trauma cognitive impairment (memory, attention, concentration, learning), her physical health, her fresh asylum claim, her daughter's future, and her in-laws' threats to remove her daughter.

Essentialist ideas of emotion are incongruent with a social constructionist position, because they are often seen as reducing experience to the intricacies of biology. They have come under significant scrutiny, indicating that the cross-cultural and linguistic research methods and the data on which they base their ideas of universality are significantly flawed and 'bereft of support'. On review, in fact, much of these data 'suggest the plausibility of the social constructionist theory' (Ratner, 1989: 211). However, I argue that we cannot afford to exclude the biological, because the body is often the site of cultural co-construction of emotion and impact, or, as Ahmed (2014) suggests, the body is the surface or thoroughfare through which connections and boundaries are created. Therefore, it is central to how we individually experience coherence in the world. Consideration of the biological does not require that we hold an essentialist position; it merely indicates that we are building inclusive, even robust, formulations that account for all the experience presented to us.

Therefore, we must consider subjective experiences and understandings of the bodily experience of shame if we are to arrive at systematic understandings of how survivors conceptualise their experiences in the context of culture.

Recommendations for practice 3

Figure 4 (overleaf) outlines a possible model for formulating and tracking the embodied experience of shame with survivors of torture. While they are not included here, it is particularly important to consider cultural aspects of locus of control, which may influence self-efficacy and sense of agency, depending on the degree of collectivistic versus individualistic values survivors hold.

Figure 4: Formulations of shame

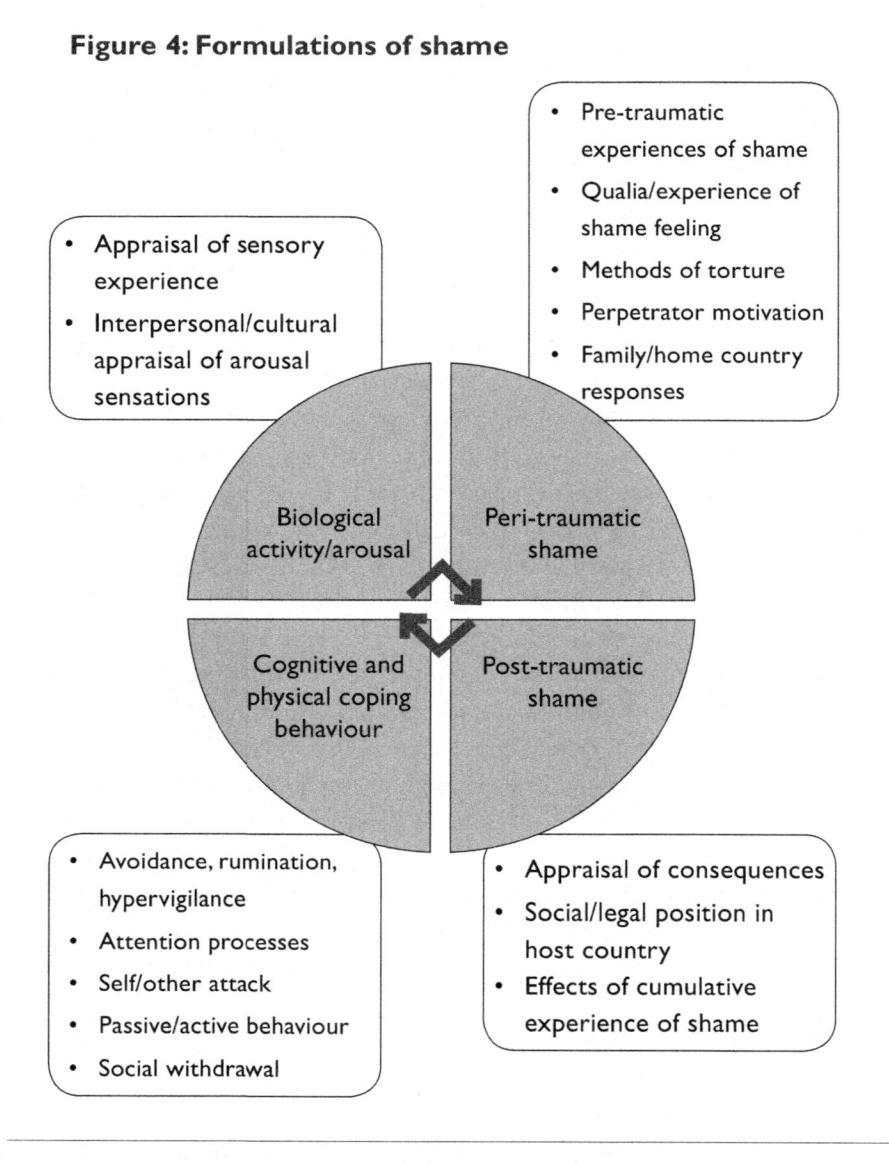

Quadrants (clockwise from top-right): Peri-traumatic shame; Post-traumatic shame; Cognitive and physical coping behaviour; Biological activity/arousal.

Peri-traumatic shame:
- Pre-traumatic experiences of shame
- Qualia/experience of shame feeling
- Methods of torture
- Perpetrator motivation
- Family/home country responses

Biological activity/arousal:
- Appraisal of sensory experience
- Interpersonal/cultural appraisal of arousal sensations

Post-traumatic shame:
- Appraisal of consequences
- Social/legal position in host country
- Effects of cumulative experience of shame

Cognitive and physical coping behaviour:
- Avoidance, rumination, hypervigilance
- Attention processes
- Self/other attack
- Passive/active behaviour
- Social withdrawal

Psychological applications of shame theories

Psychological applications build on affect theories and neurobiological and evolutionary perspectives, and often continue to privilege an intrapsychic, and therefore incomplete, account of shame and its effects. The task of this section is not to provide an exhaustive summary of psychological accounts. Background information on shame is best accessed from specialist textbooks – for example, Akhtar (2016), writing from a psychoanalytic perspective, or Gilbert and

Andrews (1998). The latter is a relatively interdisciplinary text examining the effect of shame on social behaviour, social values and mental states, which has informed Gilbert's development of compassion-focused approaches to shame and depression. I recognise that practitioners will have preferred therapeutic modalities that conceptualise shame experiences in unique ways. It is relevant and appropriate to consider these narratives, with an understanding that they may, at best, be culturally bound, intrapsychic accounts of shame, or, at worst, impose imperialistic or deterministic positions that disregard the socio-political context of self, emotion and therapeutic interventions. I argue for a standpoint of curiosity, where clinicians critically appraise the central assumptions of these often individualistic understandings of self, self-representation and self-conscious emotions to build and develop more sophisticated models that account for why, if and how such experiences differ across cultures.

Herman, among others, places shame in a biopsychosocial developmental context (2012). She suggests we come to know shame and begin to internalise it through the attachment bonds that shape our first internal working models of human intimacy. These attachment bonds are mediated through attunement with the caregiver. Threatened attachments will obviously cause fear; more subtle disruptions that threaten loss of relationship or lead to feelings of isolation will, by the child's second year of life, result in shame, which shapes neuropsychological development (see Schore, 2001). In particular, Herman argues that profound fragmentation in disorganised attachment is related to the primary attachment figure being the source of 'unremitting shame... In this case, the child is torn between need for emotional attunement and fear of rejection or ridicule... [and] forms an internal working model of relationships in which her basic needs are inherently shameful' (2012: 158). Herman, quoting Schore's (2001) work on affect dysregulation and its attachment-based origins, notes that shame is 'mediated by the parasympathetic nervous system [rest and digest, de-arousal system] and serves as a sudden brake on excited arousal states' (2012: 160).

Schore summarises the long-term implications of unresolved, unsoothed attachment disturbances where 'the regulatory failures are manifest in the individual's limited capacity to modulate... the intensity and duration of [sympathetic nervous system arousal leading to] affects like terror, rage, excitement, and elation, or parasympathetic-dominant affects like shame, disgust, and hopeless despair' (2001: 226). This has implications for interpersonal self-efficacy and our ability to self-soothe or regulate affects in the long term. Herman (2012) suggests that catastrophic shame states are inherently self-disorganising, resulting in defences in which shame is amplified because of our relationship with it and its inter-connectedness to the self and others. Catastrophic shame, particularly relevant to the torture context, results from extreme disruptions indicative of abusive and violent relations, where people who expected 'special' recognition are instead treated as objects.

Gilbert (2003) builds on attachment-based models to focus on the ongoing social effects of shame. He sees shame as originating in evolutionary processes, where it is a significant aspect of the self-focused social-threat system related to competitive behaviour and the need to prove oneself acceptable/desirable to others to maintain or further group position and rank. Within a social group context, shame has the function of alerting us to evolutionary aversive situations that may render us inferior, subordinate, or socially rejected. In this context, shame is an automatic protective/defensive response constituting inner warning signals of threat to the self and active communication signals to others, evident in the bodily signifiers of shame. Subsequent 'displays', or defensive behaviours, include escape, submission, anger, and/or concealment. This evolutionary position views shame as having a function in shaping social roles and social functioning, and in particular influencing co-operative versus competitive behaviour for the purposes of adaptation and, ultimately, social rank. Gilbert (2016) argues that, as a result of an evolutionary necessity to respond to social systems to meet our attachment/survival needs, human beings have evolved 'social mentalities'. Social mentalities refer to internalised models of how other 'minds' have and will react to us, which will influence how we process social signals, evaluate the self in relation to cultural norms, and experience and modulate emotional and behavioural reactions. Gilbert (2003) acknowledges that the role of shame is therefore environmentally influenced and the goals and values of a given society (for example, collectivistic versus individualistic) will in part lead to the social construction of what is shameful and therefore deserving of stigma.

Gilbert and Andrews (1998) delineate external and internal shame. External shame describes how one exists in the minds of others, and connotes stigmatisation of the self in the eyes of the other. External shame is regulated by the threat system, which signals that others will withhold care/be abusive, unco-operative/non-reciprocal, spurning of care or affiliation, competitive and hierarchical, or sexually rejecting (Gilbert, 2016). Gilbert argues: 'People can even risk death and serious injury in order to avoid shame and 'loss of face' (Gilbert & Procter, 2006: 353). Internal shame, correlated with external shame because it results in awareness of how one is externally perceived, results in global thoughts about the self as incompetent, inferior, bad, unacceptable, flawed, unwanted, unworthy or unattractive. Importantly, with internal shame, processes of self-directed attention result in global self-judgments that lead to further self-devaluation and self-criticism. Under these conditions, 'in an episode of shame, the person experiences the outside world turning against him or her, and his or her own self-evaluations and sense of self (internal world) also become critical, hostile and persecuting... the self can feel overwhelmed, easily fragmented and simply closes down – there is no safe place either inside or outside the self to help, soothe or calm the self' (2006: 354).

This has significance in relation to refugee survivors of torture, who are in resettlement situations that are highly cognitively demanding and necessitate a sense of agency and belief in one's problem-solving skills. Lee and colleagues (2001) summarise these in their proposed clinical model of shame and guilt-based PTSD, suggesting that shame can be seen as a current threat in that it attacks the person's psychological integrity, resulting in feelings of inferiority, social unattractiveness and powerlessness, which has implications for working with PTSD flashbacks. Taylor (2015) provides a useful multi-dimensional consideration of the role of shame in PTSD, tracing both the peri- and post-traumatic reactions that contribute to primary/secondary and internal/external shame, which may be useful for our formulations.

Thus far, we have described experiences of shame that are easily evident in the experiences, accounts and body language of survivors of torture. However, the psychodynamically informed literature argues that, despite the pervasiveness of shame, it is often invisible and goes unrecognised. Scheff (2014) elaborates on the manifestations and consequences of this unacknowledged and bypassed shame. He draws on the broad socio-historical analysis of shame by Elias (1939) and the systematic psychodynamic review of therapeutic dialogues by Lewis (1971) to explain how shame is a central mechanism in the 'civilising' process. He describes how the process of socialisation necessitates that humans learn to be 'ashamed' of shame, to hide it and hide from it, which results in bypassed and unacknowledged shame. This 'taboo of shame' manifests from interpersonal appraisals that in part link to Gilbert and Andrews' idea of social mentalities (1998). Scheff (2014) explains this in terms of the intersubjectivity of the self and how this leads to either pride or shame. He indicates that we are represented subjectively in the mind of others and that the self is constituted as we react to this awareness. Thus, some unexpected social cue alerts us to the idea that we exist in the other's mind and we begin to imagine how we might appear and how that self is judged. He suggests that our reactions to shamed positions result in 'impression management', in an attempt to rectify or challenge how we imagine we appear in the mind of others.

For example, Fila was held in an Iranian prison and raped. On leaving prison, it was evident that she had been mistreated. During the rapes, the messages of the perpetrators were that, by daring to protest against the regime, she clearly held reprehensible self-beliefs that she was equal to them and entitled, or perhaps even superior to them for holding a human rights-based perspective. In fact, the regime viewed the ordinary (especially female) citizen as inferior and unentitled: someone who should never think she had a right to demand social change. Her actions resulted in a situation where either they accepted that they/the regime were wrong and therefore 'shameful', or that she was. Thus, the rape and other shaming tactics used were designed to make her yield to the latter position and ultimately reinforce the regime and its foot soldiers' positions in being rightful in maintaining the status quo. These tactics were supported by the cultural, legal and social sanctions against women who had been raped, which meant that Fila could not speak about her shame, let alone the violations. The ultimate aim of these tactics was to completely silence her and destroy the will that had led her to protest. On release, the violations were self-evident to her family and she confirmed them, hoping for support, because her family 'surely' held a rounded view of her in their minds as a good person, mother and citizen. However, her in-laws' rejection and labelling reinforced the idea that she *should* feel shame for thinking it was acceptable for her to protest (as a woman, mother and wife); therefore, she had placed *herself* in a position where she could be raped, and they simultaneously reshamed her for revealing her shame. Ultimately, she had brought shame on her family, her body and her nation.

Lewis (1971) suggested that, when there is a risk of exposure, shame is bypassed intra-psychically through defensive manoeuvres of repression and conversion in order to distance oneself from the threat of shame, thereby suppressing awareness of shame affect. As the support dwindled, and Fila's perceived image of how others held her in their minds grew ever-more negative, she crumbled into mental defeat and withdrew from discussing the details of her torture. She attempted to redeem herself by acting like the 'perfect citizen' in her new context (impression management). Lewis also argued that witnesses, within and outside of therapeutic spaces, are ordinarily required to turn away from evidence of shame (1971). Fila's asylum screening by the Home Office forced her to reveal the details of her mistreatment in situations that were re-traumatising and in themselves shaming, because she was seeking asylum. The Home Office officials' disbelief about her torture brought with it an additional layer of shame about her country's 'unbelievable' treatment of women and the shame of having to ask for sanctuary. We can also begin to see how further shaming and damaging the therapist's position becomes when we ignore shame and label Fila's experiences as individual 'cultural' artefacts, rather than deliberate tactics by those responsible for her imprisonment and torture.

Scheff (2014) describes how unacknowledged and bypassed shame becomes evident to the observer (or therapist), despite the person themselves remaining unaware that shame is a feature of their psychic distress. He suggests overt, unidentified shame is accompanied by painful feelings, whereas bypassed shame is evident in rapid thought and speech, with little feeling content. Lewis (1971) identifies a 'spiral of shame' in which shame results in 'humiliated fury' or 'shame–rage'. Scheff and Retzinger (2000) delineate these spirals further, arguing that shame is a reflexive emotion that 'gives rise to long-lasting feedback loops of shame: one can be ashamed of being ashamed… angry that one is ashamed, ashamed that one is angry', and this is manifest within as well as between people. They link these feedback loops to gendered displays of reaction. They argue that shame–shame loops are more likely in women and lead to silence and withdrawal, which are depressive positions. Shame–anger loops result in bypassed shame, which, through defensive processes of denial, leads to reaction formations of anger and aggression. They attribute this kind of shame-proneness to hyper-masculinity and view it as the emotional basis of 'machismo', and as stemming from personal and social insecurity.

Thus, Fila worked hard to hide her 'shame' from others by appearing as well as possible. Therapeutically, I would argue that seeing the shame she experienced as simply an intra-psychic phenomenon carries the risk of evoking further shame. We have already seen how shame results in distancing and de-collectivisation. It is through a collaborative position of mutual curiosity that we begin to uncover and understand the layers of shame and the interaction between the interpersonal and intrapsychic elements of shame spirals, so that we can support the survivor to draw away from distancing from the self and others and see the value in reconnecting. Herman (2012) argues that addressing and normalising shame reactions are central to helping clients to contain and understand them and to mitigating the effects of shame–shame and shame–anger loops.

Concluding remarks

We have navigated a speedy route through various disciplines and how they view shame and its social and psychological importance. Figure 5 summarises the contextual layers of experience of a survivor's journey, as well as the evolving interiority of shame across a refugee survivor of torture's trajectory to safety from home to host country.

In navigating across disciplines, we have established how we can trace the dissolving of the self during torture by examining the moment-by-moment peri-traumatic impressions of survivors of torture, both from their field (in

Figure 5: Tracking the cumulative effects of shame

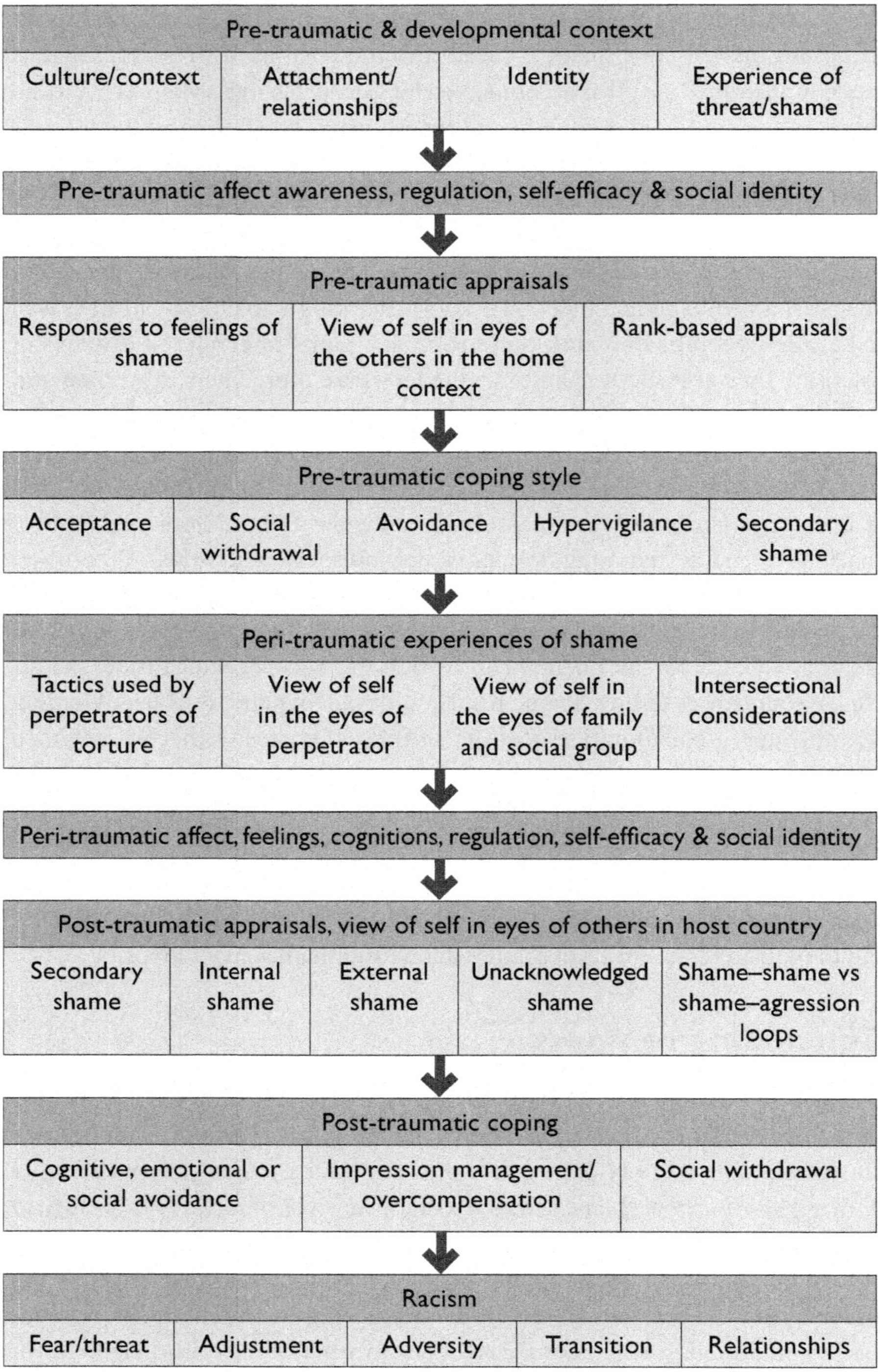

Pre-traumatic & developmental context				
Culture/context	Attachment/ relationships		Identity	Experience of threat/shame

⬇

| Pre-traumatic affect awareness, regulation, self-efficacy & social identity |

⬇

Pre-traumatic appraisals		
Responses to feelings of shame	View of self in eyes of the others in the home context	Rank-based appraisals

⬇

Pre-traumatic coping style				
Acceptance	Social withdrawal	Avoidance	Hypervigilance	Secondary shame

⬇

Peri-traumatic experiences of shame			
Tactics used by perpetrators of torture	View of self in the eyes of perpetrator	View of self in the eyes of family and social group	Intersectional considerations

⬇

| Peri-traumatic affect, feelings, cognitions, regulation, self-efficacy & social identity |

⬇

Post-traumatic appraisals, view of self in eyes of others in host country				
Secondary shame	Internal shame	External shame	Unacknowledged shame	Shame–shame vs shame–agression loops

⬇

Post-traumatic coping		
Cognitive, emotional or social avoidance	Impression management/ overcompensation	Social withdrawal

⬇

Racism				
Fear/threat	Adjustment	Adversity	Transition	Relationships

the experience itself) and observer (disembodied gaze) perspectives. The tactics used by perpetrators of torture move people from seeing themselves as worthy, capable human beings to shamed incapable bodies. The gaze of the perpetrator, their threats and verbalisations, the search for the most degrading torture, the handling of the survivor's body, specific violations, the proximity of bodies, the smear of bodily fluids and human waste of omnipotent perpetrators communicate that the survivor is an immaterial object – ie. 'nothing' – and that their inhumane treatment is ultimately a consequence of their own existence and actions. The verbalised threats and insults that degrade and dismantle the psychic space where a sense of integrity might still exist give rise to the compound 'materiality' of shame. For example, Fila held onto the fact that she was someone's respected daughter, mother, wife, teacher, friend, and an activist. The complexity of shame and its multi-faceted nature results in disempowerment and social exclusion, interpersonal disconnection and distance, poor attachments, destruction of the self, destruction of existing relationships, ongoing vulnerability, lack of participation and pleasure, and manifold problems with functioning and establishing a new life.

In Fila's experience, the perpetrators referred to legal, social, national and international sanctions that would prevent her from seeking redress. Such references were tactics aimed at destroying any sense of agency and control she might be harbouring on release from imprisonment, thereby attacking any underlying defences that might enable her to remain psychically intact or recover post-torture. The torture continued until they were satisfied that she had accepted herself as shamed, unacceptable and unworthy and irrevocably destroyed. Post-detention experiences reinforced these shamed narratives, and the need to leave her home and country offered further proof of the destruction of self. Her husband's response, coupled with the cumulative effects of shame, resulted in a final separation from all that had connected her to herself – role, family, culture, country and familiarity – and, on the face of it, appeared impossible to traverse. Furthermore, her reception in the host country, the inhumane processing of refugees and people seeking asylum, and national and global narratives of migration fed into powerful experiences of rejection, which thickened shame beliefs and narratives.

Engaging systemically with shame requires much energy and concentration on the part of practitioners and can leave us exhausted as we attempt to work through and untangle valuable insights. Furthermore, the detrimental effects of shame on families and communities may be irreversible, often because we are working with individual survivors rather than engaging in community-based interventions that might result in social change. This can be demoralising for practitioners, and the value of support and supervision can never be underestimated.

An understanding of the power differential and how it is managed is essential in reaching through the miasma of shame that blocks connection and prevents the development of a trusting bond and, ultimately, the transformative potential of the therapeutic relationship. Practitioners will have their own tools and techniques to manage the continued threat that survivors experience because of ongoing and pervasive shame and shaming tactics. My hope is that this chapter offers a framework that will help practitioners to identify the range of interdisciplinary writing that can inform their thinking about how shame is constructed. I hope that the practice points will serve as triggers to direct readers' curiosity, reflexivity and questioning so they are better able to support individuals and communities to rebuild their resilience and develop the resources that will enable them to reconstruct themselves in new, ever-challenging contexts.

Acknowledgement

The author would like to acknowledge the invaluable discussions with Dr Suryia Nayak (Programme Leader, MA Social Work, University of Salford, psychotherapist and activist) that originally shaped our initial explorations of shame and its entanglements in cross-cultural, trauma-focused and therapeutic work with refugees.

References

Ahmed S (2014). *The Cultural Politics of Emotion* (2nd edition). Edinburgh: Edinburgh University Press.

Akhtar S (ed) (2016). *Shame: developmental, cultural and clinical realms*. London: Karnac Books Ltd.

Bhavnani KK, Phoenix A (1994). Shifting identities, shifting racisms. *Feminism & Psychology* 4(1): 5–18.

Boiger M, Mesquita B (2012). The construction of emotion in interactions. *Emotion Review* 4(3): 221–229.

Crenshaw K (1991). Mapping the margins: intersectionality, identity politics, and violence against women of color. *Stanford Law Review* 43(6): 1241–1299.

Dearing RL, Tangney JP (2011). *Shame in the Therapy Hour*. Washington, DC: American Psychological Association.

Doyle McCarthy ED (1994). The social construction of emotions: new directions from culture theory. *Social Perspectives on Emotion* 2: 267–279.

Ekman P (1973). *Darwin and Facial Expression: a century of research in review.* New York, NY: Academic Press.

Elias N (1939). *The Civilizing Process: the history of manners.* London: Blackwell.

Ferguson T, Brugman D, White J, Eyre H (2007). Shame and guilt as morally warranted experiences. In: Tracy JL, Robins RW (eds). *The Self-Conscious Emotions: theory and research.* London: Guilford Press (pp330–350).

Fischer W, Tangney J (1995). Self-conscious emotions and the affect revolution: framework and overview. In: Fischer W, Tangney J (eds). *Self-Conscious Emotions: the psychology of shame, guilt, embarrassment, and pride.* London: Guilford Press (pp3–22).

Fontaine J, Luyten P, de Boeck P, Corveleyn J, Fernandez M, Herrera D (2006). Untying the Gordian knot of guilt and shame: the structure of guilt and shame reactions based on situation and person variation in Belgium, Hungary, and Peru. *Journal of Cross Cultural Psychology* 37(3): 273–292.

Fontaine J, Luyten P, Estas C, Corveleyn J (2004). Scenario-based and frequency-based approaches towards the measurement of guilt and shame: empirical evidence for unique contributions. In: Shohov SP (ed). *Advances in Psychology Research, vol 30.* New York, NY: Nova Science Publishers (pp141–154).

Franks DD (2010). *Neurosociology: the nexus between neuroscience and social psychology.* New York, NY: Springer

Gilbert P (2016). A biopsychosocial and evolutionary approach. In: Tarrier N, Johnson J (eds). *Case Formulation in Cognitive Behaviour Therapy: the treatment of challenging and complex cases.* Hove: Routledge (pp52–89).

Gilbert P (2003). Evolution, social roles, and the differences between shame and guilt. *Social Research* 70(4): 1205–1230.

Gilbert P, Andrews B (1998). *Shame: interpersonal behavior, psychopathology, and culture.* Oxford: Oxford University Press.

Gilbert P, Procter S (2006). Compassionate mind training for people with high shame and self-criticism: overview and pilot study of a group therapy approach. *Clinical Psychology & Psychotherapy* 13(6): 353–379.

Gregg B (2011). *Human Rights as Social Construction.* Cambridge: Cambridge University Press.

Harré R (1986). *The Social Construction of Emotion.* Oxford: Blackwell.

Herman JL (2012). Shattered shame states and their repair. In: Yellin J, White K (eds). *Shattered States: disorganised attachment and its repair.* New York, NY: Karnac (pp157–170).

Kinouani G (2015). *Shame and Marginalisation: an intersubjective formulation model.* [Online.] Race Reflections. https://racereflections.co.uk/2015/10/18/shame-and-marginalisation-an-intersubjective-formulation-model/ (accessed November 2016).

Lee D, Scragg P, Turner S (2001). The role of shame and guilt in traumatic events: a clinical model of shame-based and guilt-based PTSD. *British Journal of Medical Psychology* 74(4): 451–466.

Leeming D, Boyle M (2004). Shame as a social phenomenon: a critical analysis of the concept of dispositional shame. *Psychology and Psychotherapy: Theory, Research & Practice* 77(3): 375–396.

Lewis HB (1971). *Shame and Guilt in Neurosis.* New York, NY: International Universities Press.

Liddell B, Jobson L (2016). The impact of cultural differences in self-representation on the neural substrates of posttraumatic stress disorder. *European Journal of Psychotraumatology 7*: 10.3402/ejpt.v7.30464

Misheva V (2006). Shame and guilt: the social feelings in a sociological perspective. In: Jern S, Näslund J (eds). *Interaction on the Edge: proceedings from the 5th GRASP conference, Linköping University, May 2006*. Lund: Lund University (pp128–142).

Morling E, Kitavama S, Miyamoto Y (2002). Cultural practices emphasize influence in the United States and adjustment in Japan. *Personality & Social Psychology Bulletin 28*(3): 311–323.

Munt S (2007). *Queer Attachments: the cultural politics of shame*. Farnham: Ashgate.

Nathanson DL (1992). *Shame and Pride: affect, sex and the birth of self*. New York, NY: WW Norton & Co.

OHCHR (1984). *Convention against Torture and Other Cruel, Inhuman or Degrading Treatment or Punishment*. New York: United Nations.

Ratner C (2002). *Cultural Psychology: theory and method*. New York: Kluwer/Plenum.

Ratner C (1989). A social constructionist critique of naturalistic theories of emotion. *Journal of Mind and Behavior 10*: 211–230.

Scheff T (2014). The ubiquity of hidden shame in modernity. *Cultural Sociology 8*(2): 129–141.

Scheff T, Retzinger S (2000). Shame as the master emotion of everyday life. *Journal of Mundane Behavior 1*(3): 303–324.

Scheff T, Retzinger S (1991). *Violence and Emotions*. Lexington, MA: Lexington Books.

Schore AN (2001). The effects of early relational trauma on right brain development, affect regulation and infant mental health. *Infant Mental Health Journal 22*(1–2): 201–269.

Stammer N (1999). Social movements and the social construction of human rights. *Human Rights Quarterly 21*(4): 980–1008.

Tangney JP, Dearing R (2002). *Shame and Guilt*. New York, NY: Guilford Press.

Tangney JP, Steuwig J, Mashek D (2007). Moral emotions and moral behaviour. *Annual Review of Psychology 58*: 345–382.

Taylor T (2015). The influence of shame on posttrauma disorders: have we failed to see the obvious? *European Journal of Psychotraumatology 6*: 10.3402/ejpt.v6.28847.

Tomkins S (1962). *Affect, imagery, consciousness. Volume I: the positive affects*. New York, NY: Springer Publishing.

White M (2007). *Maps of Narrative Practice*. New York, NY: WW Norton & Company.

9. The application of cognitive behavioural therapies with survivors of torture[1]

Colsom Bashir

As a psychologist, I am often asked about my preferred therapeutic modality, and my short answer is 'integrative'. The start of my long answer is that I use a variety of approaches, underpinned by a social constructionist framework. As a therapist whose lived experience crosses the intersection of minoritised positions of race, gender and sexuality, I am familiar with the social and psychological effects of structural and everyday oppressions, as well as the historical exclusionary nature of traditional psychological models and research, the consequences of which have often been a sense of alienation and continuing isolation, particularly in the context of adversity. This has become a driver for my commitment to ensure that therapeutic approaches are accessible to people whose voices and participation are frequently marginalised in the mainstream, both in their communities of origin and in British society. Having developed strong feminist sensibilities from childhood (albeit without the capacity or opportunity to express them), I am driven to use my experience and position to create the conditions that allow marginalised voices to emerge, and also to strive to actively challenge oppression. I seek to learn from clients about the multiplicity of ways in which not just women, but all people negotiate oppression and discrimination, and to understand the costs (or benefits) for resilience and coping. My commitment to social justice and human rights has been strengthened by my work with people who are the least structurally privileged and who therefore are unlikely to (be able to) access mainstream services.

---

1. Parts of this chapter are taken from or adapted as identified in the text from: Bowley J, Bashir C (2016). Working with people seeking asylum. In: Tarrier N, Johnson J (eds). *Case Formulation in Cognitive Behaviour Therapy: the treatment of challenging and complex cases* (2nd edition). London: Routledge. Reprinted with permission from Taylor & Francis.

A social constructionist framework opens up the therapeutic space to help me consider how the social and political dimensions of lived experience, particularly structural oppression, can influence how we construct understandings of ourselves, our experience, our relationships and the world at large. This necessitates a critical psychology standpoint that allows me to deconstruct and destabilise received wisdom from mainstream psychological narratives and to consider these alongside marginalised client accounts. This allows me to take a systemic perspective, within which I view cognitive behaviour therapies as one set of discourses or narratives about how we come to internally represent and interact with the world in ways that are often reductionist and self-defeating. Such beliefs are themselves powerfully maintained by prescriptive social and political meta-narratives[2] and their associated practices.

I have found the most practical way to meet these challenges and to integrate a social constructionist standpoint with survivors of torture is by engaging Judith Herman's three phases of recovery from socio-political trauma (establishing safety, remembrance and mourning, and restoring connections) as an integrating psychotherapeutic tool, which has shaped the practice elements of this chapter. Herman politically, socially and diagnostically deconstructs torture, gender-based violence and the notion of trauma to elicit the core narratives in people's accounts of their experience to determine recovery processes (Herman, 1992).

Working with survivors of torture demands a situated partisan stance in its avowal of the human-rights framework as the all-encompassing lens through which we conduct our practice. It is one that sits well with my own commitment to social justice. This standpoint affords a clear ethical route into thinking about the politics of power. It involves deconstructing meta-narratives entwined with oppressive social, legal, political and therapeutic practices, and how they parallel processes between survivors of torture and oppressive regimes. It inevitably results in the raising and collectivising of marginalised voices as a means to bring about change, nationally and internationally. These are consistent with my human rights commitment to bearing witness as a therapist and my political commitment to offering accessible models of recovery. The challenge is to continue to resist individualistic, heteronormative, psychiatric, imperialistic, ethnocentric and exclusionary meta-narratives while also gathering the courage to address culturally bound oppressive understandings specific to survivors' countries of origin and appreciate the effects of experience on our biopsychosocial development. Practising with integrity from such a perspective implies that we

---

2. Over-arching dominant or ideological stories that set parameters for personal, local and national stories (eg. science, Marxism) and make claims to be the best or only way to understand reality.

must endeavour to open up the collectivising space between us and our clients. In doing so, we must address the layers of power and oppression that create separation in the therapeutic context, throughout the client's history, socially and politically. The *engagement* phase of therapy therefore becomes a deliberate, politically oriented activity, which provides the starting point for understanding human rights violations, advocacy and collectivising experience, and also for ensuring survivors have access to reparation through rehabilitation services.

CBT and survivors of torture

The proliferation of CBT-informed service provision in the NHS emanates from the development of bodies such as the National Institute for Health and Care Excellence (NICE), which, from the early 2000s, began publishing guidelines based on research evidence about the best treatment for specific health problems, including mental health. Since then, the drive towards randomised control trials and high-quality evidence, which now shapes service delivery in mental health in the UK, has resulted in a spread of diagnostic 'conditions' (eg. post-traumatic stress disorder (PTSD), depression and anxiety), which are treated using various CBT protocols delivered through Improving Access to Psychological Therapy (IAPT) Step 3 programmes in the UK (eg. Royal College of Psychiatrists, 2013).

Unfortunately, these approaches fit within a 'modernist' tradition, which reifies the objectivist individualistic stance (Sherif, 1979), positing essentialist truths about human functioning and internalised pathology (Foucault, 1965). Dogged by these meta-narratives, adult psychotherapy in NHS primary care has increasingly become concerned with 'condition management', with experts who hold the power formulating linear CBT storylines and meting out standardised treatments that ignore the social and political 'conditions' of human experience (Lyotard, 1979).

The complex sequelae that characterise the experience of survivors of torture are not easily amenable to the demands of quantitative, evidence-based research. Nor is it possible to approach the multi-faceted, life-changing experiences of this population using condition management protocols. The relatively straightforward interventions showing the effectiveness of CBT with PTSD, for example, are not particularly useful for therapists working with survivors, and in fact pathologise the expected impact of torture (eg. overwhelming fear, hypervigilance to threat, intrusive memories).

> Cognitive models of PTSD assume that both the intrusive phenomena and distorted appraisals of risk and danger are a

result of insufficiently processed sensory memories... For people, however, who remain at risk of being returned to the dangers from which they escaped, intrusive and anxious appraisals about past torture and the prospect of being tortured again will be an entirely appropriate response... Such models do not address treatment issues for people who remain at risk, whose trauma is ongoing, or continuously triggered by processes outside of their control, such as ongoing asylum cases. (Bowley & Bashir, 2016: 328)

Similarly, the cognitive biases seen in generalised anxiety (Blackburn & Davidson, 1990), where the self is seen as vulnerable, the world as dangerous and the future unpredictable, are not biases but realistic possibilities for survivors of torture in a refugee context. Likewise, depression might be seen as an appropriate response for refugee survivors, because of the multiple losses experienced, lack of language, unfamiliarity with their environment, inability to work, and also the freezing, seizing or limiting of assets, denial of access to work, and lack of choice of lifestyle and accommodation inherent to the asylum experience.

The evidence for interventions with survivors of torture is limited, and restricted mainly to treatments for PTSD, which is only part of the rehabilitation package. People who have experienced torture continue to present with complex comorbid problems in ongoing difficult circumstances. Therapists are therefore required to adapt the theoretical information processing underpinnings of CBT, which help to conceptualise how experiences might be psychically represented and guide our understanding of how individuals continue to relate to experiences of torture and their sequelae within current and expected life trajectories. One premise of this chapter is that practitioners will have trained to at least diploma level or equivalent in CBT, so I do not need to explain it. Further, this chapter is aimed at clinicians who have completed foundational training in fields that enable a holistic assessment and formulation-driven approach (eg. clinical psychology, psychotherapy or psychiatry) and who seek to integrate this within a human-rights framework.

The evidence base

McFarlane and Kaplan (2012) conducted a comprehensive review of psychosocial interventions with survivors of torture and confirm that most of the evidence is limited to how such interventions target psychiatric symptomatology (see also Bhui & Morgan, 2007; Nickerson et al, 2011). There is much detail in the paper and readers are encouraged to read it for themselves. However, it is evident that CBT-driven approaches are effective in working with a significant number of the expected effects of torture. Practitioners are most likely to encounter survivors in an asylum and refugee context, and there is increasing evidence that adapted CBT models are effective with this population, despite their disparity. For example, in a review of this literature, Regel and Berliner (2007) demonstrate the applicability and flexibility of the CBT model in different cultural contexts, despite its perceived cultural limitations. Bowley and Bashir (2016) also provide an overview of CBT approaches and evidence about their effectiveness with people seeking asylum. Their findings are summarised below:

- *Single session exposure treatments* designed to enhance control over trauma-related fear and distress in earthquake survivors were effective in reducing PTSD and depression in over 85% of cases (Başoğlu et al, 2005) and showed efficacy with female survivors of war trauma and gang rape in a series of case studies (Salcioğlu & Başoğlu, 2011). Furthermore, cognitive and behavioural coping skills strategies have shown effectiveness with refugees with PTSD (Snodgrass et al, 1993), indicating that providing strategies for symptom control may have therapeutic effects.

- *Testimony therapy* (TT) originated from the collation of human rights testimony to document the atrocities committed during the Pinochet dictatorship in Chile. It thus evolved out of the necessity to find interventions driven by a social justice agenda, and is perhaps most relevant to our work with survivors (Cienfuegos & Monelli, 1983). The evident secondary psychological benefits of TT were attributed to the contextualising and collectivising of individual suffering, as well as the public and political uses made of testimonies. Interestingly, the therapist's ethical standpoint as a witness is central and TT has been used for over 20 years in a range of contexts (Raghuvanshi & Agger, 2008).

- *Narrative exposure therapy* (NET) continues to show efficacious outcomes with refugees in the unstable context of threat and conflict in, for example, refugee camps (Schauer et al, 2011). NET is informed by the narrative and political elements of TT as well as CBT. Results from treatment trials with adults and children in refugee camps demonstrate the superiority of NET in reducing PTSD symptoms compared with other therapeutic approaches, with changes sustained at follow-up, even in the context of ongoing threat or insecurity (Neuner et al, 2010; Robjant & Fazel, 2010).

A brief, structured trauma module, given the wellspring of evidence, is an essential component of a multidisciplinary approach to the refugee's right to rehabilitation from the effects of torture. Bowley and Bashir (2016) argue that the central processes involved in TT and NET align with traditional CBT models that target post-traumatic presentations. The emphasis on politicising the actions and experience of survivors of torture offers a framework in which to reappraise identity and experiences, which bears a resemblance to examining trauma-related meanings and appraisals in CBT. The drawing up of a complete and precise testimony contains elements of exposure. The role of integrating fragmented narratives to form a coherent inclusive account, and linking the affective to the previously dissociated cognitive aspects of trauma, is paramount in treating PTSD in NET, which first facilitates habituation through prolonged exposure to traumatic hotspots, as well as using testimony to pursue justice for clients (Mueller, 2013).

Cognitive process-driven models

Arguably, all psychological therapies will offer some conceptualisation about how people process and understand their experiences. Cognitive models are explicitly informed by theories and scientific evidence from the neurocognitive and cognitive psychology fields and are particularly relevant to developing social constructionist CBT formulations. It is important to consider the advantages of traditional developmental cognitive formulations, but it's also important to look at process-driven third wave or transdiagnostic CBT approaches that have emerged over the last two decades (Table 1).

Table 1: Trends in behavioural, cognitive and information processing therapies

	Examples	Mechanisms of change
First wave	*Behavioural psychotherapies:* behaviour modification, exposure therapies, systematic desensitisation	Classical, operant and behavioural learning.

Second wave	*Cognitive therapies:* rational emotive behavioural therapy, cognitive therapy, cognitive behaviour therapy	Cognitive appraisals and restructuring of dysfunctional/irrational cognitions
Third wave	Heterogeneous approaches with a trend away from cognitive content towards cognitive and information processing and therapeutic integration: • narrative exposure therapy (NET) (Schauer, Neuner & Elbert, 2012) • compassion-focused therapy (CFT) (Gilbert, 2010) • schema therapy (Young et al, 2003), acceptance and commitment therapy (ACT) (Hayes, Strosahl & Wilson 2012) • mindfulness-based cognitive therapy (MBCT) (Segal, Williams & Teasdale, 2002) • metacognitive therapy (MCT) (Wells, 2009) • eye movement desensitisation and reprocessing (EMDR) (Shapiro, 2001) • dialectic behaviour therapy (DBT) (Linehan, 1993)	A range of models influenced by insights from the metacognitive psychology field, with attention to the individual's relationship to their experience, the linguistic and social construction of experience, learning, information processing, thinking and reasoning, memory formation and a renewed interest in the role of emotions and biological mechanisms (eg. the body, the brain) in maintaining disturbance

These have led to a spectrum of models with varying degrees of empirical support for working with particular conditions or certain client populations. Evidence increasingly demonstrates the effectiveness of such approaches, in particular for people who have failed to benefit from conventionally available models. Harvey et al (2004) offer a useful introduction to how information is processed transdiagnostically, bringing to the forefront not just models of therapy practice but the broader field of cognitive psychology as well. There is much to digest in third-wave CBT; however, there is much more to harness that will benefit survivors. Such models offer more flexible and integrated ways of working with survivors with multiple problems or whose difficulties cross diagnostic categories.

David and Hofman (2013) provide a helpful classification of trends in cognitive therapy that have been adapted and extended in Table 1. Models tend to offer a unifying approach that targets cognitive and behavioural processes that are shared across disorders and contribute to the development or maintenance of symptoms (Table 2). Heterogeneous, transdiagnostic CBTs reflect a trend away from cognitive content and towards metacognitive processes. Self-referential positions and torture survivors' responses to their changed selves, capacities, bodies, worlds, emotions or coping are essential for effective formulation in a social constructionist CBT model. The intention here is to encourage practitioners to apply the same underlying treatment principles across psychological problems without tailoring the protocol to specific diagnoses, which may be helpful with this population.

Table 2: Examples of transdiagnostic cognitive and behavioural processes

Attention	Memory and imagery	Reasoning	Thought	Behaviour
Flexibility of attention Selective attention to internal or external cues (based on expectations of (eg) failure or threat) Attentional avoidance Threat monitoring	Explicit selective memory Recurrent memory Recall of specific memories or over-general memory (not encoded by time or place) Belief-related or 'self-script'-related narrative memory or imagery Autobiographic, narrative, and episodic memories	Interpretation bias (eg. thought event fusion) Expectancy bias Emotional reasoning	Recurrent thinking Future-focused thinking (worry) Past-focused thinking (rumination) Metacognitive positions: • rumination and worry seen as helpful strategies • beliefs about the origins of thoughts • beliefs about the harm/ helpfulness of thoughts	Avoidance Safety behaviours Thought suppression Distraction Vigilance Dissociation

| | | Fragmented memories and flashbacks | | • beliefs about the controllability of cognitive phenomena and mental events | |

Cognitive processes in PTSD

Explanations of PTSD focus on the way the mind is affected by traumatic experiences and the processes that occur that interfere with the mind and body's ability to process information as they usually would. Current understandings indicate that it might be more appropriate to consider PTSD primarily as a memory-related disorder. Nijdam and Wittmann (2015) offer a comprehensive overview of the current neurocognitive theories underlying the development of PTSD, a summary of which is beyond the capacity of this chapter. However, there are some important starting points to consider, because they will shape transdiagnostic CBT assessment and formulation.

Peri-traumatic reactions are the person's responses to overwhelming perceptual and sensory information at the time of a traumatic event. Life-threatening stressors, such as those that have confronted survivors, demand that all bio-cognitive resources are directed towards survival and away from higher order cognitive functions (for example, complex thinking and decision-making processes, mental flexibility, attention, values and reasoning), which influences how the trauma is attended to at the time and therefore coded in our memories.

Brewin (2006, 2007) and colleagues (2010) have advanced his dual representation theory (DRT), which indicates that two parallel types of memories are peri-traumatically coded:

1. the encoding of sensory and affective (emotional) aspects of the trauma – (sensory-bound representation or S-rep)
2. the encoding of contextual aspects of the trauma, which includes structure, spatial and personal information – (contextual representation or C-rep).

In healthy memory, C- and S-reps are thought to be tightly linked so that sensory representations are retrieved from contextual (C-reps) and sensory (S-reps) cues at will. Involuntary flashbacks in PTSD arise when there is a dissociation between these sensory-bound and contextual representations during the trauma, because the S-rep has been more powerfully encoded.

Therefore, flashback memories are not linked with contextualising information (for example, a date and time stamp, which happens with C-reps), which gives rise to re-experiencing sensory aspects of the trauma as if it were happening in the present.

Thus, in DRT, recovery is conceptualised as working to (re)associate the S-rep with its corresponding C-rep, so that the sensory and affective/emotional representation of the traumatic event can be contextualised and brought under voluntary control.

NET incorporates a DRT model and develops this idea of a fractured memory process further to explain the effects of cumulative trauma. NET takes as its starting point neurocognitive memory theory, which predicts that powerfully elicited sensory, cognitive, emotional and physiological elements of overwhelming trauma and internalised threat are encoded as fragments of information that are not contextualised in autobiographical memory. Thus, separate sets of sensory perceptual fragments are associated into networks that result in connections between multiple traumatic events to form generalised 'fear networks'. Similarly, the contextualising of these fear networks to an autobiographical memory narrative is the main agent of change in NET (Neuner et al, 2008).

Assessment – the expected effects of torture

The *Istanbul Protocol* describes torture as the systematic, state-sanctioned infliction of 'cruel inhuman and degrading treatment', with the aim of terrorising, dehumanising and creating a sense of powerlessness in order to psychologically and physically break the human will. Torture dehumanises, objectifies and *others* the individual. The powerful psychological impact (and, indeed, the purpose of torture) may include depletion of resilience and eventual psychic disintegration. The social impact is to set survivors apart from cultures and families that have served as buffers against persecution and discrimination: 'Torture can profoundly damage intimate relationships between spouses, parents, children, other family members and relationships between the victims and their communities' (OHCHR, 1999: 45).

For those who have managed to survive torture, the effects may be conceptualised as annihilating the spirit while keeping the body alive, albeit not intact. The consequences may be that the mind, or the personality, has been 'modified' by unrelenting, prolonged and overwhelming cruelty. Despite having survived, the individual's peri-traumatic (during the torture) survival mechanisms, activated by the expectation that the torture will continue and death may be imminent, may consequently maintain and reinforce its already debilitating effects.

The IP describes a range of psychological and emotional consequences, most of which are characteristic of PTSD and depression as defined in DSM-5 and ICD-10, but also include temporary coping reactions that may become entrenched if trauma-focused therapy is delayed. Reactions may include but are not restricted to those outlined in Table 3 below.

Table 3: Expected effects of torture

Expected effect	Explanation
Re-experiencing the torture	Flashbacks, intrusive memories and nightmares result in re-experiencing sensory physical and emotional responses as if they were happening in the present. These result in physiological and psychological stress and anxiety on exposure to cues that resemble or symbolise the trauma.
Avoidance and emotional numbing	These might include avoidance of cognitive and affective phenomena, affiliations, places and imagery that cue recall of torture, often related to fear of re-experiencing and becoming overwhelmed. Coping responses may result in profound detachment or social withdrawal, feelings of helplessness, mistrust and restricted affect.
Hyperarousal	The physiological symptoms of anxiety and acute stress affect sleep, working memory, the ability to process new information, learning, concentration and attention. Overwhelming, physiological responses may result in acute stress reactions that impact on recall and current functioning. Attention may be 'hijacked" and result in hypervigilance to threat. This contributes to excessive worry and a perpetual expectation of harm, which may result in an exaggerated startle response.
Depression	Symptoms that may maintain depressed mood include learned helplessness, mental defeat, hopelessness, fatigue, guilt, self-blame and suicidal intent, ideation and plans.

Mental defeat and learned helplessness	Individuals may have experienced a complete loss of identity, autonomy and volition peri-traumatically, which may continue to be enacted as a post-traumatic symptom. This might include the conviction that the pre-torture self, values and beliefs have been destroyed, and an enduring conviction that torture has resulted in permanent and intractable personality change. Consequences include profound helplessness, passivity, inability to reclaim one's post-torture life, alienation, or catatonic responses indicative of severe and complex PTSD.
Damaged self-concept and foreshortened future	A subjective feeling of having been irreparably damaged, being defective or having undergone an irreversible personality change (overlaps with/is particularly relevant if there is a sense of mental defeat), often reinforced by overpowering PTSD symptoms that impair day-to-day functioning. These may be reinforced by a deep sense of shame. There may be a sense of foreshortened future, where the person cannot comprehend that they will have a normal lifecycle and lifespan.
Dissociation and depersonalisation	These can be temporarily helpful as survival responses to overwhelming danger during torture. However, extreme or prolonged dissociative coping in response to traumatic recollection often results in loss of sense of time and place, memory problems, confusion, disorientation and inability to experience or relate, and may provoke extreme fear or profound detachment. Depersonalisation is often a coping response at times of extreme trauma that might be likened to the 'freeze' in the 'fight, flight or freeze' response in the face of extreme danger, and therefore may manifest as a sensory flashback of the torture, or may be a reaction to re-experiencing.
Difficulties understanding the motivation to torture	Survivors may ruminate on the incomprehensibility of acts of torture and the motivations of perpetrators, which challenge their beliefs about human nature, resulting in difficulties adapting and integrating these

	into their post-torture identity and functioning. Grey and Young (2008) offer a comprehensive model for assessing and understanding the role of torture in state-sanctioned violence that may be helpful to guide cognitive and behavioural rehabilitation.
Interpersonal difficulties	Inability to trust others, connect to trusted others, resume intimate relationships or participate in ordinary community activities.
Somatic complaints	These vary in accordance with the original torture and its continued effects. Typically, they might include headaches, sexual dysfunction, traumatic brain injury, physical pain and musculoskeletal problems. Chronic pain is exacerbated by a vicious circle of inactivity, inability to find appropriate activities or occupation (due to refugee status), loss of usual coping mechanisms, insomnia, inappropriate living conditions, financial hardship and inadequate access to medical resources.
Neuropsychological impairments	This is an important aspect of post-torture rehabilitation, where symptoms might easily be missed or misdiagnosed because of the comorbid challenges of PTSD, depression, displacement, transition, change of language and unfamiliarity.
Psychotic reactions	Visual and auditory hallucinations and paranoia might be epiphenomena of the re-experiencing characteristic of PTSD (flashbacks and hypervigilance). However, these will require careful assessment to rule out predominant psychotic disorders that require multidisciplinary team approaches.
Co-morbid difficulties	Substance abuse, eating disorders and other post-torture coping reactions.

It is imperative, then, that clinicians conduct a timely, full and contextualised assessment of the individual's pre-, peri- and post-torture biopsychosocial functioning. This would include impairments, but also protective factors, resilience and resources, in order to provide survivors with the best chances of recovery.

For some survivors, the act of escape and exile may serve as a protective factor, reinforcing narratives of agency that help to preserve identity and psychological coherence. The next section considers how we use psychological formulations to build a comprehensive model of rehabilitation and recovery.

Using a dynamic formulation-based approach with survivors of torture

Bowley and Bashir (2016) provide an extensive review of recovery-based formulations to guide clinician interventions, particularly with survivors of torture who are seeking asylum. These are summarised here. They include:

- the phased approach to recovery outlined by Judith Herman (1992)
- Stirling Moorey's work around adjustment (Moorey, 1996)
- resilience models (eg. Amering & Schmolke, 2009)
- transdiagnostic models (eg. Mansell et al, 2009).

Phased recovery formulations

Judith Herman (1992) provides a framework to guide psychotherapy work with the common patterns of distress associated with atrocities, whether they are domestic violence, physical or sexual assault or political terror. Her model captures the primary tasks associated with the ongoing process of healing and recovery for survivors, and drives not only work with PTSD but also social constructionist and human rights-based interventions.

Herman identifies three stages (1992):

- safety, where the restoration of control and establishment of safety are vital
- reconstruction, where traumas are explored and transformed
- reconnection, involving developing activity and relationships.

Establishing safety and control is the guiding principle in recovery work. It is often a primary task, but one to which we return repeatedly, as the survivor's circumstances oscillate between post-trauma experiencing and the acute stress of exile. It covers all the features of an individual's experience, from physical and psychological health (from destabilising intrusions to self-destructive or risky behaviours), outward into environmental, financial and social situations.

Key tasks include anchoring oneself in a safe present and developing autonomy, which might be particularly impaired as a consequence of torture and displacement.

The second stage incorporates ongoing processes of remembrance and mourning. The retelling of the trauma and the facilitating of emotional expression, aimed at contextualising traumatic memories, provides the means by which individuals accommodate incomprehensible experiences, regain control of their experiences, and, in doing so, ameliorate the intrusive and uncontrollable nature of associated distress.

Finally, individuals work towards reconnecting with wider social and interpersonal worlds. The task is to begin to inhabit their lives in the present. Developing a new vision of the future and reinstating resilience are part of the continuing process of recovery.

Adjustment formulations

Working with survivors requires the therapist to consider the cognitive and emotional tasks of major life adjustment. Stirling Moorey (1996: 450, 2010) argues that adverse life events can be summarised as when 'bad things happen to rational people', which moves us to consider how we might partially formulate the therapeutic goal as one of 'adjustment' to the consequences of torture and exile.

This is perhaps more useful in considering post-traumatic consequences and the acute stress of negotiating the mounting challenges of transition. It allows client and therapist to accept distress, without pathologising it, and allows the opportunity to accommodate and assimilate the sensory-perceptual aspects of recent events into an autobiographical narrative. As such, it may apply to a range of processes of grief, trauma, displacement and exile, reflecting the profoundly distressing experience of refugee survivors of torture.

CBT formulations help clients to identify their immediate thoughts, appraisals and feelings, as well as understand the environmental factors that maintain distress. Standard techniques, such as managing excessive and hypothetical worry, reinstating or increasing tolerance of uncertainty, coping with PTSD symptoms, and problem-solving are used to develop appropriate coping strategies within clients' capacity and competence. Alternatively, a skills-teaching approach, consistent with a resilience model, will help survivors to incorporate new narratives of the mind, body, trauma and transition that will open up the possibilities for recovery or reintegration.

Resilience formulations

Prevalence rates indicate that PTSD is not an inevitable consequence of trauma. Disorder-specific models are inherently pathologising, fail to account for multiple, prolonged and complex trauma, and pathologise non-western or collectivist coping styles. These models might lead us to fail to ask what a 'normal' or ordinary response might be to the extensive range of stressors, losses and transitions experienced by survivors. The factors that maintain resilience in the face of abnormally adverse life events such as torture, trauma and displacement are important considerations in rehabilitation formulations.

Amering and Schmolke (2009), in their comprehensive sourcebook, argue that it is a clinical responsibility to incorporate resilience as a dynamic recovery factor. Bowley and Bashir (2016: 27) regard resilience as the ability to resist and regain mental stability following a stressful event or period. What it is *not* is a biological invulnerability; what it *is* is a flexible psychological competency involving processes of 'protection, repair, regeneration'.

Most survivors will have already endured extensive threats at the level of individual, family, community, culture and country. The aim of a resilience approach would be, first, to enable survivors to bring their historic resources helpfully into their present reality, and second, to begin to confront and integrate the impact of adverse life events, trauma, torture, loss and transition.

This approach provides clinicians with a range of resources and strengths to consider in their collaborative formulations and is represented pictorially in Figure 1. Bowley and Bashir (2016) suggest that resilience-based formulations, especially in relation to the torture, migration and trauma trajectory, aim to enable clients to:

- recount pre-existing resources (eg. positive history of attachments, self-agency/esteem, self-efficacy, active coping, socio-economic resources, political activism, spirituality, locus of control)
- consider new mechanisms that are a necessary part of migration and resettlement in a new culture and country (eg. knowledge of health/social care structures, familiarity with the culture, adjusting to an individualistic vs collectivist culture, developing new social networks, appropriate engagement and participation, renewed activism)
- consider how pre-, peri- and post-traumatic *and* migration, social, political and psychological processes continue to deplete pre-existing

protective factors and resources (eg. loss of identity, class, role, self-esteem, family, access to culture and language, reduction in personal agency as a consequence of restrictions during the asylum process or of reduced quality of life)
- consider how these pre-, peri-, and post-traumatic and migration processes present barriers to developing new resources and attachments.

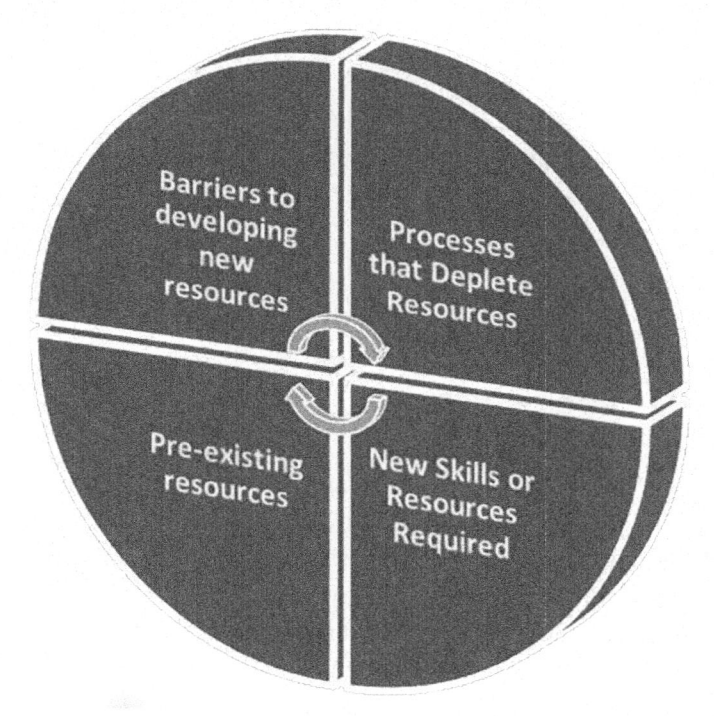

Figure 1: Resource-based formulation of resilience

Furthermore, the field of positive psychology offers a comprehensive set of ideas about what it might mean to live a satisfying life, which are useful in considering how we might support survivors to re-remember their resources, values and ideals and incorporate them into a new model for living that resists meta-narrative pressures. Seligman (2011) provides the acronym PERMA (Positive emotion, Engagement, Relationships, Meaning and purpose, Accomplishment) to connote the five measurable elements of wellbeing that can form the basis of a review of resources and sources of positive feelings in exile, with a view to helping set personal goals and helping survivors reconstruct their lives in ways that are consistent with their values.

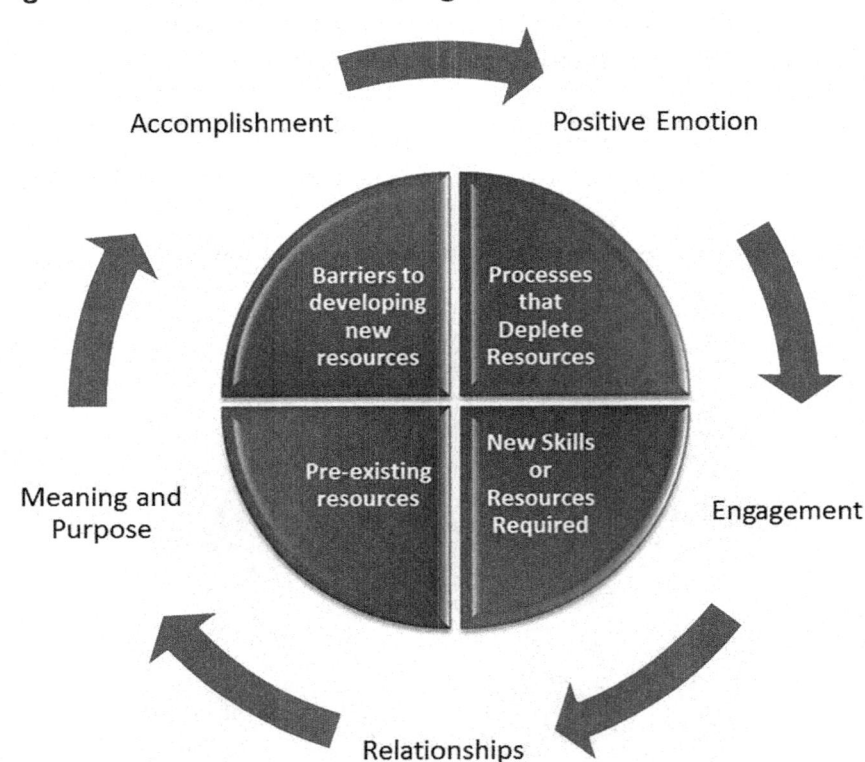

Figure 2: Resilience and wellbeing formulation

```
           Accomplishment        Positive Emotion

                  ┌─────────────┬─────────────┐
                  │ Barriers to │ Processes   │
                  │ developing  │ that        │
                  │ new         │ Deplete     │
                  │ resources   │ Resources   │
Meaning and       ├─────────────┼─────────────┤    Engagement
Purpose           │             │ New Skills  │
                  │ Pre-existing│ or          │
                  │ resources   │ Resources   │
                  │             │ Required    │
                  └─────────────┴─────────────┘

                        Relationships
```

Bowley and Bashir (2016) argue that resilience-based formulations offer the potential to consider post-traumatic growth (PTG) (Calhoun & Tedeschi, 2013) and adversity-activated development (AAD) (Papadopoulous, 2007) as responses to the adversity of torture, trauma and exile. While PTG examines positive developments following trauma, AAD assumes adverse experiences will influence the trajectory of individual development in positive, neutral and negative ways.

Culturally contextualised transdiagnostic formulations

Hinton and colleagues (2012) detail how a culturally bound therapy like CBT must be led by clients' cultural understandings if it is to be accessible and effective. For example, culturally held beliefs about knowledge, experience, the mind, the body and change will influence clients' causal attributions, as well as their engagement and recovery. In a thought-provoking study, Liddell and Jobson (2016) demonstrate that there is a culturally contingent variation in neuro-expression of PTSD symptoms. Their neural evidence shows that for people living in collectivist cultures there is a tendency to focus on background/contextual details during the trauma, as opposed to the focus on specific and central detail in individualistic cultures that we are usually directed to expect in PTSD responses. They propose five aspects of PTSD experience modulated by cultural variables: '... fear perception and regulation, attentional biases (to threat), emotional and autobiographical memory, self-referential processing and attachment systems' (2016: 1). However, lived cultural contexts are much more dynamic than the static polarities of collectivist versus individualist social systems. Nevertheless, this review has implications for how we might need to refine our assessments and interventions to capture this perceptual information.

Hinton et al (2012) offer a helpful protocol for culturally adapted CBT (CA-CBT) for trauma in refugees, which is summarised by Bowley and Bashir (2016) and extended here to consider transdiagnostic processes for survivors of torture and the social construction of selfhood. Considerations for practitioners from transdiagnostic models include:

- the approach/relationship of the individual to cognition/experience, which is particularly relevant to diverse culturally embedded understandings of the mind
- linguistic, narrative and social constructions of experience that are often culturally bound, particularly in relation to understandings of sexual violations and shame
- socio-cultural, environmental and familial factors, which influence causal attributions, locus of control, attitudes to and opportunities for change
- the role of biological mechanisms (eg. the body, the brain) in maintaining disturbance, relevant in most psychological presentations, especially trauma, anxiety and depression
- learning processes that are dependent on social, environmental, linguistic, and cultural variables, a clear assessment of which might help tailor interventions improving effectiveness
- memory formation, especially relevant to PTSD flashbacks and fractured memories
- thinking, reasoning and information processing, which are relevant to how experience is understood and processed across presenting difficulties
- psychological flexibility, which is heavily tasked by the multiple adaptation processes required when establishing a new life while accommodating experiences of torture *and* managing PTSD symptoms

- renewed interest in the role of emotions, appraisals of which are influenced by social and cultural values
- role of positive affect, relevant for self-soothing strategies or to address shame, guilt or anger underpinning trauma, loss and transition.

Practice

The model of practice outlined here is an adapted, modularised version of one produced for Bowley and Bashir (2016) and is represented pictorially in Figure 3. A strong working relationship with interpreters is the bedrock of good service delivery and is covered in other chapters in this book.

Reflexive human rights practitioners

A human-rights standpoint forces practitioners to look beyond survivors' individual needs and take action to support their rights as human beings. Respect for universal human dignity underpins human rights law. A human-rights standpoint identifies the 'duty bearers' (in this context, the therapist) who hold the responsibility to ensure these rights are honoured. The duties of those in the clinical sector will be not only to provide the right to rehabilitation for survivors of torture, but also to bear witness, document, and advocate for their clients, including the provision of medical and psychological documentation for legal, housing or forensic purposes.

Furthermore, practitioners are tasked to consider what they themselves are doing, why they adopt one course of action over another, and to continually reflect on how they can improve the services they provide. Here, reflexivity, a concept originating in systemic theory, offers a protocol for the continuous development of one's therapeutic practice (Dallos & Stedmon, 2009). A reflective practitioner is one who uses careful mental reflection to consider their practice. A reflexive practitioner, on the other hand, is one who considers from moment to moment how his/her own interests, position, standpoint, reactions and assumptions influence what is happening at any given point in his/her practice, and uses this to improve practice in the moment and afterwards. This ability to notice and understand is used 'reflexively' in and out of session to build formulations and interventions that embed a right to redress within a human-rights framework alongside the key psychological components of the intervention.

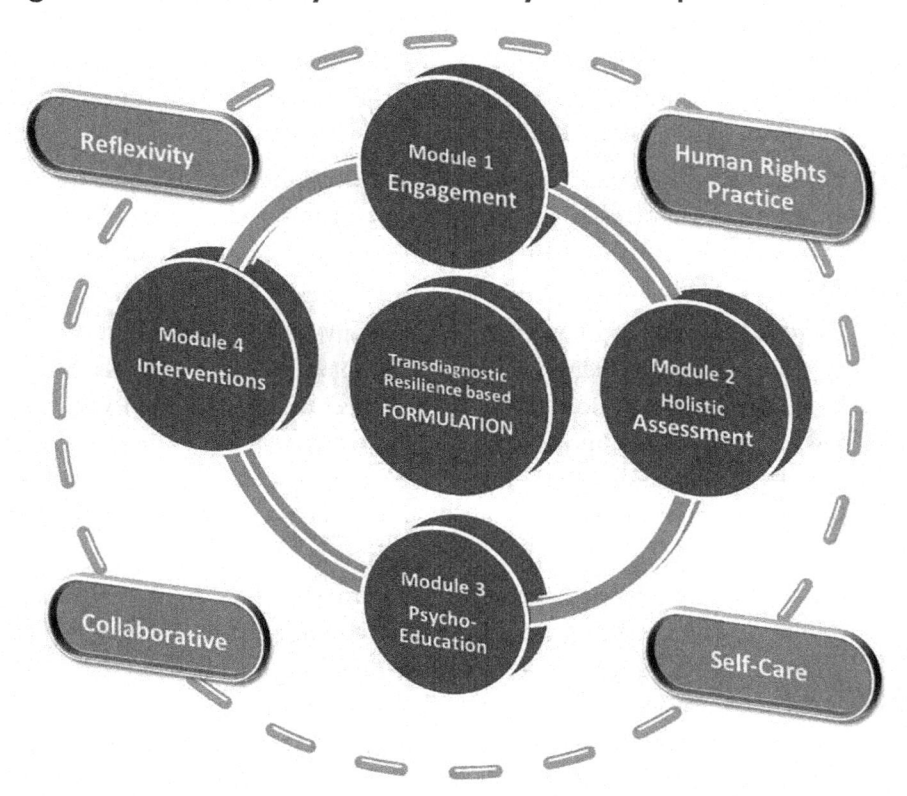

Figure 3: overview of dynamic recovery model of practice

Modules shown: Module 1 Engagement; Module 2 Holistic Assessment; Module 3 Psycho-Education; Module 4 Interventions; Transdiagnostic Resilience based FORMULATION. Surrounding principles: Reflexivity, Human Rights Practice, Self-Care, Collaborative.

Module 1: Engagement

Engagement falls within Herman's safety stage, and is about 'establishing safety in the relationship and with the goals of the relationship' (1992). While attention to the relationship between therapist and client is essential throughout, attention to how engaged a survivor is within the discourse is paramount at the outset. The issue of trust is vital with survivors and should be addressed at the beginning. Bowley (2006) and Bowley and Bashir (2016) argue that establishing the helping role and explaining confidentiality is important, especially when working with interpreters, as their commitment to confidentiality needs to be explicitly shared with the survivor. Informing clients that you are not connected with the Home Office is useful, and many therapists choose to make their commitment to human rights explicit. The tasks central to engagement include:

- *meet*, contract and brief the interpreter before meeting the survivor using a standard protocol such as that offered by Bashir and Bowley (2014)

- *introduce* the interpreter and their confidentiality obligations. Briefly, introduce self, human rights or other standpoint, separating your service from the Home Office. If relevant, discuss how interpreting will work – for example, using short sentences, and the importance of feedback when interpreting/interpreter difficulties arise
- *contextualise* the service so survivors understand the rationale for the appointment and also where it fits into their healthcare. Elicit and acknowledge differences to their home country experience of accessing and using healthcare
- *socialise* the survivor to psychological therapy by explaining what therapy is and how it might help. Survivors may not be familiar with therapy or have very idiosyncratic views as to the object of the meeting. Explaining the reason for the appointment and rationale for therapy is extremely important. Explaining the limits of one's role is useful (ie. with regard to prescribing medication or involvement in processes such as benefits and accommodation)
- *present* the therapeutic contract and parameters (length, regularity and number of sessions and confidentiality) in straightforward terms. It is important for engagement to acknowledge that this may be an alien or particularly western construct. It may be useful, when the survivor is able absorb the information, to explain the limits of psychological therapy: eg. how psychological models differ from the medical model and the ways in which working with the mind is different from treating disease processes. Explain what their responsibilities are: eg. effort, punctuality, cancellation policies, participation, between-session tasks
- provide positive *normalising* rationales for your role and reiterate the message of concern for the survivor's safety and autonomy. For some, the idea of therapy may be threatening, or associated with ill health or weakness
- offer short-term *practical assistance,* if other sources of support are unavailable. This is often a very effective way to develop engagement and trust. However, this may challenge a purist therapist's boundaries. While it is paramount that the main focus should be on enabling the client to engage in a therapeutic encounter, it may be impossible for them to do so if they are under acute stress that could be easily resolved with the appropriate support, signposting or skills development.

Module 2: Assessment

The assessment process will extend over a number of sessions, because survivors may present with multiple stressors. This is a challenge to practitioners using brief models who need to assess and formulate quickly. Persons' (1989) problem-list approach to assessment is particularly helpful if we want to develop an appreciation of the transdiagnostic processes contributing to a client's overall psychological presentation (eg. working memory difficulties as a result of PTSD, acute stress or adjustment). The problem list should include an overview of medication, other health concerns, accommodation, experience of racism, and legal difficulties. Therefore, this would form part of Herman's initial safety stage, because it offers an insight into destabilising factors for the client.

Bowley (2006) notes that the assessment of wellbeing is similar to that with other client populations, but the intensity of distress due to the effects of torture or current stressors means the sense of crisis with which people present makes it less straightforward. Fears and anxieties could have an intensity that seems delusional but are consistent with an individual's experience.

However, the assessment must cover various practical and therapeutic tasks, as outlined in Table 4 below. For example, when people report suicidal ideation, therapists need to be prepared to assess risk. It is common for survivors seeking asylum to say, 'I'll kill myself rather than be sent back,' and there is evidence that this is a real possibility. Fear of removal is often associated with the possibility of return to further torture, which may trigger or heighten PTSD symptoms. The subsequent re-experiencing results in threat-focused cognitive impairment, which may influence decision-making about acting on suicidal ideas. In such cases, if a person is threatened with removal, risk should become an imminent concern.

In assessing ideation, it is important to remember that shame, stigma or culturally bound or PTSD-related experiences might result in non-disclosure. Here, acceptance of distress and contextualising it as an understandable biopsychosocial response to overwhelming events may provide a normalising rationale. This is helpful because it enables the survivor to understand their symptoms and perhaps reduce their sense of personal responsibility, shame, guilt or worry, which often heighten distress.

Implicit in this is the idea that we need to pay attention to the survivor's appraisal of their PTSD symptoms. Nightmares or flashbacks may be seen as premonitions about the future, or all symptoms may be seen as evidence of permanent damage. There is the possibility that talking about the torture may be viewed as damaging and unhelpful because of the associated anxiety.

This is when psychoeducation about the evidence for trauma-focused talking therapies is paramount. However, as noted in Table 4, survivors may need to be encouraged to pace themselves, rather than rush into telling their history of torture, which can be retraumatising if they have not yet developed resources for coping with PTSD anxiety.

Assessing different socio-cultural interpretations of wellbeing is useful, both in eliciting beliefs about the cause and nature of problems and in socialising clients to the CBT model. When socialising clients to the model, use straightforward examples and imagery and/or metaphors that are relevant to the client's current frame of reference. Asking clients about the traditional or local name of a problem, its signs, causes and how it was addressed, will help with engagement and the development of a shared goal.

When working with survivors, it is important to be sensitive when assessing their history, especially if their coping strategy is avoidance. A pitfall during the assessment is to elicit memories, thoughts and feelings that people have been suppressing, which may lead to unmanageable levels of affect. It is important to identify the extent to which clients have talked about their experiences, the impact and their strategies for managing immediate and ongoing anxiety. It is important to prepare avoidant clients for the possibility of increased symptomatology at the outset of therapy, and to balance this with your expectations about how a trauma-focused approach will eventually reduce the impact of symptoms.

Gaining an understanding of a client's history, as outlined in Table 4, can seem difficult when their country of origin or culture is unfamiliar. If country information is necessary to help you understand the survivor and their experiences, you can find it on websites such as Human Rights Watch (www.hrw.org) or Amnesty International (www.amnesty.org.uk), who provide brief but detailed summaries of most relevant countries. It might also be helpful to conceptualise background and history in three stages:

- pre-torture – childhood years pre-torture/the time leading up to initial experiences of torture
- torture – experiences and reactions during the torture; consequences for them, their families and communities
- post-torture – experiences of release or escape, displacement, separation, transition and adjustment.

Table 4: Assessment tasks (adapted from Bowley & Bashir, 2016)

Task	Content
Contracting	Initial contract and outline for the continuing therapy process
	Consent form to contact relevant agencies eg. solicitor and social worker, where clinically indicated
Collect general relevant information	Legal process, living arrangements and financial circumstances
	Current friends, networks and activities
	Education and literacy levels in all languages (relevant for giving homework tasks, self-help materials, psychometric measures)
Introduce the model	Explain what CBT is in simple terms
History, problems, protective factors and resilience	Assess ability to concentrate/understand you and interpreter
	Begin to gather the client's problem list, in their words. Consider using loss, transition and journey into exile as categories to organise the problem list
	Encourage clients to pace themselves and not launch into descriptions of traumatic events by suggesting the time and space to do this slowly will be available. This is to prevent retraumatisation
	Consider extent of collectivist and individualist cultural influences and how they have shaped perception of self, others, adversity, trauma and resilience (See Hinton et al (2012) and Liddell and Jobson (2016)
	Determine what is going well
	Determine clients understanding of psychological difficulties (eg. cultural understandings, stigma and as well as fears of 'going mad' or being irreparable psychologically damaged)
	Physical health-related concerns
	Appetite and sleep difficulties, including nightmares
	Risk and safeguarding issues
	Chronology to include resilience and pre-morbid resources (eg. flowers and stones lifeline, as in NET)

Trans-diagnostic processes and changes since adverse life events or transition	Attention, concentration and mental flexibility
	Memory and imagery
	Understanding of the mind, brain and its functioning
	Thoughts and understanding of thinking
	Reasoning and understanding of emotions
	Behaviour, safety behaviours, avoidance
	Expectations and attributions about wellbeing

Module 3: Psychoeducation

Assessing and formulating are not separate or artificial processes, and in themselves may contain or necessitate elements of intervention, particularly those that focus on establishing safety, control and trust. Implicit in Herman's first phase of establishing safety (1992) is restoring a sense of control (often achieved through the normalising processes of formulation), which is difficult when confronted with the threat of repatriation and when one's life is externally controlled by legal, financial, and social constraints.

Furthermore, Bowley and Bashir (2016) argue:

> Prompt presentation of a general normalising recovery formulation with explicit trust and safety requirements is helpful... Using an adjustment model, distress [is seen as] an appropriate part of the individual's emotional processing and may mean they do not need formal support... a normalising rationale [alone] can alter appraisals, reduce anxieties, and allow individuals to continue on the process of recovery without formal assistance.

Psychoeducation is a process of finding a shared language to understand profoundly damaging and overwhelming experience and can be seen as preparation for the reconstruction phase of the work with survivors. The tasks are often quite significant and might best be conceptualised as a series of process-based *interventions*, where a shared understanding becomes the scaffolding for or 'backbone' of therapy. Through psychoeducation, we achieve shared formulations, align client and therapist goals, provide evidence-based information about the expected effects of trauma, torture, displacement and exile on presenting difficulties, and thereby ensure that survivors have a thorough rationale for the content and process of formulation and therapy. This also necessitates that survivors understand the role of trauma and peri-traumatic anxiety in the development of PTSD flashbacks, intrusions and hyperarousal if they are to effectively engage with interventions or trust that there are, indeed, beneficial aspects to connecting with powerful material. Other psychoeducation tasks include the physiology of anxiety, the role of thinking, emotion and behaviour in psychological wellbeing, and condition-specific models (eg. panic), if appropriate. The key tasks for this 'module' are presented by Bowley and Bashir (2016) and adapted in Table 5 below.

Table 5: The tasks for psychoeducation (from Bowley & Bashir, 2016)

Task	Content
Signposting	Provide information about the psychosocial context, including legal aid solicitors, drop-ins, destitution and rights-based projects
Loss, transition and adjustment	Normalise and empathise – accept loss of culture, language, family, community and familiarity as understandably overwhelming or stultifying
	Normalise how limited opportunities in current settings might impact on wellbeing or worsen PTSD
	Accept that there is not one way to overcome such adversity or bridge such transition. Rationale for why this is a joint endeavour
The anxiety cycle	Body's normal response to mild and extreme stress Role of the brain and hormones
	Memory formation and threat (eg. one analogy for explaining this is to indicate that the sensory parts of the brain perform harder and the thinking and higher-order functions are suppressed during extreme danger, which results in fragmented sensory memories)
	The flight, fight and freeze response to extreme stress and internal or external triggers
	Reasons for symptoms such as dizziness, feeling hot or cold, sweating, blurred vision, shaking, muscle tension
	Role of thinking/attention in maintaining stress response

Torture, trauma and flashbacks	Rationale for why trauma memories might persist
	Role of avoidance and other maintenance factors, including migration, ongoing threats, enforced idleness, poverty, ongoing breach of rights
	Explore, understand and accommodate the motivation for torture and persecution (see Grey & Young, 2008)
	Rationale for nightmares, dreams and flashbacks
	Hyperarousal and hypervigilance and how this impacts on daily living
	Rationale for insomnia and poor sleep
	Establish safety and control following intrusions and flashbacks using grounding techniques
	Reduce hyperarousal, reduce threat – cognitive, metacognitive and behavioural (eg. breathing, relaxation and mindfulness) techniques
The role of thinking, emotion and coping strategies	Recovery and resilience – the rationale for a skills/resource-focused approach to build resilience in new environments or rebuild resilience in the context of ongoing adversity
	Reasons why previous strategies might be less effective (eg. loss of nexus, ongoing loss and bereavement)
	Therapy as having a role in decentring/understanding our relationship to experience and how this benefits/disadvantages us
	Short- and long-term benefits of self-control and self-soothing strategies
	Protective factors in wellbeing (eg. activity, spirituality, absorption, education, stimulation, diet and sleep)
Reducing hyperarousal	Rationale for grounding, breathing, relaxation, visualisation (soothing imagery) and mindfulness techniques
Specific model of therapy to be used	Explain specific goal of therapy model and its rationale eg. NET is to help reconstruct a trauma narrative; MCT focuses on our relationship with, appraisals of and behaviour with regard to trauma

	Rationale for present oriented coping strategies
	Obtain informed consent for trauma-focused work
	Self-help or information in first language if literate (see Royal College of Psychiatrists website for resources)

Module 4: Interventions

Using Herman's concept of a process of recovery (1992), therapists can order their interventions around the three phases: safety, transformation and reconnection. Table 6, adapted from Bowley and Bashir (2016), outlines the range of possible intervention tasks for therapy. In practice, client needs and circumstances are not static; they move between these phases. Continuing adversity or stress during recovery may increase the likelihood of survivors becoming retraumatised. This then requires practitioners to return to the foundational phase of establishing safety.

Table 6: The tasks for transdiagnostic intervention (from Bowley & Bashir, 2016)

Task	Content
Managing risk	Manage hopelessness, suicide risk, or memories of previous attempts
	Strategies at points where risk could increase eg. legal processes (appeals, refusal, acceptance, detention, or removal), racism/stress/trauma in the present
	Update the GP or care providers regularly
	Assertive referrals to health and support services
Sleep	CBT interventions for insomnia or erratic sleep
	Management of nightmares, including acceptance as part of process of adjustment, or imagery rescripting
	Manage excessive worry and terminate intrusive/anxiety provoking thoughts
Depression	Indicate therapies for depression or transdiagnostic models focusing on the role of rumination, social isolation and avoidance

Trauma	Psychoeducation/grounding techniques (Table 5)
	Managing intrusions, flashbacks and dissociation
	Imagery rescripting for nightmares
	Bearing witness, validating and holding the client's experience
	Work meta-cognitively to reduce avoidance, suppression or focus on cognitive-attentional processes (Wells, 2009)...
	... or recontextualise trauma memories by developing a coherent and detailed narrative of experience focusing on resources and resilience
	Explore and develop the personal meaning of these events
	Explore/reframe feelings of shame and guilt
	Confront extreme affect eg. despair, fear, anger
	Understand and rebuild ruptured belief systems
	Focused therapeutic work aimed at altering traumatic memories, taking into account Liddell & Jobson's (2016) review of PTSD presentations as culturally contingent
	Referral and rationale for pain management interventions
Loss and grief	Allowing grief and mourning for multiple losses
	Managing ambiguous loss for the missing or lost (Boss, 2009)
	Loss of role, identity, culture and language
	Long-term strategies to manage grief
	Identify factors preventing connection and reconnection
	Develop skills or resources to enable reconnection eg. mindfulness
	Rebuild beliefs, values, religious and political convictions
	Conceptualise a new life and resume daily activities in line with values
	Establish new relationships or re-establish old relationships and family bonds
	Explore trust/interpersonal issues and long-term management strategies
	Rebuild a new life in a new country, developing goals and aspirations

Initial phase interventions focus on developing safety, control and trust, and include those already mentioned during engagement, assessment, formulation and psychoeducation. Bowley & Bashir (2016) argue that the decision about which intervention to use should reflect the formulation, but that the socio-linguistic and legal challenges might mean that simple behavioural approaches are the initial choice. However, this requires care, because it is imperative that this decision is formulation based rather than due to resource constraints, otherwise we might be seen to be in breach of the survivor's rights to rehabilitation from the effects of torture, which would be, at the least, inconsistent with a human-rights model.

Nevertheless, some survivors may feel unable to continue beyond the foundational/stabilisation phase of therapy. Clients have awareness of their limits and often return for more specific therapy after managing acute psychosocial stressors, such as migration or transition. For example, with survivors seeking asylum whose appeals rights are exhausted, who are detained, or who are awaiting removal, we may need to carefully consider whether continued processing of the trauma will be of benefit or likely to cause harm. An evolving formulation based on these circumstances might lead us to redirect our efforts to provide practical support, counselling or psychological support to reinforce earlier anxiety management and grounding interventions. The construct of continuous traumatic stress (CTS) places significance on regulation of anticipatory anxiety in the context of realistic threat and may also be a helpful formulation (Eagle & Kaminer, 2013; Murray et al, 2013).

Phase two interventions correspond to Herman's stage of reconstruction of experiences. These centre on the transformation of clients' experiences, and in practice closely match the active therapeutic components of transdiagnostic cognitive processes in PTSD and depression, and for emotional problems of guilt and shame. This is especially true if clients' difficulties are discrete and reflect specific traumas or losses. However, people may have had a lifetime of trauma, and in these cases, the adoption of specific interventions is augmented by consideration of the human-rights testimony approach, or NET, which reinforces the notion of bearing witness to clients' experiences.

Phase three interventions focus on reconnection and involve moving from the past into an active present and future. Here, the task for survivors is to negotiate their engagement and participation in an often unfamiliar and sometimes hostile, alienating world. Often contextual issues counteract the benefits of phase three interventions, because survivors seeking asylum are unable to work, are usually financially restricted, and, through migration and dispersal, are isolated from social networks. Education, voluntary work, reinstating professional accreditation in the present context, or reconnecting with activist ethics and other pre-torture values will play a major role in shaping which activities an individual chooses. As therapy draws to a close, this might be a matching cue to previous endings or losses, and care needs to be taken (Bowley & Bashir, 2016). Statutory services are unable to offer ongoing support beyond complex trauma intervention, so therapy may end while an individual remains in an uncertain situation or is still experiencing symptoms. This can be a difficult process for therapist and client alike, and Bowley and Bashir emphasise the necessity of supervision and self-care (2016).

Conclusion

This chapter has outlined how existing CBT models can be used in non-pathologising, transdiagnostic ways to meet the many rehabilitation challenges facing survivors of torture. In particular, this chapter has considered the usefulness of social constructionist frameworks embedded within a human-rights perspective to adapt and integrate a comprehensive CBT model of assessment and rehabilitation.

Understanding the survivor's position at the outset of therapy, which might reflect a sense of alienation or mental defeat, is vital in shaping how we pitch our earlier modules to maximise the likelihood of engagement. Engagement is considered a deliberate, politically oriented aspect of therapy that seeks to resource clients to raise their voices and exercise their right to rehabilitation. Formulation is more likely to be an organic, evolving process that is inclusive of survivors' experiences, rather than an attempt to fit their symptoms into a neat trauma model.

Practice and intervention involves an appreciation of the socio-political, cultural, contextual and therapeutic power dynamics to help combat therapist bias and oppressive processes that are endemic for survivors of torture seeking asylum and/or seeking psychological help. A commitment to human rights directs us to pay attention to power and process and address barriers to progress for survivors of torture.

Being authentically present with the survivor throughout the therapeutic contact demands reflexive practice, which is a prerequisite when using social constructionist frameworks. Therapist intention includes moment-by-moment attention to the power differential within therapy and its parallels across the survivor's life trajectory, individually, within the family, and within various oppressive contexts (including home and host countries).

Evidence indicates that torture has pernicious and pervasive biopsychosocial effects, particularly in the context of loss of nexus and social support. In these contexts, the tasks to psychically and socially integrate are served well by a range of transdiagnostic, resilience-oriented, CBT-informed interventions provided by well-trained and well-supported practitioners who have a commitment to a human rights approach.

References

Amering M, Schmolke M (2009). *Recovery in Mental Illness: reshaping scientific and clinical responsibilities*. Chichester: John Wiley & Sons.

Bashir C, Bowley J (2014). *Briefing Guidelines for Interpreters in Psychotherapeutic Settings*. [Online.] www.academia.edu/7301736/briefing_guidelines_for_interpreters_in_psychotherapeutic_settings [accessed 19 July 2016].

Başoğlu M, Salcioğlu E, Livanou M, Kalender D, Acar G (2005). Single-session behavioral treatment of earthquake-related posttraumatic stress disorder: a randomized waiting list controlled trial. *Journal of Traumatic Stress* 18(1): 1–11.

Bhui K, Morgan N (2007). Effective psychotherapy in a racially and culturally diverse society. *Advances in Psychiatric Treatment* 13: 187–193.

Blackburn IM, Davidson KM (1990). *Cognitive Therapy for Depression and Anxiety: a practitioner's guide*. Oxford: Blackwell.

Boss P (2009). The trauma and complicated grief of ambiguous loss. *Pastoral Psychology* 59(2): 137–145.

Bowley J (2006). Working with asylum seekers. In: Tarrier N (ed). *Case Formulation in Cognitive Behaviour Therapy: the treatment of challenging and complex cases*. London: Routledge (pp330-348).

Bowley J, Bashir C (2016). Working with people seeking asylum. In: Tarrier N, Johnson J (eds). *Case Formulation in Cognitive Behaviour Therapy: the treatment of challenging and complex cases* (2nd ed). London: Routledge (pp322–351).

Brewin CR (2007). Autobiographical memory for trauma: update on four controversies. *Memory* 15(3): 227–248. doi:10.1080/09658210701256423.

Brewin CR (2006). Recovered memory and false memory. In: Heaton-Armstrong A, Shepherd E, Gudjonsson G, Wolchover D (eds). *Witness Testimony: psychological, investigative and evidential perspectives*. Oxford: Oxford University Press (pp89–104).

Brewin CR, Gregory JD, Lipton M, Burgess N (2010). Intrusive images in psychological disorders: characteristics, neural mechanisms, and treatment implications. *Psychological Review* 117: 210–232.

Calhoun LG, Tedeschi RG (2013). *Post-traumatic Growth in Clinical Practice*. New York, NY: Routledge.

Cienfuegos A, Monelli C (1983). The testimony of political repression as a therapeutic instrument. *Amercian Journal of Orthopsychiatry* 53(1): 43–51.

Dallos R, Stedmon J (2009). Flying over the swampy lowlands: reflective and reflexive practice. In: Stedmon J, Dallos R (eds). *Reflective Practice in Psychotherapy and Counselling*. New York: McGraw Hill (pp1–22).

David D, Hofman SG (2013). Another error of Descartes? Implications for the 'THIRD WAVE' of cognitive behaviour therapy. *Journal of Cognitive and Behavioral Psychotherapies* 13(1): 115–124.

Eagle G, Kaminer D (2013). Continuous traumatic stress: expanding the lexicon of traumatic stress. *Peace and Conflict: Journal of Peace Psychology* 19(2): 85–99.

Foucault M (1965). *Madness and Civilization*. New York, NY: Pantheon Books.

Gilbert P (2010). *Compassion-Focused Therapy: distinctive features*. London: Routledge.

Grey N, Young K (2008). Cognitive behaviour therapy with refugees and asylum seekers experiencing traumatic stress symptoms. *Behavioural and Cognitive Psychotherapy* 36: 3–19.

Harvey A, Watkins E, Mansell W, Shafran R (2004). *Cognitive Behavioural Processes across Psychological Disorders: a transdiagnostic approach to research and treatment*. Oxford: Oxford University Press.

Hayes SC, Strosahl KD, Wilson KG (2012). *Acceptance and Commitment Therapy: the process and practice of mindful change* (2nd ed). New York, NY: Guilford Press.

Herman JL (1992). *Trauma and Recovery: the aftermath of violence – from domestic abuse to political terror*. New York, NY: Basic Books.

Hinton D, Rivera E, Hofmann S, Barlow D, Otto M (2012). Adapting CBT for traumatized refugees and ethnic minority patients: examples from culturally adapted CBT (CA-CBT). *Transcultural Psychiatry* 49(2): 340–365.

Liddell B, Jobson L (2016). The impact of cultural differences in self-representation on the neural substrates of posttraumatic stress disorder. *European Journal of Psychotraumatology* 7(1): 10.3402/ejpt.v7.30464.

Linehan M (1993). *Cognitive-Behavioral Treatment of Borderline Personality*. New York: Guilford Press.

Lyotard JF (1979). *La Condition Moderne: rapport sur le savoir (The Postmodern Condition: a report on knowledge)*. Paris: Les Editions de Minuit. Published in English in the UK (trans G Bennington, B Massumi) by University of Manchester Press, 1984.

Mansell W, Harvey A, Watkins E, Shafran R (2009). Conceptual foundations of the transdiagnostic approach to CBT. *Journal of Cognitive Psychotherapy: An International Quarterly* 23(1): 6–19.

McFarlane C, Kaplan I (2012). Evidence-based psychological interventions for adult survivors of torture and trauma: a 30-year review. *Transcultural Psychiatry* 49(3–4): 539–567.

Moorey S (2010). The six cycles maintenance model: Growing a 'vicious flower' for depression. Behavioural & Cognitive Psychotherapy 38(2): 173–184.

Moorey S (1996). When bad things happen to rational people: cognitive therapy in adverse life conditions. In: Salkovskis PM (ed). *Frontiers of Cognitive Therapy*. New York: Guilford Press (pp450–469).

Mueller M (2013). The role of narrative exposure therapy in cognitive therapy for traumatised refugees and asylum-seekers. In: Grey N (ed). *Casebook of Cognitive Therapy for Traumatic Stress Reactions*. London: Routledge (pp265–282).

Murray LK, Cohen JA, Mannarino AP (2013). Trauma-focused cognitive behavioral therapy for youth who experience continuous traumatic exposure. *Peace and Conflict: Journal of Peace Psychology 19*: 180–195.

Neuner F, Catani C, Ruf M, Schauer E, Schauer M, Elbert T (2008). Narrative exposure therapy for the treatment of traumatized children and adolescents (KidNET): from neurocognitive theory to field Intervention. *Child and Adolescent Psychiatric Clinics of North America 17*: 641–664.

Neuner F, Kurreck S, Ruf M, Odenwald M, Elbert T, Schauer M (2010). Can asylum-seekers with posttraumatic stress disorder be successfully treated? A randomized controlled pilot study. *Cognitive Behaviour Therapy 39*(2): 81–91.

Nickerson A, Bryant R, Silove D, Steel Z (2011). A critical review of psychological treatments of posttraumatic stress disorder in refugees. *Clinical Psychology Review 31*: 399–417.

Nijdam MJ, Wittmann L (2015). Psychological and social theories of PTSD. In: Schnyder U, Cloitre M (eds). *Evidence Based Treatments for Trauma-Related Psychological Disorders: a practical guide for clinicians*. New York, NY: Springer International (pp41–61).

OHCHR (1999). *Istanbul Protocol: manual on the effective investigation and documentation of torture and other cruel, inhuman or degrading treatment or punishment*. Geneva: OHCHR.

Papdopoulous RK (2007). Refugees, trauma and adversity activated development. *European Journal of Psychotherapy and Counselling 9*(3): 301–312.

Persons JB (1989). *Cognitive Therapy in Practice: a case formulation approach*. London: WW Norton & Company.

Raghuvanshi L, Agger I (2008). *Giving voice: using testimony as a brief therapy intervention in psychosocial community work for survivors of torture and organized violence*. Manual for community workers and human rights defenders. Varanasi, India: PVCHR.

Regel S, Berliner P (2007). Current perspectives on assessment and therapy with survivors of torture: the use of a cognitive behavioural approach. *European Journal of Psychotherapy and Counselling 9*(3): 289–299.

Robjant K, Fazel M (2010). The emerging evidence for narrative exposure therapy: a review. *Clinical Psychology Review 30*: 1030–1039.

Royal College of Psychiatrists (2013). *Psychological Therapies/IAPT workstream: evidence based practice update*. [Online]. Royal College of Psychiatrists www.rcpsych.ac.uk/pdf/May%20Update%20-%20Full%20version.pdf (accessed 19 July 2016).

Salcioğlu E, Başoğlu M (2011). Control-focused behavioural treatment of female war survivors with torture and gang rape experience: four case studies. *European Journal of Traumatology 2*(s1): s192.

Schauer M, Neuner F, Elbert T (2012). *Narrative Exposure Therapy: a short-term treatment for traumatic stress disorders* (2nd ed). Cambridge, MA: Hogrefe & Huber.

Schauer M, Neuner F, Elbert T (2011). *Narrative Exposure Therapy: a short-term treatment for traumatic stress disorders* (2nd revised and expanded edition). Gottingen: Hogrefe.

Segal ZV, Williams JMG, Teasdale JD (2002). *Mindfulness-based Cognitive Therapy for Depression: a new approach to preventing relapse*. New York, NY: Guilford Press.

Seligman M (2011). *Flourish: a visionary new understanding of happiness and well-being*. New York, NY: Simon & Schuster.

Shapiro F (2001). *Eye Movement Desensitization and Reprocessing: basic principles, protocols and procedures*. New York, NY: Guilford Press.

Sherif C (1979). Bias in psychology. In: Sherman JA, Beck ET (eds). *The Prism of Sex: essays in the sociology of knowledge*. Madison, WI: University of Wisconsin Press (pp93–133).

Snodgrass LL, Yamamoto J, Frederick C et al (1993). Vietnamese refugees with PTSD symptomatology: intervention via a coping skills model. *Journal of Traumatic Stress* 6: 569–575.

Wells A (2009). *Metacognitive Therapy for Anxiety and Depression*. New York: Guilford Press.

Young J, Klosko J, Weishaar M (2003). *Schema Therapy: a practitioner's guide*. New York: Guilford Press.

10. Queering the pitch: sexuality, torture and recovery

Ashley Fletcher

For all survivors of torture, protection is the fundamental prerequisite to recovery and rehabilitation. The symptoms of trauma are the response to exposure to jeopardy, the interface with a life-and-death situation. So long as this jeopardy continues through the asylum system, with the threat of return to the survivor's country of origin, the other goals of therapy can remain elusive. The therapist has a responsibility, a duty, to address the issue of protection effectively in order to work towards rehabilitation. For the survivor, safety in therapy is key.

Many of the chapters in this book articulate the principles, approaches and experiences of psychological therapy with torture survivors. Many issues influencing the therapeutic relationship, recovery and rehabilitation will, through those chapters, be conveyed to the reader. My contribution is the exploration of the role of sexuality in the process, and how it affects the survivor's experience of torture and, perhaps more importantly, their capacity for recovery.

My work over the last 35 years has been with 'sexual minorities': specifically, men who have sex and relationships with other men, but don't necessarily identify as 'gay' or 'bisexual', although many do. The standard collective research term for these men is 'men who have sex with men'. This term has been in use in the public health discourse since at least 1990.

This has been my focus in both the NHS and in voluntary sector HIV services, private practice and, for the last eight years, in a human rights organisation, working specifically with survivors of torture. This chapter focuses on the experience of this group of survivors, although some aspects will be relevant to lesbian, transsexual and other sexual minority communities.

For all torture survivors, there are three key elements to recovery that need to be addressed: first, protection and how to address risk; second, trauma and how to manage symptoms, and third, rehabilitation, a return to normal functioning. For most survivors in the UK, the asylum process itself is a major inhibiting factor in work to address these issues. For survivors from lesbian, gay, bisexual and transsexual (LGBT) communities, their very identity is placed at the centre of this process.

Verification of 'I am what I am' supersedes their story of their struggle to survive (Gaynor, 1984). It is my aim in this chapter to explore discursive (dialogic) rather than interrogative (empirical) interviewing techniques as a means of securing the principle requirements for recovery: ie. how an understanding of the transnational and cross-cultural aspects of a marginalised sexuality can secure protection and therapy for LGBT survivors. I also outline the interviewing techniques I have used with gay male survivors to enable me to write a psychological report, when requested by their legal representatives, to support their goal of securing protection in the UK.

The terms sexuality and sexual orientation can be distinctly different or interchangeable in their meanings, depending on which of the many nuanced definitions you are reading. Some say sexual orientation is the 'who and how' of attraction, and sexuality the 'what and where' of sexual activity. Others define sexual orientation as the direction of sexual identity, and sexuality as the innate nature of desire. Whichever is used will be debatable. Reflecting these nuances, and following my own view and experience, I have chosen to use both of these terms throughout.

It is important to draw a distinction between a 'gay-identified' man, which refers to a shared set of points of sub-cultural reference and an identity based on these, and 'homosexual', which refers primarily to same-sex sexual preference and behaviour.

While the lexicon of gay terminology is both contemporary and fluid, this needs to be understood to comprehend how gay men, forced to hide the public expression of their relationships and sexuality, are, by sharing these points of reference, able to identify each other without attracting the attention of others. The terminology, though, is perhaps irrelevant: survivors are not necessarily tortured because of their identity or label, but because of their same-sex activity or desire, however they describe it. For the purpose of making the chapter more human, I will mostly use the words 'gay' or 'gay men' throughout, as an inadequate but convenient shorthand, rather than reduce everyone to initials or research labels.

There is, of course, no objective measure of an individual's sexual orientation or the identity they might attach to or associate with it. Desire, orientation and identity are highly subjective (although inter-subjectively negotiated), as are the assumptions, attitudes and consequent judgments they may attract. As a gay man, I can only refer to my own experience, and the 35 years in which I have specialised in the experiences and physical and psychological health and wellbeing of what might broadly be termed 'sexual minorities', with a variety of self-concepts, whatever identity is claimed by the individual concerned. For the last 15 years I have worked (though not exclusively) with sexual minorities facing the specific challenges of asylum, trauma and recovery – a context that has necessitated objective measures of these experiences to judge, believe or disbelieve.

The Home Office itself finally recognised this and issued an Asylum Policy Instruction (API) on sexual orientation in asylum claims in August 2016, which was a great step forward. The API states: 'In other cultures, this term [LGB] or even the term homosexual is not used as a form of self-identification by people with a same-gender physical, romantic and/or emotional attraction. The term may exist but have very different connotations and may not imply any shared social identity or particular community affiliation based on sexual orientation' (Home Office, 2016a: 6).

This goes a long way to meet the Yogyakarta principles on the application of international human rights law in relation to sexual orientation and gender identity, which '... is understood to refer to each person's capacity for profound emotional, affectional and sexual attraction to, and intimate and sexual relations with, individuals of a different gender or the same gender or more than one gender' (Onufer Corrêa et al, 2007: 1).

This chapter navigates its way through the complexity of terminology, identity and experience in an attempt to address the asylum system's focus on 'evidence' of the survivor's story as the route to decision-making. This evidence is largely located in the documented experience of sexuality and identity in western culture. This chapter aims at evidencing non-western experience and accounts through cross-cultural comparisons.

I must openly declare my partisanship. I am committed of course to human rights, but, perhaps most importantly, I am opposed to human wrongs. However, I hope that I bring both insight and understanding of this client group, who in my experience are the most excluded, even within the marginalised communities of which they form a part.

I also hope in this endeavour to offer practical approaches to both validation (the acceptance and belief of the client's story), and verification (the capturing and documenting of this story as evidence that will help build the therapeutic relationship and contribute towards securing a pathway to protection).

Psychosocial dislocation

People fleeing from persecution due to their sexual orientation have one other thing in common: homosexuality, or same sex activity, is illegal in almost all the countries of origin of people seeking asylum in the UK. In the top five countries of origin in 2015, homosexuality is a punishable offence, and it carries the death penalty in two of them: Iran and Sudan (Home Office, 2016b).

In many cases, regardless of political, legislative or social repression, the persecution, criminalisation and even execution of sexual minorities receives widespread public support or acquiescence. For the gay person, this represents a unique degree of psychosocial dislocation from their nation, home culture or 'meta-tribe', compounding issues of isolation and inhibiting disclosure when seeking protection, as well as when seeking understanding, support or solidarity towards redress, recovery and rehabilitation.

It might seem counterintuitive, given the current culture in the UK, that until very recently the Home Office was not sympathetic to survivors of this near-global persecution, preferring instead (up until a Supreme Court ruling in 2010) to reject their initial asylum claims. A report by the UK Lesbian and Gay Immigration Group (UKLGIG, 2010) found that, while 73% of all initial asylum were rejected in 2009, the refusal rate was 98–99% among the claims made by lesbians and gay men that were brought to UKLGIG's attention. In the majority of these refusals, it was argued that the persecution was somehow invited and that the applicant could conceal their sexuality by behaving discretely and thus avoid bringing upon themselves unwanted attention (often implying that they could relocate to a different area, where their sexuality was not known).

This approach was challenged by the Supreme Court, which ruled that:[1] 'To pretend that it [the immutable characteristic of the particular social group's sexual orientation or sexuality] does not exist, or that the behaviour by which it manifests itself can be suppressed, is to deny the members of this group their fundamental right to be what they are', and this was in breach of the 1951 Refugee Convention.

This decision, however, has merely shifted the goalposts, as the culture of disbelief that pervades the asylum system has now shifted, and credibility is now the main focus (Held, 2016). As Paul Dillane, former Amnesty expert and former CEO of UKLGIG commented: 'Consistently, we see cases where the answer the Home Office is giving is "No, you're lying, you're making it

---

1. See *HJ (Iran) and HT (Cameroon) v Secretary of State for the Home Department* [2010] UKSC 31

up"... in practice, years after the Supreme Court's judgement, we're still seeing cases that raise serious concerns about how the credibility assessment is taking place' (Batchelor, 2015). He highlighted 'inappropriate, shocking and highly sexualised questions', adding that the 'Home Office find it bizarre that (on £5 a day) they're not going clubbing in their local community. There are assumptions about what it is that a "good" gay applicant should be doing'. Initial decision-making is still weighted very much against the applicant.

We can see and understand that the experience of gay men and other sexual minorities of exclusion, repression, torture, exile, trauma, recovery and rehabilitation has significant implications both for the relationship and the responsibility that the therapist must assume when working with survivors from these communities.

The price of identity

For survivors, whether detained at a demonstration, seized off the street or abducted in a dawn raid, a hole is punched through the normality of their life, and a world of certainties, assumptions and familiarities ends. Most survivors I have worked with feel their old world ends there, to be replaced by the surreal space of powerlessness and dread – like death itself, almost unimaginable and impossible to prepare for.

Torture takes place for many different reasons and takes different forms, but at its heart, universally, is an attack on an individual's sense of self. The aim of the abductor and the torturer is to remove from us our sense of entitlement. It is a state where we are no longer a citizen; where there are no rights; where our education, skills or status count for nothing. Points of reference, past and future relationships, disappear into an arbitrary, lawless, relentless present, free of restraint or morality. The construct of identity is shattered. Survival begins here. 'The primary aim is more to break down the identity of the victim. The pain consists in particular in this breaking down and in the destruction of the personality' (Elsass, 1997: 10).

This dissembling experience varies in length and content, but key to surviving are the survivor's resources and resilience. For many, the connections and structures from which they have been taken give them the strength to endure and the goal to which to return. It is here that the departure from commonality of experience often becomes evident for clients who are LGBT. In most cases (in all that I have worked with), if the person is known to be gay, then ostracisation and exile follow, at best; prosecution, torture or murder (judicial or otherwise) at worst. If their sexual orientation is not previously known, then public exposure, with the same consequences, invariably follows arrest. Traditional sources of resilience are either missing or imperilled by the event. The cost to identity is already huge.

It is also here that a commonality of experience with LGBT communities in the west emerges, which can form the basis for evidencing and verifying the client's experiences. What gay people have in common is often caricatured as imagined sexual practices by non-gay people. In reality, what they share is a fear of the consequences of the relationships to which they are drawn. The term 'closet' has become commonplace in western understanding of the lives of sexual minorities, denoting a sexuality that is kept secret, hidden from the family and wider society.

This is not a space in which to thrive, but one that already requires an instinct for survival. Rarely do gay men see their sexuality as normal and that society around them is at fault. Cultural norms inform them that they are profoundly damaged, wicked and not entitled to acceptance or belonging. It is a cause of shame, and a product of fear that can traumatise, independently of any torture event. The closet is a means of survival in a world where heteronormative values are so taken for granted that only in our current political generation have stigma and prejudice become considered worthy of challenge. 'It is practically impossible for a lesbian, gay or bisexual person who has grown up in British society *not* to have internalised society's negative images about their sexuality' (Davies, 1996: 55).

What is unique to being gay is the experience of living with a clandestine identity and the cultural 'bilingualism' that enables you to seamlessly fit into the majority society around you and develop sub-cultural points of reference that connect and enable you to communicate with others in the same situation – an experience that cuts across cultures, even if the specifics do not.

Western concepts of identity often revolve around cultural specifics that may be known to other cultures through the diffusion of international travel or social media. These western beliefs about the lives of gay men are often erroneously used as the benchmark to verify sexuality. The benchmark should be the commonality of experience of clandestine sexuality and its consequences. This is the marker on which we should base our assessment.

Where the person's sexuality is known to the torturer, the form that abuse takes can become quite specific (though by no means exclusive) for sexual minorities. Rape is endemic in the experience of torture survivors, but the disclosing of sexuality to other inmates makes the survivor the object of abuse from guards and other prisoners alike ('The guards would laugh and encourage the other inmates to rape me'). Genital abuse and ritual humiliation are common punishment ('They tied a cord to my penis and paraded me through the police station, calling me a pede [pederast]'). Visible scarring and disfigurement are commonly used, generally signifying the torturer's sense of impunity ('They slashed at my face saying "Now no one will ever touch you"'). Other tactics include photographing or filming the assault to humiliate and control the survivor ('They filmed me on mobile phones. They said they would show it to my mother and put it on the internet') – I have paraphrased examples I have heard. Sexuality, identity and disclosure are indelibly stamped with danger and humiliation. This has consequences when seeking asylum.

Many torture survivors, whatever their orientation, are reluctant to disclose torture in their initial screening and substantive interviews with the Home Office in the UK, fearing that they will be seen as having merited it in some way, or be seen as troublemakers. They may fear that disclosure will bring retribution on family or friends, or cannot face recounting what they have been through. In many cases, their narrative is so disordered through trauma that coherent recall seems impossible (an aim of torture – if you cannot tell the story you won't be believed; if you aren't believed, you will not have a case; without a case, there can be no redress or retribution). This often leads to disbelief when torture is brought up late in a claim for asylum, on grounds that, if it were true, it would have been disclosed earlier. Changing your story can be seen as a sign of a lack of credibility, and tends then to be extended to cover all aspects of the case.

This also applies to disclosure around sexuality. In my experience, sexuality isn't disclosed for the same reasons, and others. Invariably, the sexuality of the survivor is a criminal offence in the country they have fled from and, in my experience, many survivors have no idea that it is legal in the UK. Sexuality has associations with being judged and abused, and the Home Office interviewer is a stranger who possibly shares this view, and if not the interviewer, then the interpreter, who may come from a similar cultural background to the survivor. Many clients have described hostility from interpreters when talking about their sexuality and abuse: 'I'm not going to translate that, you bring shame to our community'; 'You're a disgrace to your family.' In some cases, the interpreter is seen to be sharing a joke with the interviewer, or simply not translating at all. Barriers to disclosure can continue in consultations with legal representatives: 'I didn't tell my first solicitor; she seemed very busy and didn't look at me. I didn't feel comfortable.' The key issue of credibility then comes in when sexuality is later disclosed.

At whatever stage of disclosure, as mentioned above, the default position of the Home Office is to disbelieve, and the process of verification becomes of key importance to whoever is taking the account. For the legal representative, this is central to the success of the asylum claim; for the therapist, this is the key to protection and achieving the other therapeutic goals.

The Home Office approach seeks answers, rather than understanding. An interrogative approach that addresses the curiosity of the questioner is framed from their perspective (and consequently, their assumptions and prejudices.) By seeking factual verification, this empirical approach, in my experience, is founded on a perception of homosexuality that is deeply rooted in a medical model, and seeks evidence of it as a pathology. Homosexuality was only removed from the *Diagnostic and Statistical Manual of Mental Disorders* (DSM) in 1987.

This pathology-based practice has deep roots in western understanding. Up until 2014, the Czech Republic was using a pseudo-scientific method called phallometry to evidence sexuality in asylum cases. This is the attaching of electrodes to the genitals to measure stimulation during exposure to erotic images. Now roundly condemned, its roots lie in the development in the 1960s of electric shock treatment as aversion therapy (Tatchell, 2016).

While such barbaric practices have ended, the interrogative approach still seeks verification by using forensic techniques that are at times crudely sexual and explicit. In 2014, John Vine, the then Independent Chief Inspector of Borders and Immigration in the UK, investigated what he called 'intrusive and unsatisfactory' questioning that invited LGBT applicants 'to give sexually explicit responses that were likely to be irrelevant to their asylum claims'. Assessing that this occurred in about 10% of cases, he added that the questions 'appeared to be formulated to make claimants feel uncomfortable... implying their sexuality was a deviance...' (Travis, 2014).

The parameters of the interrogative approach adopted by Home Office interviewers has changed following his report, but the binary formulations of who, how, what, when, where and why continue to fail to capture an unfamiliar context that eludes the questioner's understanding. It not only fails in its own aim to gain verification of sexuality, but could open itself up to abuse, and at the same time trigger the experience of detention and interrogation for LGBT people seeking protection.

Breaking the boundaries

A more damaging outcome of the interrogative approach is that it inevitably produces the very contradictions it seeks as evidence of lack of credibility. During my time working with gay survivors, I have seen the consequent conclusions drawn both in initial Home Office decisions and also by tribunal judges in their appeal determinations for gay men from a wide range of cultural backgrounds. The following are typical examples:

> Iran: 'If you were as discrete as you say you needed to be, you and your boyfriend would not have known each other were gay.'
>
> Egypt: 'Why would you have taken the risk with your boyfriend in a public place when you knew that it would be so risky?'
>
> Pakistan: 'Yet you allowed the arrangements for your wedding to continue for two years despite knowing you were gay.'
>
> Uganda: 'Homosexuality is illegal and it is therefore unlikely that a prison officer, an upholder of the law, would have raped you.'
>
> Cameroon: 'You responded that you were happy as a teenager whilst [quoting a US LGBT study] states that you LGBT people are unhappy in their teenage years.'

In one case, the judge accused the claimant of 'conflating homosexuality and abuse' when the survivor was recounting that his first sexual experience had been with an adult while at school. This represents a minefield, not just for the client but for the Home Office too, which mires itself more and more in guidance that limits but does not illuminate the parameters of questioning.

In contrast, the therapist needs to have a completely different aim and approach: that of exploration and evidencing through validation. As will be shown, validation elicits verification, which in turn can be documented in a report for the person's legal representative, citing the parallels with western culture and literature that are already noted and understood. This documentation can assist with the key need of survivors of torture for protection within the asylum system. The therapist is in a unique position to enable this as a natural enhancement of the therapeutic relationship that seeks to build safety and psychological contact. To some practitioners, this may initially seem counter-intuitive, changing from 'being' in therapy to 'doing', and so breaking the boundaries of traditional western therapeutic concepts.

Indeed, 20 years ago, when I worked for an HIV charity, a counsellor at a hospital clinic called our centre to ask if our welfare fund could give £5 to an impoverished client who had just finished a session. In response to the answer 'yes', the counsellor then asked if we would pay for a taxi for the client to come and collect it, at a further cost of £15. When asked if the counsellor had £5 that they could give the client (which we would reimburse later from our welfare fund), the response was an emphatic refusal: 'That would break the boundaries of the client-therapist relationship.'

For the therapist not to see the link between action and the outcome for the client is a dereliction of duty. The paradigms we work with have changed, as have the lives of so many of our clients. Hardship is now destitution, and the stakes for thousands have never been higher. 'Protection', for the therapist, must change from a noun that describes the need of the client to a verb that secures it. This is the essence of a human-rights approach to psychotherapy with torture survivors.

Voice of authenticity

The starting point, as always, is the relationship – one that is thought through and prepared for by the therapist, and is transparent and congruent, not just a 'meeting' in a therapeutic space. Relationship and trust play a part in all therapeutic encounters as a crucial enabler of intimacy and disclosure. For many sexual minorities, though, relationship itself may be problematic.

In my experience, gay men do not seamlessly come to an awareness of their difference and conclude that they are right and society around them is wrong. They sense disapproval, disdain, hatred or danger, which will be powerfully absorbed and internalised. With this comes the experience that acceptance and safety are highly conditional on being perceived as 'normal' and conforming. This can undermine a sense of entitlement in every aspect of life and activity, within the family, at school, work, in institutions, in the street, café or shop. This is key to survival with clandestine sexuality in a hostile culture, whether it is explicitly so, or otherwise.

Building trust and connection on this basis is a conscious task of demonstrating openness, receptiveness and accessibility to disclosure of sexuality and history. If the therapist is from a sexual minority, their own disclosure should be considered an optimising opportunity. If the therapist is not from a sexual minority, they should give thought to how they will receive, reflect on and understand such disclosure by the client. In both cases, supervision will be a crucial means of processing impact, transference and countertransference issues for the therapist.

While sexual disclosure is not central to verifying sexuality, the therapist must be congruent about their feelings towards the client. It is axiomatic in therapy that both respect and understanding of the client's internal frame of reference are core conditions for working successfully. A sense of repulsion is a block to these conditions being realised. The fact that the client's context may be unfamiliar to us is not the key issue: there are very many client circumstances and experiences that will be new to us, but that is not the route to verification. While there are always new contexts, arguably there are no new feelings; I might have no capacity to imagine being tortured in an Iranian prison, but I can still empathise with shock, despair and hopelessness. It is the client's understanding and feelings about that experience that are the voice of authenticity, which in turn, through its western parallels, can then be documented.

Therapy

A sense of safety or entitlement, the right to respect, and to openness and authenticity in relationships are often absent in the lives of gay men in their home societies. This doesn't mean that they have not found imaginative and creative ways of surviving, or even thriving, in their absence, although this may have been undone by detention and torture. It does mean that they may have no expectation of anything different from the therapist.

The asylum system itself, with its institutional default to disbelief of the survivor, will, in my experience, have disappointed the expectations of the gay man seeking protection. It is crucial, then, that, as well as being open to disclosure, as described above, the therapist must be conscious of not appearing to replicate the priorities or processes of the Home Office. Naming and labelling detail is not the most important part of identity, but they can be potentially demeaning red herrings.

This openness must involve an awareness of the potential for homophobia and heterosexism, inadvertently mirroring the Home Office. The client's experience of this from the Home Office may frame his expectations of the therapist. In other words, the approach to verify an individual's sexual identity should take into account the 'presumption' of heterosexuality within the dominant culture. This is the basis of 'heterosexism': 'a presumption of heterosexuality which is encoded in language, in institutional practices and the encounters of everyday life' (Epstein & Johnson, 1994: 198).

Understanding a client's feelings of shame could be of crucial importance. Shame and guilt often feature highly for survivors in any circumstances, but in relation to sexuality, it has often been an internalised response to cultural expectation and blame, irrespective of a torture event. Belief and validation are what the therapist should aim for. The therapist should use a discursive (dialogic) approach, exploring the experience of the client, framed from their perspective, thus enabling an exploration of content that has a contextual authenticity.

The course of therapy itself is, in my experience, the same as with other torture-survivor clients. My approach is consistent with the three-stage model that Judith Herman elaborates (1992). Here she asserts: 'The central task of the first stage is the establishment of safety. The central task of the second stage is remembrance and mourning. The central focus of the third stage is reconnection with ordinary life' (p155).

Essentially, this is stabilisation, processing and rehabilitation. What can be important in its difference is its content, and, indeed, the significance of that content. As already emphasised, effective therapy rests on the quality of the relationship, its components being safety, intimacy and trust. This relationship is initiated in a contract that conveys these essential conditions. With vulnerable clients, undertaking practical casework tasks or advocating for a survivor, where required, can be an important part of helping this relationship grow, and can demonstrate both care and containment.

Powerlessness is political

One of the healing goals of therapy, for survivors, is not just to talk and reprocess the torture experience, but to reconnect with a sense of self, repair the hiatus in their personal story, and regain a sense of entitlement and respect. It is to belong again. For most gay survivors, the barriers and starting points for this can be quite different to those of other survivors. Often they have never formed or articulated an acceptable personal narrative; they have only the socially constructed one they have created in order to conform. If they have, it is only within a narrow, specific context (among a few other contacts or intimates in the same circumstances).

Telling 'their' story has never been an option for most gay survivors. Consequently, the prospect of continuing relationships following such disclosures may seem anathema to them, and very risky. Thus, the focus is less on regaining a sense of entitlement and more on working to help the client discover one. This requires a solidity of respect and the availability of new connection that doesn't reproduce the limitations of past encounters. Passive 'non-judgmentalism' may be insufficient. Power is political, powerlessness is political too, and a partisan commitment to that right, to validation, is essential as the manifestation of acceptance and respect. If the personhood of the gay client is to be fostered, it cannot be as a restored, closeted, social pariah, but as a grounded and acceptable identity or self-concept, as far as the client is able. Without this, there is neither respect, entitlement nor an authentic relationship.

This recounting can be a genuinely liberating process for the client. For the therapist, it demands a commitment to its consequences. Acceptance and recognition as a gay person finally cuts off a return to the past, to a closeted re-immersion in a hostile and potentially violent home culture. For the client, it will be clear that there is no going back from here. This is where the difference is of great significance. A new story made possible through validation can provide its own verification in its authenticity. The documentation of this in the form of a written report, using verifiable parallels with what is already known and understood of the experience of clandestine sexuality in western society, may contribute to securing protection.

Talking through these issues allows the client to find an experiential narrative that expresses who they are, allowing a unique contextual authenticity to emerge that is hard to counterfeit and difficult to refute. It can empower the client with a new confidence and ability to provide verification for their case for protection. Unlike the interrogative Home Office approach, it establishes the language, terminology and significance that can be documented against well-researched sub-cultural parallels in western culture.

My practice has evolved over the years as a form of reflexive praxis. Representatives have identified that such reports have played a significant part in successfully overturning negative Home Office decisions at appeal in the Asylum Tribunal, where the case has rested on sexual orientation.

It is not my intention here to change the practice of the Home Office towards more just and therefore more effective outcomes (though that would be welcome), as justice is not their brief. It is their role and culture to control and limit successful outcomes, as evidenced by the number of cases successfully challenging initial Home Office decision-making on appeal to the Asylum Tribunal. The proportion of asylum appeals allowed in 2015 increased from 28% in 2014 to 35% (Refugee Council, 2016).

However, Home Office guidelines change, as will be shown later, and asylum applications continue to be met with disbelief. It is my suggestion that, in response to this, attention to the quality of a survivor's testimony and its recording for possible report writing will continue to be a key responsibility of the human-rights therapist and practitioner.

To preserve the confidentiality of survivors I have worked with, I am using fictional case studies that are composites from my work with gay men over the last 20 years. I aim to give an accurate portrayal of the results and benefits of this discursive, as opposed to interrogative, approach, and the process from there to verifiable documentation in the form of a therapy report.

Feeling heard can be transforming

Interrogative approaches focus on facts and detail, as in this typical sequence of questions from a Home Office substantive interview, which generally elicit answers of a few words, and mainly yes or no:

> When did you come to realise you were gay? What happened that made you realise you were gay? Was there a particular thing that happened or experience that made you aware you were gay? Did that [sexual intercourse] make you realise you were gay? The question I asked is was there a particular thing that happened or experience that made you aware of being gay?

A discursive approach focuses on experience and meaning, such as this sequence of questions from a therapy session:

> How did you feel being asked the question, 'When did you first know you were gay?' When did you first have a sense that the difference you felt made you feel unsafe? Were you aware of words used for people having a secret like yours, or did you have a name or words for it yourself? Between yourselves, and amongst other people like you, did you have words/use a language to describe each other that was distinct from how others might describe you?

This elicits explanations, emotion and reminiscence, which could come from nowhere else but experience. For example, a response brought out by the first Home Office question, 'When did you come to realise you were gay?' was: 'When I was 13 or 14 years old.'

And this was the answer to the first dialogic question, 'How did you feel being asked the question "When did you first know you were gay?"':

> How am I supposed to answer a question like that? Who is he to ask a gay man a question like that when he didn't even look at me? I said 13 because I felt pressured and that was when I was first involved with someone, but it could have been six or 10. I knew a long time before that I wasn't interested in girls but I have no idea what age I 'knew' I was gay. I didn't use that word for a long time. How did I feel about it then? I am nearly 40 now,

how am I supposed to remember my feelings from when I was a child? A lot has happened since.

The first type of question brings out a response that anyone could give, and is followed by questions that open the door to apparent contradictions. Was it 13 or 14? Which experience or event? Why the lack of answers when the clear question is being repeated? It ends up questioning the validity of the survivor story. For example:

Why did you not tell your friends and family or work colleagues you were gay? Did you know how homosexuality was viewed... before you were caught? Why then would you take such a risk?... You were engaged in a gay sexual act in public, I don't understand why you would take such a risk knowing the possible consequences.

The question gives rise to defensiveness, embarrassment and shame: 'It was only a moment and I paid a big penalty for it. It was night time and it was dark. It was two minutes and we weren't expecting those people.'

The second type of question gives an emotional, social, experiential context, which could only be given by one person, the one with an authentic experience. The difference that this makes is that it opens other pathways for the testimony to unfold. Being listened to is important; feeling heard can be transforming. For example, the question: 'Can you help me understand about your early realisations of attraction, sex and recognition of difference?' brings forth a rich narrative that is spontaneous and remembered, suggesting real experience:

At primary school, we were all doing it. It seemed natural. No one called it gay and it wasn't sex, it was just a little naughty and fun. Showing each other things and boys playing with each other, we all did it. What changed is that others seemed to grow out of it, but I didn't. That's when I began to realise things were different for me. I realised girls fancied me but I wasn't interested like other boys. I felt ashamed and hoped it was a phase but it didn't change. I tried to hide it and became more secretive, what could I do? By 13 or 14, I began having sex with my best friend, but it would always be while we were pretending to do our homework together, so people didn't think anything of it.

In this account, the client demonstrates an intimate and personal relationship to the experience of growing up gay and living clandestinely in a hostile dominant culture. He talks of feelings, not just sex, and describes shame at his early discoveries. He expresses frustration with a simplistic understanding of his dilemma in relation to the concept of sexual exploration, of the morally imbued question of relationship rather than sex. His account of early sexual exploration before forming a gay identity is coherent and consistent and rarely a connection that is made in the context of a 'heterosexual' identity.

Vignettes of lives lived

Continuing with this benign, open curiosity about the experience, rather than a fixation on the detail, invites the unfolding of a narrative of what it is like to experience a clandestine relationship within a hostile culture, from which words, phrases, concepts and structures emerge that allow cross-cultural comparisons to be made. The common threads with western cultural concepts can then be documented as facets and attributes of the lives of sexual minorities. Here are examples of how that documentation can be applied.

A Francophone client used the French term 'sortir de la noir' ('out of the night') as his cultural expression of 'coming out of the closet', a familiar subcultural concept in the west. To the question, 'Among those you were familiar with, how were you able to express "mutuality" or community, or how did you refer to yourselves/each other?', he responded: 'We didn't use community, that means church or meeting. We used a street language of "pigeon" English. "Boy" was our word for ourselves and each other, whether the person was a "boy" or not.'

'Gay' was not a term they used with one another, but they did use the word 'boy'. This use of colloquial references among themselves, as distinct from people 'not like us', has its documentable parallels in western gay culture. I then asked for help in understanding how he would know who was gay and who wasn't: how did men manage acknowledgement and communication?

> You got to hear where 'those' [he used derogatory words to describe 'those' people] hang out. I went to check it out. It was dangerous and all very subtle. Gestures, winks, catching someone's eye. Bars were full of dangers, toilets too, but sometimes you just knew. Not even names or 'dates'. That was too dangerous, but you just know.

In the west, a common expression for the community to be able to 'read itself' is 'gaydar', a phenomenon now being widely researched in the US and Europe. Dr Lorenza Colzato and colleagues of Leiden University in the Netherlands have stated (2010): 'Scientific proof has been found for the existence of a gaydar mechanism amongst homosexuals. This perceptual skill allows homosexuals to recognise other gay people faster and we think it's because they are much more analytical than heterosexuals.' This phenomenon has importance in this case. It is never easy for an 'outsider' to become an 'insider' in any distinct community, especially one alert to its own concerns about marginalisation and safety. The client added:

> Sometimes women would hang out with us. Friends. They didn't seem to mind so much. They would hang out with us and we looked like we fitted in. We would say 'Elle est ma choucha'. Figuratively, 'She is my vagina.'

These relationships with women for appearance sake have their equivalent in the west, where the term 'beard' emerged in the 1960s to describe a female companion of a gay or bisexual man, '... to provide that person with a heterosexual "disguise", usually for marriage or career purposes'. PinkUK, the online gay slang dictionary, puts it thus: '... a beard is used to make the world think the gay partner is straight. Sometimes the beard knows they are a beard, sometime they are being deceived.'

This is the response from another client to the same questions:

> Between us we played with nicknames. With feminine names. Everyone had one, like a girl or a woman, but it might depend on what role you play: for example, who was the man and who was the woman in bed. Or 'the man' (insertive partner) would be called 'plus', the woman (receptive) would be called 'minus'. My nickname was 'mother', the woman in the relationship is always called 'mother of', as wives and mothers are called in my country.

Role play, the subcultural subversion or incorporation of classic gender role stereotypes, is a subcultural feature we are familiar with in our own culture. A western parallel might be the concept of 'camp', and the roles of butch and femme, and men addressing each other as 'she' or 'her'. Also important is the mention of sexual roles. Research into the sexual practices and identities of communities described as men who have sex with men (primarily in the field of HIV with reference to transmission and prevention, or in academia, concerning social constructionist 'queer theory' and identity) place great significance on the roles of active (insertive) and passive (receptive) partner roles in anal sex. The passive role in such activity is often seen as unacceptably 'feminising', while playing the role of 'active' partner preserves a sense of masculine or heterosexual identity.

Such candidness would only come from someone with a lived experience in that community, as the implied taboos are too great. These are a few examples of the success of the discourse approach in drawing out both circumstantial and contextual authenticity and producing documented parallels that verify sexual identity in reports requested by legal representatives.

This approach has contributed to overturning decisions where there have been issues of credibility and disbelief about the professed identity of a survivor.

From account to action

There are various ways in which this kind of work with survivors can be used for their protection in the asylum process. For the client, there is a renewed sense of entitlement and also an awareness of what has been missing from their case. This can empower and equip survivors to re-instruct their legal representatives to make further submissions, or, in the case of appeal rights exhausted (ARE) survivors, a fresh claim for asylum. If a survivor is unable to do this, an alternative would be for them to inform their legal representative that fresh disclosures of material significance have been made. At this stage, a survivor's legal representative may write to the therapist to request a clinical letter or psychological therapy report that describes what has taken place in therapy.

Report writing is a necessary part of the responsibilities of the human-rights therapist if they are mindful of their duty to protect and witness. This is a shift of focus and responsibility for the therapist, and as such should be preceded by familiarisation with the *Istanbul Protocol* (OHCHR, 1999). This sets out the internationally recognised standards for the documentation of the physical and psychological evidence of torture.

In all cases where protection is an issue, therapy notes should be accurate and detailed. If a clinical letter or report cannot be assembled from the notes taken in sessions, or further information is needed, structured interview time can be arranged outside of therapy for the account to be taken.

For report purposes, the approach remains the same: keep to the principle that the survivor's voice is an authentic testimony that will ultimately speak for itself. The therapist's role is to draw out the common parallels that emerge from the account. I have already used some examples of the types of questions that enable the story to unfold. If this is a focused interview, it is best to have considered what other questions will be most likely to illuminate the client's experience. Here are other suggestions that could be used in specific interview contexts:

Relationships and language. Can you help me understand your sexual relationship(s), whether it was different from what you had with other men/boys? Did your relationship feel different and did you know of any other gay men? How long had you been with this partner and how would describe your relationship?

Others and safety. How did you and your partner(s) both realise each other was gay and that you liked each other? Were there places you might go where you would know there were other people like you? Were you able to find a place that was safe to be in relationship and be together?

Expectations and clandestine life. At home, was there ever any pressure to meet women or have girlfriends? What are your feelings about the expectation that you would or should have sex/relationships with women? Were you ever able to tell your family what was happening for you?

Identity and feelings. Were you aware of other people like you, gay, who feared the consequences of it and how would you know where they were or how to find them? Have you ever felt responsible for being gay or that you had 'chosen' it? Is there any one thing you could do to change things around your sexuality?

Life in exile. How has life been for you now in the UK and how could it be different? Can you help me understand what other obstacles might exist to more freely explore your sexuality here? How do you feel about the idea/question that you could be more involved with relationships and LGBT groups since being in the UK than you have been?

Dilemmas and consequences. Did you feel it was possible to carry on like this? What had got in the way of your experience and caution that had led to taking that risk? How do you feel about the possibility of return and how your family would react?

This list is not exhaustive or prescriptive, and the therapist should adapt it to meet the requirements of the instructions from the legal representative. It is the approach and methodology that are important.

Eye of the regime

Trends are difficult to gauge, as the Home Office does not publicise statistics on asylum claims related to sexuality, despite a longstanding commitment to do so. It has become more widely recognised by LGBT activists that the interrogative approach of the Home Office continues to fail LGBT people in the asylum process, including torture survivors (Held, 2016).

For the last few years, the London-based human rights barrister S Chelvan has been developing a model for interviewing sexual minorities, the Difference, Stigma, Shame, Harm (DSSH) model (Chelvan, 2014), for use by legal representatives and report writers. This is an important and innovative guide, but it also needs to capture identity, memory, relationships and their understanding of their experience.

This, as already referred to above, is now recognised to some degree by the Home Office in its current API on sexual orientation in asylum claims (2016a: 6).

It does, however, still beg the question as to whether it is the guidance or the culture of disbelief that is the main issue that needs to change. I know of a gay survivor who was refused asylum after being asked many questions about a sexual act in public that had led to his discovery in his home country. The interviewer, applying a mechanical and formulaic interpretation, in line with the guidance, subjectively concluded that the client had talked too much about sex and not about the emotional content of the relationship, and was consequently not gay.

The API itself still explicitly states: 'Any perceived lack of contact with the LGB community is a relevant area of investigation to explore and they should be considered on a case-by-case basis, in the round with all other evidence' (Home Office, 2016a: 23). The API also makes explicit that, if an individual has been found to be LGB and from a country where LGB people are persecuted, there can be no presumption that the person making the application will not be removed or that the Home Office can automatically grant protection. If the Home Office thinks the applicant has the intention to remain discrete and not act (for whatever reason) in a manner that may bring their sexuality to attention, there is no case of risk on return and consequently no need for protection.

Moreover, the ban on basing decisions on stereotyping, explicit questioning or explicit images (such as photographs of sexual intimacy) is driven by current EU law and directives. This raises the question of the implications for future decision-making when the UK leaves the European Union.

The interviews I draw from above, where disbelief of the client's sexuality has been of key importance to their asylum claim, are conducted in a two-hour session, based loosely around a framework of 25 questions. I have used this approach for both report writing and to help the client formulate their own coherent narrative to relate to their legal representative.

The current system continues to retraumatise torture survivors from all communities through its default to disbelief. This disbelief is shocking for people who see their core and formative experiences forensically shredded in front of their eyes, with potential fatal consequences. If the issue of their sexuality were not in the eye of their home country's authorities before the asylum case, it will be after.

One client mocked this process by asking, if he was not believed, would he at least be given a certificate of his non-gayness to take back with him for protection?

Personal in every sense

The approach I take, and the way I apply it, is not a sudden discovery; nor is it entirely new. I lay no claim to any 'exceptionalism' over to whom it should be applied and how. Indeed, it has gradually condensed over time, from my life, my experiences and my practice, into a solid and structured approach that optimises the benefit of therapy and ensures the best outcome for the client in terms of usable evidential testimony.

Writing this chapter has been a valuable opportunity for me to give a coherent account of my experience. This has progressed from my own anecdotal recounting to documenting and evidencing. All the gay clients I have worked with now have refugee status, despite their initial (and sometimes subsequent) refusals, after an average wait of three years. Many other gay people seeking asylum wait much longer; many are still refused.

The outcome for me as a therapist, when a report or clinical letter has helped a client, is immensely rewarding. It also takes its toll.

I am a gay man of a certain age and I grew up in a period of relative prohibition and near total admonition. My lived experience has been that all my attachments were not real, but intensely conditional; that the family might not be the safe haven it is supposed to be; that my adolescence and its youthful exploration were unavailable to me, and that the resolution might result in society's total rejection of me, or worse. This gives me insight into and empathy with a context that is resonantly familiar. It also makes me wonder at times whether the great distance the lives of gay people seem to have come is at times illusory – a transient period of affordable tolerance in an evaporating liberal moment.

For me, and for the non-gay therapist, the interface with such a Kafkaesque concept of justice – that is to say, injustice – is a gnawing challenge. The dance between human rights on the one side and the asylum system on the other is both energetic and tiresome, especially when the choreography keeps changing and you do not call the tune.

In the face of stories of torture, abuse and institutional coldness, it is hard not to see society at large as cruel and undeserving. Society is neither of these things, of course, as our clients, who are also a part of it, constantly teach us. For each disappointment I encounter that makes me a little more indifferent to the comparatively minor tribulations of friends and colleagues around me, there comes an inspiration that motivates and re-energises me.

The impact is not just professional and ethical but personal in every sense. For this to be manageable, self-care must also be attended to, through good supervision, training and attending to the quality of my own life and relationships. The eye on the prize for me is that I have learned to thrive, and I passionately aspire to this for my clients too.

References

Batchelor T (2015). Guilty until proven difficult: the trial of LGBT asylum seekers detained in the UK. *New Statesman*; 10 March. www.newstatesman.com/world/2015/03/guilty-until-proven-innocent-trial-lgbt-asylum-seekers-detained-uk (accessed July 2017).

Chelvan S (2014). *DSSH Model and LGBTI Asylum Claims*. Powerpoint presentation. No5 Chambers. www.no5.com/cms/documents/DSSH%20Model%20and%20LGBTI%20Asylum%20 Claims.pdf (accessed July 2017).

Colzato LS, van Hooidonk L, van den Wildenberg WPM, Harinck F, Hommel B (2010). Sexual orientation biases attentional control: a possible gaydar mechanism. [Online.] *Frontiers in Psychology* 7 May. https://doi.org/10.3389/fpsyg.2010.00013 (accessed July 2017).

Davies D (1996). Towards a model of gay affirmative therapy. In: Davies D, Neal C (eds). *Pink Therapy: a guide for counsellors and therapists working with lesbian, gay and bisexual clients.* Maidenhead: Open University Press (pp24–40).

Elsass P (1997). *Treating Victims of Torture and Violence: theoretical, cross-cultural and clinical implications.* New York, NY: New York University Press.

Epstein D, Johnson R (1994). On the straight and narrow: the heterosexual presumption, homophobia and schools. In: Epstein D (ed). *Challenging Lesbian and Gay Inequalities in Education.* Maidenhead: Open University Press.

Gaynor G (1984). I am what I am. In: Gaynor G. *I am Gloria Gaynor.* [Album.] London: Chrysalis Records.

Held N (2016). What does a 'genuine lesbian' look like? Intersections of sexuality and 'race' in Manchester's gay village and in the UK asylum system. In: Stella F, Taylor Y, Reynolds T, Rogers Antoine (eds). *Sexuality, Citizenship and Belonging: transnational and intersectional perspectives.* London/ New York, NY: Routledge (pp131–148).

Herman JL (1992). *Trauma and Recovery: the aftermath of violence – from domestic abuse to political terror.* New York: Basic Books.

Home Office (2016a) *Asylum Policy Instruction: sexual orientation in asylum claims v 6.0.* London: Home Office. www.gov.uk/government/uploads/system/uploads/attachment_data/file/543882/Sexual-orientation-in-asylum-claims-v6.pdf (accessed July 2017).

Home Office (2016b). *National Statistics: asylum.* [Online.] London: Home Office.

www.gov.uk/government/publications/immigration-statistics-october-to-december-2015/asylum (accessed July 2017).

OHCHR (1999). *Istanbul protocol: the UN manual on the principles of the effective investigation and documentation of torture and other cruel, inhuman or degrading treatment or punishment.* Geneva: OHCHR. www.ohchr.org/Documents/Publications/training8Rev1en.pdf (accessed July 2017).

Onufer Corrêa S, Muntarbhorn V (co-chairs) et al (2007). *The Yogyakarta Principles: principles on the application of international human rights law in relation to sexual orientation and gender identity.* [Online.] www.yogyakartaprinciples.org/wp/wp-content/uploads/2016/08/principles_en.pdf (accessed July 2017).

PinkUK (undated). *Gay Slang Dictionary.* [Online.] pinkuk.com/stayingin/slang.aspx (accessed July 2017).

Refugee Council (2016). *Top 20 Facts About Asylum.* [Online.] London: Refugee Council. www.refugeecouncil.org.uk/latest/news/4548_top_20_facts_about_asylum (accessed July 2017).

Tatchell P (2016). *Aversion therapy exposed.* [Blog.] Peter Tatchell. www.petertatchell.net/lgbt_rights/psychiatry/aversion.htm (accessed October 2016).

Travis A (2014). Gay asylum seekers face 'intrusive' sexual questions. London: *The Guardian*; 23 October. www.theguardian.com/uk-news/2014/oct/23/gay-asylum-seekers-sexual-questions-uk-immigration (accessed July 2017).

UK Lesbian and Gay Immigration Group (UKLGIG) (2010). *Failing the Grade.* London: UKLGIG. http://uklgig.org.uk/wp-content/uploads/2014/04/Failing-the-Grade.pdf (accessed October 2016).

11. You are here with us now (we have changed): systemic therapy with families who have survived torture

Emma Roberts

> Torture never happens to one person.
> It taunts the woman: now you can never go home.
> When the man disappears, it warns: you must never do what he did.
> It teaches the children: you won't grow up to be like them.
> Torture reaches through the branches of family, friends, colleagues, villages and cities saying: this has happened and it could happen to you.
> Now we are all changed.

In my work with survivors of torture, there is rarely just one person's experience in the room. Both torture and recovery happen in relationship with others. People have died, are missing, are travelling towards us, are struggling to survive with us, or leaving us, and we have all changed. Because of this, systemic work is often a useful approach.

The world is changing quickly too. We see the human impact of political decisions made far away from the populations they affect. We hear stories of the resulting terror, flight and life in exile for millions. We try to understand something of the huge, physical and cultural distances travelled, the opportunities and challenges for those who often never predicted that this journey would be necessary.

I hope that I will read these words one day in the future, and feel that I have made great changes in my approach, my working methods and the techniques that bring them to life in-session. I make these permanent by writing about them here, but they are never really complete: 'Solutions are only dilemmas that are less of a dilemma than the dilemma one had' (Mason, 1993: 193). Having acknowledged that my work will always be developing, I am grateful for the opportunity to set down some tentative ideas for now.

In this chapter, I will describe two families' positions regarding safety and certainty in their adjustment to life post-torture as they undergo the UK asylum process. I will use the theoretical frame of drawing distinctions and/or making connections for the systemic therapist within the family system. The case studies are fictional and based on amalgamated examples from my practice.

I have worked with survivors of torture for the past 14 years. I began working with families before I knew that systemic therapy existed. Women brought their babies and young children to therapy sessions because there were no alternatives, and, of course, the children joined in.

At that time, my taught theoretical approach was that children should be protected from their parents' experiences and traumatic responses, and that optimal psychological therapy for recovery was the private, adult dyad. At the same time, when I sat among conversations and interactions between family members, I often felt their powerful momentum towards recovery, even – perhaps especially – with the fragmented, traumatised families who had survived torture.

Seeing family members together while striving to maintain an individual focus is a common challenge for those working in the asylum-seeking world. It is not ethical or appropriate to ask children or family members to interpret, but professionals with little time or resources might ask one family member to interpret for the others, or might speak with one person while the rest of the family is present. The lack of physical space in many drop-in centres can make private conversation impossible. Newly arrived children may have to be with parents during difficult conversations because they are not yet enrolled in school, or the family has no home, or no access to childcare. Children usually learn English more quickly than their parents, and so become the voice of the family in many situations. Shamefully, officials at our borders often interview parents about their torture while their children are present.

Some settings, such as substantive interviews for asylum claims, or medical examinations for forensic evidence or healthcare, should offer privacy and confidentiality. Women and girls in any culture will require a confidential space to disclose sexual violence that could place them at risk of being shamed, ostracised or at risk of further violence or abandonment by their family or community. However, family therapy with a professional who is alert to the different requirements of all the family's members can be helpful if they are to work through the trauma of torture together.

When I contracted to undertake individual therapeutic work with women who brought their young children with them to therapy, I had to develop new techniques. The things I said and did in the room came to feel incongruous with my taught model of individual therapy, and this oriented me towards a systemic approach. My interest in systemic work grew more concrete with training and support from others in this field.

As I later learned, this pattern of development fits very well with the systemic idea that changes made at the ground level of working technique can then alter the orientation of one's approach (theories and values), and vice versa (Burnham, 1992).

I find this aspect of systemic theory very useful in work with survivors of torture – a therapeutic setting that is characterised by rapid change. Everyone involved can feel overwhelmed by an unexpected letter threatening homelessness, detention or even forced return to the site of the original torture. The potential for removal is usually held constantly in mind, and is often especially hard to bear for those who have already suffered multiple, sudden, violent losses. For professionals, the sense of unsafe uncertainty (Mason, 1993) relies heavily on innovation in technique, and can be exhausting and shake your sense of competence. I have found that being able to work collaboratively with families during crisis draws on the resilience of everyone involved and often leads to deeper therapeutic connection.

Drawing distinctions (when nothing is changing)

My first experience of systemic working was with a mother and her two-year-old daughter.

Amrha, a survivor of torture from Somalia, was sure that her fragile mental health had harmed her two-year-old daughter, Sara. She presented me with an inflexible belief that their lives were damaged beyond hope. This had become her fixed position. She often spoke of 'always' and 'never' when describing their lives: 'We are always unhappy, we never play.' Their everyday circumstances in the asylum process were punishing, and there appeared to be little space for creativity, optimism or change. Systemic theory suggests that families often come for help in this position of unsafe certainty (Mason, 1993), knowing that things are very bad and thinking that they have no power to change them. They may doubt that change is possible or have a certain belief in just one course of action.

Amrha had only one solution in mind: 'If they decide to send us back, I could kill myself and then Sara would have another family here. Would you find her another family?' A heartbreaking solution. As Mason says of unsafe certainty: 'I guess that all of us, in periods of great stress, have wanted someone to just take the burden of responsibility for change away from us. I wouldn't see this as an unusual request' (Mason, 1993: 194). When I read this paper, many years later, I thought of Amrha's dreadful, logical conclusion.

I worried that our sessions were too much for a small girl, watching her mum cry and talk of hopelessness and suicide. It was also upsetting for me. When I discussed this with Amrha, she qualified my worry and gave me the key for what was useful to her: 'This is all we do at home. I am not good for her. At least you are here with us now.'

It can be tempting to not talk about upsetting things when working with families, for fear of upsetting someone – usually a child – but it may be far worse for the child to experience these things at home, without support from a therapist.

'You are here with us now': Amrha identified my presence, to me a seemingly small difference, as significant to her. Might this allow the family to experience a different space, with new possibilities? We did not know what difference could emerge from being three people together with the distress, but it felt safer. Mason describes this as 'a respectful, collaborative, evolving narrative, one which allows a context to emerge whereby new explanations can be placed alongside rather than instead of, in competition with, the explanations that clients and therapists bring' (1993: 194).

Co-ordinating meaning: how did you reach this place?

Edith Montgomery describes social constructionism theory: 'A person's understanding of his or her reality has a great influence on his or her possibilities of action' (2004: 350–351). This means that we are likely to make choices within our family or other social systems based on our assumptions about their boundaries and limitations. We co-create these realities in relationship with others in the system. These could be explicitly stated laws, or they could be unwritten, even unspoken assumptions about behaviour: 'how we do things' or 'the right way'. This means that we are each creating our own subjective reality. All social systems are evolving all of the time; they adapt as the humans involved redefine unwanted and outdated boundaries, and eventually laws may be amended too.

In each part of our life, or 'context', there will be a highest priority, or 'context marker', by which that context is organised. For example, I could say: 'In my work context, my responsibility for safeguarding is my highest context marker. Ensuring that I fulfil this requirement might be upsetting for a parent; I might also stay at work late and miss a social event, and this would still feel like the right order of priority for me right now.'

Montgomery describes co-ordinated management of meaning (CMM) theory as 'a model for understanding the relationship between meaning and action, and for how change in context-dependent, socially constructed realities takes place' (2004: 351).

Different contexts co-exist in life; we all make different choices, and may even feel and behave like quite different people in each context – family, friendships, work and so on. Experiences in one area can sometimes affect behaviours in another. Systemic theory prefers to think of people as existing in any number of hierarchically related, overlapping contexts, with different customs and rules, rather than people having a single version of their 'real' self. This is a useful theory for understanding extreme human responses to extreme circumstances as symptomatic of the situation, not the individual. In this way, systemic family therapy can help families move towards possibility for recovery and away from notions of individual blame for family failure (Amrha's 'I am not good for her').

Our contexts are ranked in order of importance, depending on our understanding of our situation. The most important level of meaning to us at that time and in that place will inform our experience of the other(s): 'Two units of meaning are hierarchically related when one unit constitutes the context for understanding the other' (Montgomery, 2004: 351). For families seeking asylum, the right to remain in a safe country is very often their priority and can, understandably, overshadow other aspects of family life.

CMM allows us to see that the influence of the highest level on lower levels will be stronger than the influence of the lower on the higher, which is described as a weaker, implicative effect. For example, a parent might think: 'Why would we learn English and integrate with parenting customs here when we could be removed at any time?' The order of the hierarchy can change when new information is introduced into the system. Amrha had noticed a change when I was temporarily invited into the family. New meaning is created when this information is embedded in our experience of ourselves, using language, and language happens, of course, in relationship.

Amrha's existence as a torture-surviving mother seeking asylum demanded that her daughter's survival should be her highest context marker, more important than the survival of the family unit. The survival of the family unit would require a first-order change from outside the system (the absence of the threat of removal, further torture and death) – a change that was beyond her powers to achieve. Keeping emotional distance from her daughter made sense in a situation where Amrha expected she might have to leave her. A parent's belief that their death may ensure their child's survival, making death an acceptable, sometimes inevitable solution, has been frequently cited in media reports of refugee experiences over the past few years. To me, new to working with torture-surviving families at that time, this was shocking. Of course, it still should be.

It was useful for me to think about our contexts, how they both differed and overlapped and how my highest context marker was the safety of both mother and daughter in relationship, as a family, not as individuals.

For me, the greatest danger to both while they waited for a decision on their claim for asylum was the absence of real protection, and that their relationship could deteriorate to the point where they could lose each other – where Sara might be removed from Amrha's care, unless something changed. How could mother and daughter be more connected when the pain of potential loss was always present for Amrha? What position or perspective could Amrha hold other than despair? How could she recognise herself as essential to her daughter's wellbeing? How could she place herself back in the family?

A common feature of the refugee experience in the UK is that the years of waiting for a decision on a claim for asylum exact a price that is hard to recoup once safety is established. Children lose nurturing years; couples become estranged; families experience conflict as a consequence of being deprived of justice. People become isolated from each other by the trauma of uncertainty in exile layered over the trauma of torture. Connections that were the fabric of life become faint – more memories than realities.

For Amrha, repeated experiences of disempowerment and subsequent feelings of hopelessness had made suicide seem like a reasonable response to extraordinary circumstances. Her loving relationship with her daughter had become less valuable (implicative and subordinate) than she imagined her absence (contextual and dominant) would be. The stronger contextual effect of existing as a survivor of torture and refugee in the UK asylum process was having a potentially catastrophically weakening effect on the family.

Distinctions: questions that make a difference

Our adult conversations were often disrupted by two-year-old Sara's singing, acting and bringing us her drawings. One afternoon, we both watched her arranging flashcards on the floor. She began to trace the words with her finger: 'Bee, clock, book...' I was amazed: 'She's reading!' I imagine I looked enchanted. 'Yes,' said Amrha, 'she is teaching herself. I used to teach her too.'

Questions about this subordinate context encouraged Amrha to pay attention to and amplify the strengths in their relationship. I used:

- questions about observable behaviour –
    When you smile, what does she do?
    When she smiles, what do you do?

- questions about past traditions and influential past figures –
    Who taught you when you were young?
    What would they say if they could see your daughter now?
    How would it be if she were to be very intelligent?
    Where would that have come from?

- questions about resources, capabilities and future plans –
    Who has helped her to achieve this?
    What does she need next?
    What do you need to make this happen?

- questions encouraging empathy –
    What do you think she is thinking right now?

- questions about relationship –
    When is it easiest to connect with each other?
    When is it hardest?

Amrha revealed a family history of academic brilliance. She and her brother had been top of their class. Their aunt believed that they were especially talented and had funded their education. They had managed to study through some dreadful years of conflict, danger and hunger. Amrha missed her brother and her aunt terribly, and yes, they would have been very proud of Sara. For much of her life, education had been her family's highest context marker, valued throughout years of adversity, and a means of coping with and making sense of life in adversity as well.

These emerging memories of resilience, dedication and pride in family values revived expression of a context embedded in past generations: one in which Amrha was important not only as a generic mother who could be replaced if necessary, but as her unique self.

Reflexivity: reflections that make a difference

Both in session and in my reflections on the work, I was aware that I had never explored or questioned my own value within my family. My own assumption that no one else could be as good as me for my children was revealed to me as a consequence of the privilege of my socioeconomic status.

My personal reactions were anger, outrage, frustration, sadness and guilt about the structure of my country: 'How dare they – we – I – do this to people seeking protection?' 'What if' fantasies about safety and equal privilege featured in my reactions: 'What if we were friends, colleagues; what if our children were friends?' The idea that I would die for my children, a throwaway remark I had often heard but had never considered could be a reality, was now a real-life nightmare scenario. Strong personal reactions are inevitable in work where clients face danger and injustice. It is helpful for therapists to understand and use reflexive information in work that is politically and ethically motivated. In this way, the polarised positions of either overpowering our clients as a saviour or becoming disempowered ourselves as a victim can be avoided.

Working as a therapist with families, both as a woman and a mother with such a different, safe context, was an education for me. Dallos and Stedmon (2009: 6) believe the key to using reflection ethically is to make it reflexively useful and relevant, looping the information back into the work. Without this, my own learning in this therapeutic relationship would be purely self-serving, another layer of inequality.

By combining personal *reflection in action* (the physical sensations, emotional responses and cognitive reactions in session), and later *reflection on action* (the reflexivity of looking back on the session, and reflecting on the reflections that occurred then in the context of the knowledge and theory available now), the systemic practitioner can create useful developments for the work. The therapist becomes part of the reflexive process of creating new meaning with clients, using language.

I work in a human-rights context where clients seeking asylum can access a range of services, including casework for welfare needs. This is powerful and requires attention in the therapeutic relationship. Being in family therapy with me brought significant benefits to this family's asylum claim. This aspect of our context could be disempowering for clients and destabilising to the integrity of the therapy work. This concern has traditionally encouraged therapists to avoid 'getting involved' outside the therapy room. I believe that offering practical protection and advocacy is an authentic ethical stance if it is considered actively and carefully in the therapeutic relationship. Neutrality is not an appropriate or possible response to the dangers our clients face.

The results of my reflexive practice were a message that sounded like this: 'I can see something that might be useful for you because I am safe enough to be able to see this. The difference between our perspectives is intense and painful for me, and may be even more so for you. It is not about worth, but about context. I can see the long-term benefit of your therapy and I invite you to trust my perspective. I respect that it is a challenge, as it would be for me if our positions were reversed.'

Saying goodbye: we feel closer and safer now

Amrha began to notice Sara, and Sara began to notice being noticed by her mum. We played with the flashcards more, and read small books together. As the sessions went by, I played and read less, reflected and commented more. Sara related to me less and to her mum more in their reading together. There were more smiles, fewer tears. From the position of being valuable as a mother, Amrha was increasingly able to empathise with her child. She now held both their present danger and the value of being a nurturing, connected mother in this.

The difference that my presence had made initially – the outsider's ability to notice something different from the story being told, and to value it, be curious about it and ask for more detail – had become the new normal. This information was now part of an easy conversation that this family could have about itself: 'We are a family who value reading. We go to the library every Wednesday afternoon. We really enjoy it. There is little safety in our lives but the library is a safe place.'

Joining the family as a temporary member who is not an expert is a central concept of systemic therapy. It allows the emergence of safe uncertainty, where experimentation with change is possible when the family system has been previously stuck in difficulty. Most families come to therapy having already tried lots of solutions available to them to make their problems better. The therapist is a new pair of eyes, but cannot know which is the 'right' thing for the family to pick up and use. The therapist, by virtue of their training in, and experience of, paying careful attention (that is, expertise and experience of being alive to human systems, not expertise in any particular family), can help to create safe conditions for the family to try new things in the therapy room (reading together), and then in the world outside (going to the library). Changes need to be big enough to be useful, noticed and make a difference, otherwise therapy will be boring, but not so big that they are frightening and further entrench a sense of inadequacy. For example, Amrha would not have felt safe to take her daughter to a library when we first met.

It is also important for the systemic therapist to come up with lots of ideas in order to create the possibility of exploring a multiverse, in recognition that before the family now is a limitless set of possible, constructed realities. They can notice and ask about lots of things in a playful way, so that the family does not feel ideas are being imposed on them. They can be prepared for the family to discard ideas or aspects of ideas that do not fit with their own ideas about recovery, trusting that other, more useful notions will soon emerge and can be nurtured through the care and attention of the therapeutic relationship.

The therapist does not know what will or should happen in the move towards recovery. This is inevitable, for, in the act of providing therapy, 'the therapist becomes part of the very process that she is trying to step back from and observe' (Dallos & Stedmon, 2009: 3). We might embark on a session with a hunch, a wish or a worry about what might emerge, as we would in any human encounter, and what actually emerges is often unexpected.

From the position of valuing herself and her ability to make her daughter's life good, it was possible for Amrha to imagine how her aunt might have felt about her education and why she had striven to provide this, despite the dangerous circumstances. This came to feel part of Amrha's family tradition. In the absence of any other living family, it was strengthening for Amrha to keep her aunt's imagined intentions for Sara in mind. Keeping valued family members' influences alive in therapy is especially useful where families, and sometimes whole communities, have died or been separated.

I wondered about Amrha's plans for herself in the light of this new information. It took a great deal of courage for her to return to study, to be a beginner, to concentrate with post-traumatic symptoms and depression. Studying woke powerful grieving. Amrha had never studied without her brother and without her aunt's encouragement. While seeking asylum, she was not eligible for free childcare, or allowed onto some courses. She had no computer for studying at home and often had no bus fare. The present context was punishing in so many ways that the meaning of her intelligence sometimes seemed buried under the weight of the present injustice. I often wondered whether she would manage to continue. I imagined that I might not, if I were in her place.

The end of the story, as I knew it, was a very good one. Amrha and Sara stayed together in the UK and continued to thrive as a family. Tom Andersen, in *The Reflecting Team*, says: 'A stuck system, that is, a family with a problem, needs new ideas in order to broaden its perspectives and its contextual premises' (1987: 415).

I wonder whether we would have been able to rediscover this highest context marker if Sara had not been with us in sessions, and brought her family's tradition to life – a tradition that she could never have known about because it had never been told to her, a connection to the uncle and great aunt she had never met. My part in the system was to notice and amplify the aspects of the mother–daughter relationship that were nourishing. My own status as a mother of young children, a student and a member of an academic family no doubt played a part in what I noticed. Doubtless, other important information could also have been noticed.

Making connections (when too much is changing)

Torture draws distinctions. By this I mean that, wherever in the world it occurs, bystanders are led to believe, by powerful, vocal influences, for their own, often concealed, purposes, that survivors of torture are not like us. Media images of families in situations unimaginable to those living in safety can lead us to forget that the situations are also often unimaginable to them. We can be distanced by fear, revulsion and horror at the difficulties, and feel overwhelmed by the numbers that we are told are seeking protection. These other people, we are often told, are not like us. This can serve a politics of division. Even when the well-meaning urge us to 'imagine if this was your wife, your child', their inference is that no, we cannot imagine that. Whether torture turns people into heroes, victims, or even, more recently, pretenders and villains, there is often little space for them to be real people.

Systemic theory helps practitioners to find the confidence and skills to make connections. Some of our clients' experiences, values and ambitions will feel familiar enough for us to allow connection with torture-surviving families to whom, as with every family in difficulty, we have a duty.

Dallos and Stedmon identify 'the swampy lowlands' – an area of work where we tolerate ambiguity, the unique, the unexpected and value conflicts (2009). These will probably be familiar to professionals working with torture-surviving families. Such differences and challenges may actually be helpful starting points for us to be genuinely, respectfully curious. In fact, curiosity might be even more important when working with families with whom we feel we are culturally similar, because this is when our sense of cultural familiarity can invite us to make assumptions that might go unchecked, and these could be far from accurate.

Tolerating change: whose problem is this?

More recently, in a formal family therapy setting, I met a family who had just been reunited after nearly a year apart. They were a father who had survived torture, his wife, and four children, aged between nine and 16, who had all joined him in the UK.

Therapy was initially instigated by both parents, who wanted help to settle their children into the English school system and their new culture. In the initial assessment session, none of the family identified a specific problem or set of problems, but they did agree that their home life had changed hugely and was now unhappy. The older children were quiet and appeared less willing to talk about difficulties with strangers. The youngest boy, Fahmy, aged nine, talked about difficulties, such as family arguments, which I sensed other family members might experience as exposing.

The family had lived in poverty and as a persecuted minority for all of their lives, and for many generations. They all agreed that living in the UK brought relative security, and that this was a welcome change. They had lived through increasing violence against their community until the point at which their father was dragged from the family home one night by government agents and was not heard of for several months. Their journeys to the UK had been dangerous and traumatising for all of them, and accomplished with the aid of people smugglers and using false documents to avoid discovery. They had experienced what Montgomery describes as 'a deep change in the protecting quality of the family atmosphere' (2004: 350).

Their previous home culture had been characterised by relatively strict rules of behaviour for women and girls and autonomy for men and young boys. The father, Ibrahim, spoke of having to accept that girls could study alongside boys here, and that his wife might speak to a male housing worker, and even invite him into the family home for a meeting. This was difficult for him.

Maryam, the mother, was pragmatic about the new demands on her and her two daughters to engage with the wider world. She had never expected to speak to a man outside her family, and in her home country she never left the collection of family homes grouped around a central courtyard. She spoke of 'coping' with her stress as there was no alternative: she must survive, feed and clothe her family. She was relieved to be reunited with her husband and distressed to find that his behaviour had changed a great deal.

Ibrahim was suffering post-traumatic symptoms: flashbacks and intrusive thoughts about his torture. He was anxious and tearful, and angry and unpredictable at home. He had been tortured in prison and, after his escape, had been trapped in hiding for months. During his flight out of the country, he had been at risk of discovery and death. Then, as he was beginning to come to terms with his survival, his family had arrived and placed huge demands on him to be the father figure he had been in the past, ruling and holding the family together.

Because the children could speak and read English, they knew more than their father about welfare benefits and helped Maryam use the bank and buy food. Ibrahim had always brought home food daily from his farm work. He had no formal education and now had no visible role in the family.

The older son, Kamal, had become accustomed to leading the family through danger in his father's absence. He missed home the most; he had been popular and important in his community, which was often involved in violent conflict with the state authorities. At 15, he saw himself as a man and felt out of place in a high school. After the initial therapy session, he refused to attend. His older sisters, Naima and Khadija, reported Kamal's fights at school and aggressive behaviour at home that Ibrahim was not able to manage. The girls resented him behaving as if he were still in charge here in the UK; they felt they were older and entitled to make their own choices.

The girls began to change their dress from hijab to western clothes and to disobey rules about coming straight home from school. They now spent no time with their mother, who was busy managing the family finances and resettlement, or their father, who isolated himself. They missed both parents and described having no one to discuss their new lives with. They began to speak in derogatory ways about both parents: 'They can't speak English, they don't understand life here, they are living in the past.'

The younger boy, Fahmy, was able to connect with and be close to all family members. He thrived at school and was treated affectionately by everyone. His father and mother argued often, and neither of them spoke to his sisters, and vice versa. Kamal did not speak to anyone except his father. Fahmy spoke to everyone and was asked to pass messages between the arguing parties. He appeared to be under extraordinary stress. His parents described how he had stopped eating, except for chips. All family members now ate different foods alone, whereas before the torture, every night they had eaten together food that was brought home by their father and cooked by their mother.

Risk management: the power to undermine the system

The daughters' behaviour became the focus of the therapeutic work – the problem for the parents. Both parents reacted angrily to the girls; they tried methods of discipline that would have been effective at home – expressing disappointment, disapproval, isolation, withdrawing privileges like phone use. The girls did not respect these boundaries; they saw their brother behaving similarly and felt that they should have the same freedoms. They left the house without permission and, instead of a small community where they would be conspicuous, had a large city into which to disappear. Their parents used increasingly controlling methods to try to keep them safe. Both girls reacted to control with further disobedience. I identified a pattern – an outward moving loop of concern and control by the parents resulting in withdrawal and rebellion by the girls. Each reaction looked to provoke a bigger reaction in opposition. This cycle seemed likely to lead to harm. The girls' behaviour became dangerous, including drug and alcohol use, and other unsafe choices. Both girls eventually made allegations about violence at home, and were aware of their power over their parents to bring the police into the family home to investigate.

The parents had been able to tolerate therapy when the family briefly sat together in initial sessions and described agreed facts about the events they had survived. It was far less acceptable for different opinions and conflicts to emerge with an outsider present, and for the girls to challenge their parents. My preference to look at the system and to avoid individual blame was too big a change in perspective for all the family members to accept. Each was heavily defended against empathising with the others in the system. The parents described feeling threatened by the relentless pace of change and difference that had overwhelmed the family during torture, flight and adjustment to life in exile. They spoke often of the differences between life before and life now. The girls described their sense of injustice that they were being unfairly controlled in archaic ways.

At this point, the sessions necessarily became linear and focused on managing the risk of the girls' allegations of violence and the choices they were making outside the home. After a period of decisive intervention, child protection procedures and the involvement of social workers and police, the family stopped attending sessions together. The parents attended separately to their daughters and the boys stopped coming at all. The experience of the interventions had been too great a difference for the family to tolerate. Andersen defines this 'too great' difference as having a 'disorganising effect' on the family. He notes that: 'In such cases, the system often closes itself to those who would try to implement such a difference' (1987: 417).

The idea that the state would intervene in family life and could overrule the parents was new and alien to the family. Their past experience of the police was of violent oppression and the parents were afraid when police officers spoke to their daughters without them being present and understanding what was happening.

I had to consider the risks to the girls of 'honour'-based violence at home and sexual exploitation, substance use and illegal behaviour outside the home. As the weeks passed, each risk seemed to compete for importance, yet had to be kept separate. For example, if the parents heard of their daughters' allegations of sexual exploitation outside of the home, the girls would be at risk of 'honour'-based violence. The parents' exclusion from aspects of their children's transition to adulthood was also a painful experience for all.

One of the daughters, Naima, said she wanted to train as a vet and not to marry, which would not have been possible in their home country. She reported that her mother comforted her traumatised crying at night by saying: 'All will be well when you marry and have your own children.' Naima sometimes said that she would 'have a marriage to get out of the family stress'. I felt an ethical duty to suggest there were other ways of living independently – ways that were entirely unacceptable to the family's home culture. There was a period where I was concerned about the possibility of forced marriage.

Working with an interpreter added to the complexity. For example, quick, friendly exchanges in English between me and the older children were patiently related to their parents by the interpreter. Informal chats between family members were carefully fed back to me in English. Yet, without this rigorous approach to communicating all verbal information, there could have been increased uncertainty for everyone about what was happening in the room.

An interpreter may or may not be familiar with aspects of a family's culture. They may be perceived by the family as more similar to them than they feel they are, or less. The therapist may feel closer to the interpreter's culture than the family, or less close. The interpreter is unlikely to be trained to manage the complexity of systemic therapy, and may require support and debriefing to manage the tensions to which he or she is exposed in their role. In this situation, it will help the therapist to consider what meaning(s) the interpreter might hold for family members: what do they think she or he is thinking? Which issues can be safely discussed with someone so similar to them? What are the dangers of exposing family issues to him/her? Who does she/he remind them of? How do these aspects of the relationship change over time?

Alerting the authorities to the family's situation placed me in a position of greater power, in some respects, than Maryam and Ibrahim, in a system that was increasingly undermining their authority. It deepened the distrust and difference between me and the parents, and devalued the parents even further in their children's eyes. It also further devalued the parents' already disempowered status in their new culture. They clearly knew, as parents often do, that something was very wrong for the girls, and suspected, rightly, that I held the information. They understandably resented my relationship with their daughters, and discouraged them from attending sessions alone. They attended for the purpose of gathering information about their daughters, which I could not disclose. I was often asked to 'tell my Mum...' or 'explain to my daughters...', as though I held the power in the family and could adjudicate as an expert on life in the UK and how the family should behave here. My responses to these requests were often a disappointment to them. I resisted being on any one side, much as I was tempted to say, 'You should not follow your daughter to college' or, 'You should not lie to your parents about where you are going.' My refusal to take a stand left the family unsupported in their sense of unsafe uncertainty.

Reflections on power: inner conversation, intimacy and the not yet said

Power was conferred on me due to my profession, which was seen to give me the power to judge the family. Underpinning this, of course, was my membership of a culture that privileges white, western cultural norms as superior, preferable, the standard measure, and regards different family structures as other, and judges them against this standard. There is potential for great professional and personal development when the therapist holds this in awareness: 'As therapists, we can begin to reflect and become more available to disentangle the contradictions within our stories and develop an increased awareness of our own unconscious racism, fears and guilt' (Bains, 2010: 30).

Peggy McIntosh (1989) draws attention to the importance of questioning the larger system of oppression as well as the behaviour of individuals within oppressive structures. It is not enough to oppose isolated incidents of racism, to stand against the 'individual acts of meanness by members of my group'. One should also oppose the unfair and unearned advantage inherent in the 'invisible systems conferring unsought racial dominance'. Those in power may assume these systems are the norm and, by virtue of their dominance, make them the norm.

> My schooling gave me no training in seeing myself as an oppressor, as an unfairly advantaged person, or as a participant in a damaged culture. I was taught to see myself as an individual whose moral state depended on her individual moral will. My schooling followed the pattern my colleague Elizabeth Minnich has pointed out: whites are taught to think of their lives as morally neutral, normative, and average, and also ideal, so that when we work to benefit others, this is seen as work that will allow 'them' to be more like 'us' (McIntosh, 1989: 11).

My temporary presence in this family was complex and not always helpful. The aspects of myself that could be seen by the family – a professional, non-Muslim woman – already made me representative of an aspect of UK culture that was contentious for the family. All members asked questions about my invisible aspects: my faith, beliefs, marital status, children, social life, attitude to tattoos and piercings and many intimate matters. They asked these questions as if the answers could illuminate my rightness or wrongness to be with them, or the rightness or wrongness of their own choices. In some sessions, my personal disclosures were sought in order to attack or criticise them.

I reflected that these were reasonable questions about issues that were important to members of the family. If I sat in on their intimate lives, I should expect to be open myself. I also considered how influential and disempowering my disclosures could be for family members. I reflected on which aspects of myself I wished to keep private and why, as well as how and why family members might use information I gave and the possible consequences of this.

These issues of therapist disclosure are particularly important when working with families where there are high levels of conflict and where the therapist might be seen as a representative of the new, threatening or superior culture, in the struggle for power within the family.

The therapist cannot claim objectivity, and inevitably her dialogue with clients is influenced by her own impressions of their situation and the origins of those impressions in her own life story. While in dialogue with clients, there is also an internal dialogical process taking place for the therapist about these impressions and their usefulness at this time: the therapist's 'inner conversation' (Rober, 1999: 209).

The difficulties clients are facing may be to do with conflicts or an impasse in their family, often referred to in therapy as 'stuckness', due to issues that have been too dangerous, difficult or painful to put into words. Surviving torture leaves the people directly affected and their loved ones with memories that may seem beyond words. Torture is often described as the most extreme human experience, one inflicted by other humans. The survivor of torture may be left with a vocabulary that seems inadequate to express these extremes. Revulsion, horror, guilt or shame will require a safe-enough context to be expressed in a way that can enable recovery. Rober writes: '[By] contributing to such a safe therapeutic culture, the therapist makes space for the "not-yet-said"' (1999: 210).

Becoming a temporary member of the family is often a necessary part of therapy, as a transitional phase. In the case of Amrha and Sara, this was easily outgrown once mother and daughter reclaimed their preferred relationship. In this family, moving out of this phase was more complex. Striving to be honest and to transmit my respect, care and attempts at empathy for all family members required all of my selfhood, life experiences and taught learning.

Using self-reflexivity again to place myself in this work and to apply my personal reflections both in action (in the session) and on action (reflective collaboration with myself and others in supervision out of the session) in the family's best interest involved inner conversation. I chose to disclose aspects of myself that I thought could be useful, and managed to tolerate not always knowing the meaning of my values to the different family members. For example, discussions with the women about my identification as a feminist showed me that I had a lot in common with Maryam and I admired her a great deal. She was able to make radical changes far outside her own comfort and custom zone in order to protect her family.

My position as a mother of a teenage child helped me to empathise with the parents. I could identify with their worries about hidden risks and their wanting their teenage children to stay closer than the children wanted, and could only wonder how hard this was in a new culture and language. The risks I knew about were real: drug and alcohol use, poor friendship choices, illegal activity. I was privileged to hear some of the true stories from the girls and was able to help them negotiate their lives more safely.

I listened especially for the male voices in the family. They seemed to have been lost after the family's terrible experiences. The women's experiences involved stress and demanded rapid adjustments and outward movement that was gaining momentum. The men appeared to have lost their roles as family leader, breadwinner, protector, activist, community figure, treasured youngest son. These roles appeared too difficult to maintain in a culture that did not value their skills and life experiences. Male tradition and honour, patriarchal power and protection had relatively low value in their post-flight context, leaving the men with little meaning and a great deal of frustration. All the men seemed to be focusing inward, and felt defensive, humiliated and threatened by UK cultural ways. As a woman in the therapeutic role, sitting with their female relatives and dependants, I was limited in what I could offer to help them, and there was nothing the setting could offer that was helpful either.

With hindsight, I see potential for male children, adolescents, fathers and grandfathers to connect and support their own cultural transition to living in the UK. Amira Hassan's work with father-and-son storytelling groups in Liverpool was helpful for men of all ages in adjusting to family and community life in new cultures, and showed how this approach can link to and be enhanced by the values they have brought from home (Kagan et al, 2013). I wish I had been better equipped to address the men's experiences of loss and frustration, to acknowledge their hard work in surviving and readjusting, and to facilitate their greater understanding of each other's experiences.

Connections: questions that make a difference

I asked questions, hoping to amplify safer connections within the family; unfortunately, I was seeing the girls and the parents separately now, never together. They had no consensus about what the problem was. Each member located their problem in the behaviour of another – a situation very common in highly conflicting systems. Dallos and Stedmon also identify this lack of clarity as something that is often overlooked in therapy:

> The need to question what is so easily taken for granted, namely that we know what the 'problem' is. In clinical work this is often far from clear. Typically, we begin with a referral form from another professional or a self-referral from a client, wanting something to be done about a difficulty. But what exactly is the problem? For whom is it a problem? How has it come to be defined in this way? What is the life history of the problem? (2009:10).

I used:

- questions about behaviour, routine, possibility –
    What are the differences in daily life for each member?
    What are the differences in cultural beliefs for each member?
    Which things are possible now? Impossible now? Compared to life before?
    What are the pros and cons of each?

- questions encouraging empathy between members –
    Who do you imagine is missing home the most?
    Who do you imagine is happiest here?

- questions encouraging connections and similarities –
    Which things does everyone miss?
    Which things is everyone glad to have left?
    How do they show this?
    What might you think about what is similar?

- questions comparing attitudes –
    Where do you feel safest (home, college, friends)?
    Where do you imagine mum and dad think you are safest?

How would you like family life to be?
How do you think your children would like family life to be?

- questions remembering or imagining the situation both back and forward in time and generations –
  How is this changing over time?
  If things continue as they are, where do you imagine you will be in six months' time?
  What might any future generations of your family think about this?
  What would your grandparents have said about that?

In these conversations, themes emerged that re-awakened my sense that the family's situation was not solely due to the rupture of torture, flight and exile. Some of the challenges and risks pre-dated these events. The children had already been maturing and changing, rebelling and disobeying family and cultural rules. The parents had been arguing and under stress. Life stages and events that I could recognise in my own history had been taking place.

In the wider cultural landscape, poverty, fear and hatred of authorities had always been present. Home had been a predictably dangerous place. There had never been a time of economic, personal or cultural safety. Members of the community had disappeared, been tortured and killed. Before the crisis that prompted them to flee, the family had lived with rumours and whispered conversations about what had happened to a neighbour, which woman had been 'shamed', what had happened in the next village, which song one shouldn't sing, which clothing one shouldn't wear, and even which members of their own community might not be trusted. The possibility of torture was part of their culture; their parents, grandparents and generations beyond had all been accustomed to this terror as part of daily life.

Papadopoulos writes of home as a self-regulating system of knowable certainties: 'Whether a person experiences home as a safe place is different from the primary experience of stability that a home exists. This means that continuity itself within a certain felt space contributes to the development of a deep sense of reliability about life' (2002: 19).

The family had coped with conflict at home and the wider context of threat, and felt they were a protective-enough unit in their home country. My sense of their difficulties, and perhaps theirs too, had come in part from assumptions about cultural difference that were overstated. They had experienced torture, the disappearance of the father and separation at a time when the family was already undergoing a major life-cycle transition – the children's teenage years, where one might expect some conflict to occur between generations. At the same time, they had lost their home – a dangerous place, but known to them for generations. Although it may be reductive to apply universal themes across widely diverse cultures to the stages of the typical family lifecycle, the knowledge that other families had also been through similar difficulties allowed the members of this family to find more common ground and empathy for each other's positions.

My responsibility for safeguarding will be familiar to most professionals working with families. It is crucial to report every child or vulnerable adult protection concern to the statutory agencies. We are bound by rules and procedures to protect vulnerable people, for good reasons.

The way in which these concerns are received by the statutory services will vary. Professionals will, as we all do, see concerns through their own cultural lenses and assumptions about family life. If these are left unexamined, it is possible to make potentially dangerous decisions about who is right or telling the truth. To seek the safety and certainty of our own cultural norms can be tempting when risks are high and culturally unfamiliar: for example, when they are about 'honour' killing or forced marriage. When working with this family, I spoke to professionals, who dismissed these possibilities, perhaps because they were too awful to contemplate and they preferred to believe that the girls were exaggerating and that their parents were 'lovely' and 'caring', in the way that they might prefer to understand love and care. The reality of work with traumatised families adjusting to life in new cultures is that uncertainty and change is likely to be rapid and intensely felt. Looking out for and amplifying similarities may create enough safety for open dialogue, space for the 'not yet said'.

As well as listening to all verbal information about risk, it is also helpful to listen out for hunches, insights, bodily sensations and unconscious reactions to information – both our own and those of the family. Although, of course, you cannot refer concerns to statutory services because 'something doesn't feel right', it is important to be curious about what might be behind this feeling. If trauma is stored in these non-verbal, bodily sensations, then it is likely to be registered there too by the listener.

It is hard to accept that we can never know for sure that a situation is safe when we care so deeply for the wellbeing of those involved. By the time we have made a judgment, the reality of the situation will have evolved, and so our understanding of risk is continuously incomplete. Our intervention to protect someone from one risk will no doubt alter the intensity of a co-existing risk. Making a safeguarding referral is a powerful act and one that might make future disclosure either more or less likely. Once a therapist has taken the power away from a family to set its own course, relationships will be permanently changed. These events happen inside the therapeutic relationship, but are, of course, not therapy. Involving social services and the police has a hugely destabilising effect on the shape of any family, and may be seen as positive or negative by different members. This is especially significant for those who have suffered state violence. Once the therapist is aligned with the power of the state, rebuilding a relationship of trust is only possible if you can heal the rupture in the previous relationship and the family is able to see your actions as meant in their best interest.

Saying goodbye: we know more now

This family did not stay in family therapy. The differences between each member's priorities, values and ambitions were too great to maintain relationships with me or with each other. The necessary intrusions of safeguarding wrought further changes in these relationships that were too great for some members to accept. I hope that the therapeutic work we did together helped the family to empathise with each other's positions and stay open to the possibility of better relationships in future, even though they could not live together, or even sit down together in therapy, at that time.

When working with survivors of torture and their families, it can be difficult and painful to accept that family members may choose to leave or rearrange the pre-existing family system. In some cases, surviving torture and travelling huge physical and cultural distances to safety may provide an opportunity to live in ways that would not otherwise have been conceivable.

This is what happens in the 'swampy lowlands' – the search for patterns that connect us to the values and fabric of family members' lives, where we must also declare that we cannot sit with the risk of serious harm, as defined by our own home culture. Connecting may be the most helpful thing to do: to find where we are similar, and have similar cares and goals and wishes for ourselves and our children. How and why are things different here? And also, crucially, how are they similar? How does life here link to the stories and memories of home: those that were sustaining and positive and those that were punishing and oppressive? How might those differ for different members? How might members begin to express these differences here, now that difference is permitted? The life-threatening danger of torture is in the past. What threatens to rupture family life now is misunderstanding of difference, of what it means to each person to be here and to be safe. The values sometimes clash, different things are mourned and carried into the present, different things are discarded and gladly forgotten.

This has happened, now we are all changed

Walking home to finish writing this chapter this morning, I passed a newsagent and saw the headlines of the right-wing press claiming that 'economic migrants' are deliberately cheating our government and coming to 'destroy' our society. The headline grouped together as a threat all the people who travel to the UK, all their past histories, all their journeys and all their future intentions – a position of unsafe certainty. I wondered about the fragility of a culture that could imagine another group of people to be different enough to 'destroy' it by their presence.

When I reached home, I opened an email about some children who had formed a group to welcome child refugees into their community. They had drawn pictures and recorded messages of kindness. These messages assumed common interest and similarity: 'I would like to meet you,' 'I hope you will be OK here,' 'You can play on my PlayStation' – positions of safe uncertainty. I wondered who had explained the refugees' situation to the children and helped them to make this connection?

I suppose that groups of people have always been attracted to or repelled by those they perceive as other, depending on how welcoming or threatened they feel. The family group, as the smallest social unit, is just one part of the systemic pattern of human life, and is hugely affected by the wider social circles in which it exists.

The families I have worked with continue to be significantly affected by their perceived difference from a prescribed norm. Persecution, torture, flight into a new, often hostile culture, having to prove their suitability to remain in this host culture and find new ways to integrate with its rules and written and unspoken cultural customs all emphasise difference.

The therapists who connect with these families have many more dynamics to consider than they would when working with families who have more familiar experiences. The fragility or strength of therapeutic relationships in a context where a family could be removed from the UK at any time are considerable; perhaps each session is the last. These media headlines illustrate both the barriers to connection and the possibilities for richer connection.

As both the inward-looking, defensive aspect of our current UK culture and its counterculture of generosity look likely to intensify, I am grateful for the opportunity to connect with families who have survived torture and to be part of their journey towards safety in an increasingly hostile political and social global climate. I find this work fascinating and enriching, as well as sometimes challenging and upsetting.

While a UK politician might claim: 'If you believe you're a citizen of the world, you're a citizen of nowhere' (May, 2016), the reality of life today suggests to me that it would take an extraordinary effort of cultural impoverishment to be anything else. Global issues, such as environmental damage, disease, war and terrorism, do not respect countries' borders, and so any effective action seems likely to require mutual understanding, co-operation and a constantly evolving global approach. Language, literature, music, food, faith, custom, culture and intellectual tradition adapt and travel with their people quite naturally.

As in every cultural exchange, in family therapy, the wider our cultural lens and the more information we allow to be relevant, the richer and more truthful our experience with families can become. Of course, at some point, this requires us to let go of the illusion of certainty and understanding, when the system becomes unknowable. To navigate, we must rely on a process of curiosity and tentative connection with others. The more information our navigating systems hold, the more likely we are to flourish in our work, and, looking wider, as a species.

References

Andersen T (1987). The reflecting team: dialogue and meta-dialogue in clinical work. *Family Process* 26(4): 415–428.

Bains S (2010). Racism as trauma. In: Lago C, Smith B (eds). *Anti-discriminatory Practice in Counselling and Psychotherapy*. London: Sage (pp23–32).

Burnham J (1992). Approach method technique: making distinctions and creating connections. *Human Systems: The Journal of Systemic Consultation and Management* 3(1): 3–26.

Dallos R, Stedmon J (2009). Flying over the swampy lowlands: reflective and reflexive practice. In: Stedmon J, Dallos R. *Reflective Practice in Psychotherapy and Counselling*. Oxford: Oxford University Press (pp1–22).

Kagan C, Micallef A, Siddiquee A, Fatimilehin I, Hassan A, de Santis C et al (2013). Intergenerational work, social capital and wellbeing. *Global Journal of Community Psychology Practice* 3(4): 286–293.

Mason B (1993). Towards positions of safe uncertainty. *Human Systems: The Journal of Systemic Consultation and Management* 4: 189–200.

May T (2016). *Theresa May's Conference Speech in Full*. Conservative Party Conference 2016; 5 October. www.telegraph.co.uk/news/2016/10/05/theresa-mays-conference-speech-in-full/ (accessed July 2017).

McIntosh P (1989). White privilege: unpacking the invisible knapsack. *Peace and Freedom Magazine July–August*: 10–12.

Montgomery E (2004). Tortured families: a coordinated management of meaning analysis. *Family Process* 43(3): 349–369.

Papadopoulos R (2002). *No Place Like Home: therapeutic care for refugees*. London: Karnac Books.

Rober P (1999). The therapist's inner conversation in family therapy practice: some ideas about the self of the therapist, therapeutic impasse, and the process of reflection. *Family Process* 38: 209–228.

12. Creating a safe haven: a community-based, creative approach to working with refugee and asylum-seeking families and young people affected by torture

Carl Dutton

> Traumatized people relive the moment of trauma not only in their thoughts and dreams but also in their actions.
> (Herman, 1992: 39)

This chapter will explore and highlight the positive aspects of using creative approaches such as sport, poetry, creative writing and art with asylum-seeking and refugee families and young people who have witnessed or experienced torture.

> Creative interventions involving art, play, music, movement, or other modalities add a unique dimension to treatment because they have several specific characteristics not always found in strictly verbal therapies used in trauma interventions. These characteristics include, but are not limited to: 1, externalisation 2, sensory processing 3, attachment and 4, arousal reduction and affect regulation. (Malchiodi, 2008: 13–14)

I will explore some of the underlying theory around using these methods with people who have suffered from traumatic experiences associated with being a refugee, including those directly and indirectly exposed to torture and organised violence.

I will advocate that services should be embedded, where possible, within local communities so that access to services is available in a place and at a time that is acceptable to the individual or family who is seeking help. I will highlight the importance of the group as a healing agent, be it a formal therapy group, shared interest group, or informal get-together group.

I am a psychodrama psychotherapist and, before the project closed, co-ordinated specific trauma-focused therapies for victims of torture in the Haven, a small service in an NHS setting in Liverpool. A haven means a place of safety or refuge. The service delivered its work primarily in school settings and community venues, which allowed for early intervention to take place around assessment, therapy and identifying wider local support networks.

The ethos of the service was that every family and young person seen in these settings should have easy access to a therapist who could deliver a number of creative and trauma-focused therapies.

Liverpool has a long history of welcoming new arrivals, due to its position as a major sea port. The river Mersey is the gateway for ships to come and go, exporting trade from the UK and importing goods from all over the world. It is both an entrance for new arrivals and an exit to new places.

The Haven was developed in 2003 out of the need to provide timely and appropriate services to large numbers of refugee families who were placed in Liverpool as part of a government strategy to disperse across other cities and regions the high numbers of people seeking asylum that were accommodated in London and the south east of England.

In Liverpool, a network of statutory and non-statutory services came together in a local refugee forum to find ways to share expertise and resources to manage the situation. This included GPs, health workers, faith groups, therapy services, local authority social care providers, housing providers, and local refugee organisations and support groups.

What brought me to the Haven was my commitment to developing community-embedded support that could meet the needs of families and children without them having to negotiate the barriers that deny many refugees access to mental health and therapy services. The arrival of refugees in Liverpool also tapped into my humanity. I wanted to respond to a situation that I had not come across in other work settings.

> The victim, on the contrary, asks the bystander to share the burden of pain. The victim demands action, engagement, and remembering. (Herman, 1992: 7–8)

I wanted to take action, do something, and speak with, speak alongside, and speak up about the atrocities about which I had heard from the families and young people.

Dr JL Moreno (1889–1974), throughout his work, felt that the group was the therapeutic agent and that, for the individual to be healthy, they required skills and opportunities to be in groups that offered a chance to try something new and different, without the risk of rejection. He developed psychodrama as one of the creative solutions to such challenges, and many of the approaches described in this chapter are underpinned by his philosophy.

He saw humans as social, emotional, psychic and cosmic beings who need chances to develop these sides of themselves in a safe and contained way – a haven where they can maximise their potential and achieve a healthy state. 'The affairs of men are dynamic, they do not remain in any one particular state but are ever changing, ever responding to the bombardment of forces which alter them' (White, 1993: 14).

Dr Moreno, and later his widow Zerka T Moreno (1914–2016), encouraged us to be spontaneous and creative with each other and the wider communities we might find ourselves in, and co-create new and innovative ways to manage the many aspects of the human condition.

The idea of developing wider social support systems for asylum-seeking and refugee young people is echoed in Rousseau and Guzder's paper on school-based prevention programmes for refugee children. They cite Watters and Ingleby (2004), who highlight:

> ... the risk inherent in a victimizing perspective that portrays refugees as passive, helpless, and afflicted by psychopathology and [...] the need to co-construct services and programs with the refugees themselves to develop culturally appropriate interventions and to foster a sense of ownership and empowerment in refugee communities. (Rousseau & Guzder, 2008: 535)

We believed that, for the Haven to be successful, we needed to develop the service with the involvement of the main stakeholders, which included teachers, support agencies, children, young people and families, and professionals working in mental health and with refugees.

The stories used in this chapter are based on clients I have worked with. Names have been changed.

Getting started – warming up to develop the service

The work in which I have been involved with asylum-seeking and refugee communities has recognised the importance of creative therapies and arts, physical sports and horticulture as ways to help those affected by the traumatic effects of torture, conflict, forced removal, difficult journeys and settling into a new home and country. They offer the chance to live normally and develop connections, and provide therapy through the diverse media of the creative arts.

> When trauma hits, the self becomes psychologically disorganized. The patterns and structures of self-organization that were there, whether in childhood or as an adult, become frozen in time. Violence threatens the very existence of self physically, intellectually, psychologically, emotionally, and spiritually. (Hudgins, 2002: 11)

During the development of the Haven, we recognised early on that 'just talking' didn't seem to be enough. We wanted to develop an approach that would include everyday activities where people could meet up, do meaningful activities together, and be reconnected with wider social support systems, as well as share their thoughts and feelings, which may have become frozen by traumatic events. As Moreno emphasised: 'The body remembers what the mind forgets' (Moreno, 1993).

> Social support is of paramount importance in coping with a traumatic event. A good, extensive social network is the best comfort to one who has been through a traumatic experience. (Saari, 2005: 58)

As therapists, we also neede these networks so that we can provide the support required in our therapeutic work with traumatised individuals, families and communities. At the Haven, this included setting up and developing supervision for the team with a colleague from Freedom from Torture in Manchester, a specialist rehabilitation charity for survivors of torture. 'This work is highly stressful. It is not a good idea to attempt it without some sort of supervision' (Blackwell, 2005: 94).

We embedded regular supervision into the Haven structure when we established the service, for the team to have time to reflect, digest and refresh, so that we could deliver our work in a sensitive, creative, and empowering way that recognised the strengths and abilities in each of us and the wider system.

We also made a commitment to work with as wide a range of people, groups and organisations as possible in an attempt to develop a network of support for us and our clients – with schools, asylum and refugee organisations, arts groups and artists, sports groups, social workers, mental health workers, faith groups and a multitude of other formal and informal groups.

This reflected our view that the work is huge and could not be held by any one organisation. It was important to know who was available to work as informal co-therapists, and where to deliver support so that we could make therapy more accessible and fruitful for the individuals and families we supported.

Often in statutory settings – in the NHS and education, in particular – therapeutic care and support stays inside the treatment room. It should go beyond that space and be accessible after working hours.

Our approach was developed from observations about what was needed and from our community approach to service delivery. We consulted with survivors who would tell us about their feelings of boredom, frustration, lack of meaningful activity, isolation and fears of the past, present and future. Survivors shared the hopelessness they felt and described the daily reality of being in the asylum process, with all the uncertainties that brings.

Over recent years, there has been a growing recognition of the important role of creative therapies in healing trauma, accessing unprocessed traumatic responses and providing an opportunity for creative expression.

Van der Kolk highlights the importance of such activities (2014: 357): 'Children and adults alike need to experience how rewarding it is to work at the edge of their abilities. Resilience is the product of agency: knowing that what you do can make a difference.' He goes on to say: 'Athletics, playing music, dancing, and theatrical performance all promote agency and community.'

The service we co-created with our service users recognised the importance of self-expression, self-determination and self-discovery with the support of the therapists and others who have had similar experiences. 'For young trauma survivors with limited language or who may be unable to put ideas into speech, expression through art, music, movement or play can be a way to convey these ideas without words and may be the primary form of communication in therapy' (Malchiodi, 2008:13).

Winnicott points out the importance of play for children and adults: 'It is play that is the universal, and that belongs to health: playing leads into group relationships; playing can be a form of communication, and lastly, playing is in the service of communication with oneself and others' (1971: 41).

This idea around play and being playful feeds into an important aspect of the service. The team wanted to try things out: to explore with sensitivity what could be possible for us, in terms of our own unique creativity, for our clients, in terms of resilience and resourcefulness, and for the wider systems in terms of social/emotional support. Both the Haven therapists were trained in creative approaches: one is a psychodrama psychotherapist and the other an art psychotherapist.

We believed that creative therapies have an important role in healing traumatic experiences related to war, conflict, torture, forced migration and settling into a new place, far from home, and that our approach was transferable across cultures. Over the many years of the project, we ran, or co-ran, countless therapy sessions, groups and one-off events, as well as offering long-term, one-to-one therapy.

I shall try to give a flavour of two of the groups the Haven delivered in the community, as well as reflect on my one-to-one work with a young person, where I used a narrative exposure therapy (NET) approach. My therapeutic model has always aimed to open up to the client a world of possibilities, beyond the constraints of the illness model, the pathology model, and the one-size-fits-all model.

Here you will hear stories of struggles, frustrations, joy, fun and hope. They are just a taster and a signpost to possibilities that, with appropriate support and supervision, can make a difference to the lives of those affected by torture.

A football adventure

During the early days of the project, I used to meet up with many young, unaccompanied men from most parts of Africa at a centre that provided accommodation and educational advice. I had been invited to provide some baseline mental health screening, in the form of a simple questionnaire and some basic questions about how these young men felt.

As I got to know the group, what struck me most of all was that they were bored and frustrated by the lack of opportunity to play football in an organised way. Some told me they had played football at a high level in their home country and we shared stories of positions played, favourite players, and aspirations to play for a famous team.

We eventually got to the point where the group wanted to play football on a regular basis with each other. I explored what was possible and asked if we could use the five-a-side pitch at a local school where I already had a connection. The school was more than happy to allow this group of young men to use the pitch, and so we arranged for them to play there one evening a week.

I also took part in the sessions, as a passionate football fan. I recognised that it would be a good way to meet and talk with these young men in an informal way, before, sometimes during, and after the match. The group enabled me, as a therapist, to meet with these young men on the same level – not as someone in a position of power. Many of the young men had been subjected to abuses of power by authority figures, and, by joining in their football games, I was trying to gain their trust.

> After an acute trauma, like an assault, accident, or natural disaster, survivors require the presence of familiar people, faces, and voices; physical contact; food; shelter and a safe place; and time to sleep. (van der Kolk, 2014: 212)

These were young men who had witnessed family and friends murdered, executed, and tortured, and many were also survivors of torture themselves. What became clear was that this weekly session allowed them to be with a group, to express the joy and pain of scoring or missing a goal, to have physical contact when they celebrated a goal, and begin to develop a life that felt normal on a physical, emotional and social level.

Hudgins concludes, in her book on the treatment of post-traumatic stress disorder, that treatments 'must address the whole person: body; mind; emotion, and spirit' (2002: 22).

Football offers all these aspects. In terms of the physical, it allows players to reconnect physically with others by way of a pat on the back or warm embrace after scoring a goal. In terms of mental activity, it involves different ways of thinking, such as strategies for passing the ball or organising the team to defend or attack. Emotionally, it engenders expressions of joy and frustration, in a normal way. The spirit can be lifted by collective endeavour towards a common goal – a shared experience that can be spiritual in a simple way.

Hughes and Kaur highlight, in their narrative therapy article about the 'Team of Life', how football can have a positive effect in helping refugee young people talk, and can be a way of exploring roles, using the positions in a football team to look at strengths: 'Football offered rich meanings about personal and collective values, and their passion for the game had related to things they valued in other parts of their life' (2014: 26–27).

After six or so weeks of playing together, some of the young men asked me if they could now have some coaching from a qualified football coach. This, for me, was an example of their growing confidence. We had moved from being together on a weekly basis, to a place where they could trust each other and share some of what was happening in their lives. We would talk about immigration matters, English classes and racism in the local area. We explored what to do about not sleeping, worries about relatives left behind, and nightmares and flashbacks, as well as ruminating about the past.

Everton Football Club had a coach whose remit was to work with local communities. I spoke to him about the group and explained that some had played at a high level in their home country. He was keen to help the young men, and agreed to provide coaching. We arranged for the sessions to be at the same time and place as before, and booked six coaching sessions. The young men then started inviting other friends who were also seeking asylum to come along, and the sessions grew and grew.

Each session started with warming up and stretching exercises, followed by some skills sessions, a game, and a warm down. Having sessions that followed the same format is like a therapy session in that it has a ritualistic component that brings predictability and containment, so trust can develop.

> Traumatised human beings recover in the context of relationships with families, loved ones, AA meetings, veterans' organisations, religious communities, or professional therapists. The role of those relationships is to provide physical and emotional safety. (van der Kolk, 2014: 212)

The football coaching sessions offered such relationships, with the common purpose of learning and playing football. It offered the young men time to meet up with others who had similar, and different, experiences of trauma due to war and conflict, and to reconnect with their bodies in a physical way that was familiar from the past and grounded them in the present.

In psychodrama terminology, this was role expansion: the young men were moving from a group coming together simply to do something, to a group wanting to learn new skills. This is a good example of social role expansion, whereby the young men in the group did not want just to be participants but wanted more for themselves.

> Whether baker or farmer, lover or landlord, we are engaged in role behaviour continually. Sometimes we are quite pleased with

> how we play a role... On other occasions, we are dissatisfied with how we act in particular situations, or we get the urge to try a new role. (Sternberg & Garcia, 1994: 47)

Following these sessions, the group asked whether they could now train to be football coaches. They were not satisfied with just playing or being coached; they wanted to be leaders and give something back to others in their local communities.

I investigated how the Haven could facilitate this and, with local support, we were able to source funding to offer the group a Level 1 Football Association coaching course. The training took place over a weekend and the entire group who took part passed and qualified as level 1 coaches. This was a fantastic achievement that we celebrated with an awards ceremony to hand out the official certificates.

What can be seen from this story is that, given the right opportunities, people can grow beyond their existing roles or those in which they have been cast. The football group was a good example of how, if the conditions are correct and the therapist is open, and there is trust and optimism, then most things are possible. New roles, new connections, and new ways of being can be discovered that can enhance and maintain physical, emotional and social health. 'The ultimate goal of most therapy is not just change, but transformation, usually from lower-functioning behaviours into growth orientated ones' (Hudgins & Toscani, 2013: 100).

Football not only helped the young men to become coaches, it also facilitated conversations about the psychological effects of torture, a space to share advice on ways to manage their difficulties with sleep, anxiety and low mood, and opportunities to arrange appointments for longer term psychological therapy with me, if needed.

What started as a request by a group of young men to play football on a casual basis turned into a desire to become community coaches who could inspire others.

Healing power of poems

> Imagination and human stories are key forces in opening pathways toward integrating and organizing the highly complex realities of trauma. (St Thomas & Johnson, 2007: 22)

The Haven had been working with another, mixed group of young refugees for some time. In one of the sessions, the young people talked about how they felt unable to take part in activities in the local community because they thought no one else there would understand them. They described feeling afraid to go to new places close to where they lived, and that they often had to do homework and then chores, leaving no time for other activities in their lives.

Many complained of physical symptoms – headaches, stomach aches, poor sleep and feeling anxious and 'paranoid' around others. They were describing the symptoms of trauma that held them in a vice-like grip and often resulted in their being afraid to mix with other young people. At times, the group members would describe how frightened they were that they would be seen in a particular way: as a 'scrounger' on state benefits or someone who was 'not genuine' in seeking asylum from war or torture. Herman says: 'Chronically traumatised people no longer have any baseline state of physical calm or comfort. Over time they perceive their bodies as having turned against them. They begin to complain, not only of insomnia and agitation, but also of numerous types of somatic symptoms' (1992: 86).

These young people were describing themselves as stuck, and saying they had no place or space to express themselves in a safe and secure way. We discussed this as a team, and wondered if we could offer a creative space where the young people would have time to express themselves in different ways. We wanted it to include a variety of creative media, which could be written, art based, or a physical therapy such as dance or drama.

We again approached several projects delivering arts-based community initiatives in the city, to help facilitate the sessions, and asked the young people what they would want to do if they could get the chance to take part in a creative activity. The young people said they wanted a place where they could meet weekly, straight after school, share food and try out different creative arts. We agreed to hold several workshops, including art, music, dance and poetry.

> Writing stories, telling life stories and becoming more self-aware; this is the greatest story of all. The more you can face reality in life, the less stressful your life becomes, less even though the stressful events still exist. (Salans, 2004: 192)

The young people were encouraged to plan the sessions and what they wanted included. They wanted the sessions to be about their lives – past, present and future – and to use poems and art as a basis to explore this.

We held weekly creative writing and poetry workshops, which were co-facilitated with a local charity called The Reader Organisation. A local print artist also gave her time for free to help the young people make pictures to go with the poems they wrote. The poems explored several themes, including past, present and lost relationships, missing home and being in a new place, and thoughts and feelings about living in exile. We discussed poems that reflected their interests, such as poems about food, relationships, music and school. We would read the poems aloud to each other, and then the young people would write their own poems.

This can be seen as a warm-up to the his-and-her stories (the personal aspects of their lives that connected them) that would develop over time. As the sessions progressed over the eight weeks the group ran, so did the poems and the prints that the young people produced to illustrate them. The group went on to produce a wonderful book of personal poems with the title *Same City, Different Journeys*.

> **Humankind wishes to be heard and more importantly to be understood. (St Thomas & Johnson, 2007: 26)**

One of the poems was written by a young woman in the group about the situation in the Democratic Republic of the Congo (DRC) and highlights her on-going worries and concerns, even though she was now in a safe place.

> **Congo**
> I am from a place that's very sunny,
> My friends sometimes say I'm funny.
> Congo has a war and has lost all its money,
> That's why every night I fill with worry.

In the poem, the young woman looks and is described as very sunny and often funny in her presentation to everyone. But behind her outward shell, she continues to feel anxious about her situation. The poem articulates how her experience of being a refugee continues to affect her in the present.

Her family had had a good life in the DRC: a car, nice home, and family and friends. In the UK, she now lived in a damp house in a deprived area. Her mother had become depressed by the situation they found themselves in, and thoughts of the war/conflict were never far away for her or for her daughter. The young woman was also struggling to make new friends.

In the group, many of the young people identified with her. They shared similar stories and situations, and she developed a support system that went beyond our once-weekly sessions.

This can be seen in another poem she produced, which highlights the very important need for social support to help maintain emotional health.

Best friends

Me and my friends are always there for each other.

We're united,

We're together,

We're like one person:

We'll never be apart.

When we talk, we never stop.

We think we have the same voice.

Best Friends.

Having someone alongside us during difficult journeys to support, share, identify, care and be a witness is vitally important for healing and growth from traumatic events. 'The value of psychosocial methods of support is now widely accepted' (Kalmanowitz & Lloyd, 1997: 14).

This poem illustrates the vital importance for health of having a safe space to connect with others. Feeling isolated, rejected and alone with thoughts and feelings for a prolonged time can only compound those feelings, whereas being with others in the 'same boat' gives you the chance and opportunity to be reconnected.

As van der Kolk reflects: 'Most human beings simply cannot tolerate being disengaged from others for any length of time' (2014: 117).

Stones and flowers

Among the therapies we offered the young people were specific trauma-focused approaches, including eye movement desensitisation and reprocessing (EMDR), children's accelerated trauma therapy (CATT), and narrative exposure therapy (NET).

We recognised that trauma often disables a person's social and emotional life, and that the above therapies have a place in exploring and reprocessing trauma in a safe and contained way.

As a team, NET fitted with our creative approach, in that it uses techniques from cognitive behaviour therapy (CBT), narrative therapy and creative arts.

> In NET, the client, with the assistance of the therapist, constructs a chronological narrative of his or her life story, with a focus on the traumatic experiences. Fragmented reports of the traumatic experiences will be transformed into a coherent narrative. Empathic understanding, active listening, congruency, unconditional positive regard, and directive perseverance are key components of the therapist's approach. (Schauer, 2015: 199)

NET helps the client develop a coherent narrative of the trauma experienced in the here and now. The client creates a lifeline, along which stones and flowers are placed to represent trauma (stones) and strengths/positive moments (flowers).

The therapist guides and supports the client to revisit the trauma in the here and now. During the therapy, the therapist creates a narrative letter, which they read back to the survivor for the following session. Any changes about the understanding of the narrative are then made with the client, and a new letter is produced. This can happen many times before a coherent narrative is reached and agreed with the survivor. This process helps to create some order to memories that feel jumbled, chaotic and unmanageable.

Before starting NET, the therapist explains the process to the client, and explains trauma responses to them and the families or carers supporting them. The therapist also shares simple techniques to help the young person 'ground' themselves in the here and now. These include deep breathing, noting physical symptoms, focusing on being in the moment, and having someone with them (such as the therapist) to support them through the terrifying scenes.

One young man came to our service with severe trauma symptoms. He had fainting attacks, epileptic-like fits and visual disturbances that meant he sometimes thought parts of his body were bigger than they were. He was seen by several medical doctors, who ruled out physical causes, but his symptoms continued, and distressed him and those around him.

I explained NET to him and suggested he might find it helpful, and he agreed to give it a go. The flower moments are placed along the lifeline first, and the client is encouraged to note their strengths and positive aspects that could be helpful in managing the stone (trauma) moments.

The young man remembered being on a veranda with his grandmother, with a pet canary bird. He felt very positive about this moment, having had a good relationship with his grandmother. They would listen to the sound of the canary in the late evening sunlight. He also placed some other flower moments, such as playing with a friend in the street, and the joy and pleasure of playing for its own sake.

With the stone events, I encouraged him to describe each trauma moment in detail, and we revisited each event together. I supported him to stay in the here and now, and to recognise that he could explore the scene without his body sensations overwhelming him to such an extent that he would not be able to view the scene.

NET also has a role in documenting a coherent story of atrocities that can be used as testimony in the asylum process, and more widely in gathering evidence on torture and genocide.

> **Working through disturbing thoughts and feelings is achieved by actively thinking about them, talking or writing about them, or processing them by other means of expression. The crucial point is that difficult thoughts or feelings are confronted rather than denied or avoided. (Saari, 2005: 127)**

Eventually we came to the big stone – the event he avoided and never talked about, but always remembered in his dreams and bodily sensations. I could see that just the thought of looking at it made him breathe faster, and he became restless in his seat and was in a heightened state of arousal – a protective response to a perceived threat that he feared confronting.

I spoke directly to him, using his name and reminding him to breathe slowly, that he was here with me now, that he was not alone, and that he was safe now. He brought his breathing under control and we began the journey to the traumatic event, which he had been unable to face for many years.

He began to retell the story of being taken by his grandfather in a big car out into the desert, to a military base. He remembered the smell of the car and that he fell asleep on the journey. As he spoke, he was back at the military base; he could see the colours of the walls, and he described going down a corridor with his grandfather, who took him into a room and left him there.

His breathing again increased as he described the room and his body became tense. Again, I spoke to him about his breathing, how to bring it under control, and that we were here together to face the event that he had always avoided talking about to anyone.

He told me the room had a window onto a courtyard, and he was aware that there were others around. He saw a man being dragged across the courtyard and tied against a post. 'I knew something bad was going to happen. I wanted to shout "stop" but couldn't.'

Then he heard the shot, and the man slumped to the ground. He remembered the pool of blood on the ground. He told me that the door to the room opened and his grandfather came in and took him outside to see the shot man. 'I can smell his blood. I should have stopped it.'

He began to breathe faster and sob at what he had seen, but this time, he was not alone. I spoke directly to him, encouraging him to concentrate on his breathing and note for himself how his body felt and what his thoughts were.

He calmed down, and spoke of how his grandfather said only: 'This is how we deal with traitors,' and then he was taken back home across the desert. 'I never spoke to anyone about it. I just couldn't speak. I went straight to my room and went to sleep.'

Following this session, I developed a narrative letter that described to him the event with his grandfather. In the letter, I wrote about how he could manage his thoughts and body sensations, and then checked out with him that what we had heard was correct, and subsequently supported him with his body and emotional response to the narrative. We used breathing techniques that he had learnt in our work together for when his bodily sensations became overwhelming, and this helped him to have a sense of control over them. 'Being validated by feeling heard and seen is a precondition for feeling safe, which is critical when we explore the dangerous territory of trauma and abandonment' (van der Kolk, 2014: 303).

From that moment on, we took the same path together. He would retell the story and I would support him with his bodily symptoms and emotional response. He learned he could control his symptoms and reactions with simple breathing techniques and visualisations of the positive remembered scene on the veranda with his grandmother, in the late evening sun, with the song of the canary that brought a sense of calm and joy to him during difficult times.

Last words

Today I feel
Today I feel more powerful,
In my family and life:
Cool.

The above short verse is another young person's poem from *Same City, Different Journeys*.

Working creatively with survivors of war, trauma, torture and displacement is a worthwhile endeavour. It requires the therapist and team to see the potential of physical activities, like football, and creative approaches such as art, drama, writing and music as ways of healing the damaging effects of trauma on both the individual and collective psyche.

The work is complex and requires us to think beyond our traditional boundaries. No one person or agency can take on the enormous task of healing the individual and the collective.

JL Moreno, who worked in the refugee camps in central Europe during the First World War, commented that 'a truly therapeutic procedure cannot have less an objective than the whole of mankind' (Moreno, 1993: 3).

This statement is so true in refugee work, and reminds us that everyone can be co-therapists to others on the journey of healing from torture and trauma.

I believe that working in the ways described in this chapter can help us move towards achieving this aim.

References

Blackwell D (2005). *Counselling and Psychotherapy with Refugees*. London: Jessica Kingsley Publishing.

Herman JL (1992). *Trauma and Recovery: the aftermath of violence – from domestic abuse to political terror*. New York, NY: Basic Books.

Hudgins K, Toscani F (2013). *Healing World Trauma with the Therapeutic Spiral Model: psychodramatic stories from the frontlines*. London: Jessica Kingsley Publishing.

Hudgins MK (2002). *Experiential Treatment for PTSD: the therapeutic spiral model*. New York: Springer Publishing Company.

Hughes G, Kaur P (2014). Young men from refugee communities score goals for their future, using the team of life. *Context 134*: 25–31.

Kalmanowitz D, Lloyd B (1997). *The Portable Studio. Art therapy and political conflict: initiatives in former Yugoslavia and South Africa*. London: Health Education Authority.

Malchiodi CA (2008). *Creative Interventions with Traumatised Children*. New York, NY: Guilford Press.

Moreno JL (1993). *Who Shall Survive? Foundations of sociometry, group psychotherapy and sociodrama – student edition*. Roanoke, VA: Royal Publishing.

Rousseau C, Guzder J (2008). School-based prevention programs for refugee children. *Child and Adolescent Psychiatric Clinics of North America 17*: 533–549.

Saari S (2005). *A Bolt from the Blue: coping with disasters and acute traumas*. London: Jessica Kingsley Publishing.

St Thomas B, Johnson P (2007). *Empowering Children through Art and Expression.* London: Jessica Kingsley Publishing.

Salans M (2004). *Storytelling with Children in Crisis.* London: Jessica Kingsley Publishing.

Schauer M (2015). Narrative exposure therapy. In: Wright JD (ed). *International Encyclopaedia of the Social and Behavioural Sciences. Vol 16* (2nd edition). Oxford: Elsevier.

Sternberg P, Garcia A (1994). *Sociodrama: who's in your shoes?* Santa Barbara, CA: Praeger Publishing.

van der Kolk B (2014). *The Body Keeps the Score: brain, mind, and body in the healing of trauma.* London: Penguin Books.

Watter C, Ingleby D (2004). Locatrions of care: meeting the mental health and social care needs of refugees in Europe. *International Journal of Law & Psychiatry* 27: 549–570.

White WA (1993). Foreword. In: Moreno JL. *Who shall survive? Foundations of sociometry, group psychotherapy and sociodrama – student edition.* Roanoke, VA: Royal Publishing (p14).

Winnicott DW (1971). *Playing and Reality.* New York, NY: Basic Books.

13. Trauma, attachment and development: the impact of torture on children and young people

Ann Salter

> The combination of the words 'children and torture' is in itself horrifying and alludes to the darker sides of humankind. Yet, children do become victims of torture and the effects can be far more devastating and long-lasting than in the case of adults.
> (Tsiskarishvili, quoted in OHCHR, 2016: 8)

I have worked for more than 10 years with children and young people who have been tortured or indirectly exposed through the torture of family members or others in their communities. I work as a psychotherapist in a human-rights, third-sector organisation that provides rehabilitation to survivors of torture. I have also worked with survivors in other third-sector organisations.

During my work, I have noticed the impact of torture and other traumatic experiences on young people. I have also observed some of the protective factors, such as close contact with family. Conversely, I have noted common factors that lead to a higher degree of vulnerability in young people. This chapter will explore the ways in which the experience of torture can severely impact on a child or young person's mental wellbeing. It will also discuss how a young person's resilience can become a protective feature in their recovery and rehabilitation. The case studies described here are fictional, based on amalgamated examples from my practice.

Torture is brutal, objectifying and dehumanising. It has a devastating impact on individuals, families and communities. Children and young people are especially vulnerable. For them, it has both an immediate effect and an ongoing impact in terms of their physical, cognitive, emotional, social and spiritual development. Torture, therefore, can have a strong influence on the shaping of the adult that the child will become.

Torture causes intense fear, humiliation and shame. The capture, imprisonment and torture of a child or adolescent fundamentally undermines his or her ability to feel safe and protected. A child might feel abandoned by their carer (even though the events may have been totally out of the adult's control). The child may feel completely alone and unprotected, for perhaps the first time. A child or adolescent might also be forced to consider his or her own imminent death, and even to wish for it, as a way of escaping the intolerable pain. Even after torture has ended and the events surrounding the torture are in the past, the child's previous sense of reality and of him or herself may have been totally undermined.

Torture can have different short- and long-term effects on children and adolescents to those it has on adults. Children and young people are developing mentally, physically and emotionally, and the impact of torture can cause problems in any or all of these spheres. They need an ongoing relationship with a trusted adult (who is usually, but not always, a parent), in which they feel protected and cared for. The experience of torture can cause a huge rupture for the young person: the adult in whom they trusted was unable to protect them. This can have a major impact on their ability to feel safe in the world. Therefore, child and adolescent development and attachment are important factors to consider in relation to the impact of torture.

Anyone under the age of 18 has the right to be treated as a child in international and domestic law, due to their needs and vulnerability. At times, I refer to 'children' in this chapter, to emphasise this point. When I am writing about the developmental impact of trauma, I will refer to adolescents to highlight the particular stage of development. Otherwise, I will use the term 'young people' to describe anyone between the age of 14 and the early 20s.

I hope that this chapter will be useful for practitioners working with adults, as well as those working with children and adolescents. Many adult survivors of torture were first tortured while they were still young people. Some may not have been able to flee their country of origin immediately, and so may arrive in the UK as adults. Sometimes young torture survivors who arrive in the UK are unable to access therapeutic and rehabilitation services specifically aimed at children and young people. This can be due to a lack of specialist services designed to meet the needs of child and adolescent survivors of torture. It might also be because the young person's support workers are not aware that the young person is a survivor of torture. In these situations, a survivor of torture may grow into adulthood before they can access therapeutic services to address the torture experienced during adolescence. When this happens, it is sometimes not clear to the practitioner that the adult who they are now seeing for therapy was in fact a child or adolescent when the torture occurred. This might mean that one of the key aspects of the impact of torture could be missed: the developmental and attachment aspect of the (now) adult survivor's trauma response.

Adolescents are among the most vulnerable groups, along with young children, to the effects of war and violence: 'The youngest because of the risk of separation from parents, the adolescents by the high vulnerability and higher sensitivity for traumatisation and subsequent interference with phase-specific and identity development' (Adam & van Essen, 2004: 524).

In this chapter, I will reflect on both the adolescent experience of 'higher sensitivity for traumatisation' and its subsequent impact and interference with development, as well as explore the impact on young people of separation from their parents/key attachment figures. This might be a temporary separation, with reunion after the period of captivity and torture, or it might last for several years. It might even be permanent if the parents have been killed or have 'disappeared'. Enforced separation at a time of acute stress is likely to have a lasting effect on the young person.

Adolescents who are tortured very often develop a response of complex trauma. The ISTSS definition of complex post-traumatic stress disorder (PTSD) (ISTSS Complex Trauma Task Force, 2012) includes the core symptoms of PTSD, such as re-experiencing the traumatic event, avoidance/numbing and hyper-arousal, in conjunction with a range of other disturbances related to an individual's capacity for self-regulation. This includes the ability to relate to others, emotional regulation, dissociation and somatic symptoms. I will explore the impact that these trauma responses can have on a child and young person's development. I will also explore the layers of loss and ruptured attachments that form part of a young person's traumatic experience. The combination of these factors can mean that adolescents face a unique assault on their developing identity and sense of themselves in the world.

I will discuss the effects that the experience of complex trauma has on a child's or young person's development, and the relationship between this and their ongoing need for attachment with a trusted adult. I will consider the inter-relationship of complex trauma, attachment and development to highlight some of the particular difficulties faced by young people who have been tortured. And I will explore the impact of life in exile, where a child is separated from family and community, on the rehabilitation and recovery of children and young people who have been tortured.

Attachment relationships and their importance

One of the aims of torture is to undermine and destroy an individual's personality, relationships and sense of themselves as part of a family and community: 'The torturer attempts to destroy a victim's sense of being grounded in a family and society as a human being with dreams, hopes and aspirations for the future...Torture can profoundly damage relationships between spouses, parents, children... and their communities' (OHCHR, 1999: 43).

Young people rely on their attachment with families and communities for emotional and physical safety. The attachment relationship is fundamental to healthy development; the violent rupture of this through torture has profound consequences for the young person. This is the case even for adolescents who might be in many ways capable of living independently.

Attachment theory is often discussed with reference to babies and young children and to adult attachment style. For young people who have experienced catastrophic events such as torture and brutal separation from their families and communities, attachment is clearly highly significant. These experiences have an impact on a young person's ability to form secure and trusting relationships. This can become significant in the therapy.

One of my clients, a 19-year-old young man called Anton, from the Democratic Republic of the Congo (DRC), spent the first six months of therapy in a state of almost constant terror. His eyes would dart around the room, and he would react fearfully to any noise, such as doors closing elsewhere in the building. He barely spoke. After a few months, Anton told me that he was frightened that people wanted to kill him. I asked him to tell me more about this, and Anton was able to tell me that he also thought that I and the interpreter wanted to kill him. Anton said that when he walked into the building, people looked at him 'with mean faces'. He had been so affected that he was unable to recognise when people were expressing kindness or concern in their face, voice or body language. After a number of months in therapy, Anton was slowly able to internalise the relationship with both me and the interpreter. He then found a small number of other people with whom he felt safe. From this point, he was able to start rebuilding his life.

These primary relationships are internalised by babies and children to form internal working models of relationships, from which an individual is able to make secure relationships throughout the lifespan. Torture can therefore be seen as an attempt to destroy a young person's primary attachment relationships, and thus damage their ability to develop trusting and fulfilling relationships as they develop into adulthood.

Attachment theory is a cornerstone of developmental psychology, psychotherapy and mental health (Berry, Danquah & Wallin, 2016). It was devised initially by John Bowlby and developed in collaboration with Mary Ainsworth. This has led to a deeper understanding of the central importance of the earliest caregiver–infant relationship throughout a person's life.

This attachment relationship continues throughout childhood and into adolescence and adulthood. While attachment patterns change and develop, and the attachment between primary caregiver and child may appear to become less important during adolescence, acute stress is likely to trigger the need for the attachment bond.

The attachment system between a baby and the caregiver has at its root survival: 'Bowlby understood that the primal nature of attachment as a motivational system is rooted in the infant's absolute need to maintain physical proximity to the caregiver, not just to promote emotional security but in fact to ensure the infant's literal survival' (Wallin, 2007: 11-12).

There are three key phases of attachment described by Bowlby as part of the attachment system: seeking, monitoring, and attempting to maintain proximity to a protective attachment figure; secure base, and safe haven (Wallin, 2007:12). The attachment system is a life-or-death necessity; Wallin writes about the child 'fleeing to an attachment figure as a "safe haven" in situations of danger and moments of alarm' (Wallin, 2007: 12).

This description of the importance of the physical proximity of a caregiver to the child has been expanded to include the development of the child's internal sense of safety and security. Furthermore, this attachment system remains crucial for a person's whole life. Wallin writes that Bowlby 'came to believe that the manifestations of the biologically driven need to attach are significant across the entire lifespan' (2007: 13).

Steele and van der Hart write of the importance of secure attachment in the development of a coherent self:

> Secure attachment supports the hard wiring of the child's brain that will determine to a large degree how well he or she is able to regulate and relate to others across the lifespan (Schore, 2003). Consistent activation of the social engagement system via secure attachments help maintain a regulated psychobiological foundation that supports ongoing integration of a child's personality, that is, the predictable and consistent ways of being that define a child. The child learns not only to depend safely upon others to help soothe and reassure but also to self-regulate

and to integrate experience and a consistent sense of self across time and situations (Steele & van der Hart, 2014: 79–80)

While adults tend to develop their attachment bonds with sexual partners and friends they love, adolescents still maintain a strong attachment need for their primary caregiver, such as their mother. This can be the case even when a young person is in the process of forming new bonds with peers, sexual partners, or, indeed, their own children. Like the child described by Wallin, young people will also need to be able to seek out an attachment figure, particularly during times of stress: 'Attachment behaviour involves seeking proximity to a figure able to assuage distress... one who is older and wiser' (Steele & van der Hart, 2014: 16-17).

They may be approaching adulthood, and may have achieved a high level of competence in many areas, but adolescents may still in other ways be highly vulnerable. They still need to be able to return to the 'safe haven' of someone who is 'older and wiser.'

This is clearly not possible for young people who have been brutally removed from their family and community, and who may be living in exile in an unfamiliar country.

Cultural differences, multiple attachment systems and gender

Attachment theory is a predominately western theory and has been criticised for accepting western paradigms of parenting and parent–child relationships as the norm. Quinn and Mageo argue that 'attachment theory's claims and constructs suffer from profound ethnocentrism' (2013: 3).

Research conducted into forms of attachment and styles of child-rearing across cultures has questioned the universal desirability of a model of childcare where the mother forms an almost exclusive bond with her baby. Indeed, according to Morelli and Henry: 'Babies develop close, trusting relationships with many... of the people who care for them... babies may develop multiple representations of relationships with many, though not all, of the people who care for them' (2013: 244).

Similarly, Meehan and Hawks write of a 'growing understanding of the extent and nature of children's broader social relationships – specifically, that the mother–child dyad does not exist in isolation' (2013: 85). They continue: '... children form meaningful attachment relationships with some, but not all, of their non-maternal caregivers' (2013: 85).

It is therefore important to remember that young survivors of torture who have fled to the UK may have had a very different experience of family and community patterns of attachment than is predominant in the west. There may not be the single child–mother attachment bond, but rather a 'network of relationships' that underlies the child's attachment system: '... it makes little sense to consider close relationships in isolation of one another from either the infant's or the caregiver's perspective. Rather, they should be seen as constituting a network of relationships that engender feelings of security in babies' (Morelli & Henry, 2013: 244).

While attachment, and the resulting ability to feel safe and secure, may have developed through a range of caregiving relationships internalised by the baby and developing child, much of the research, including cross-cultural research, positions the mother as primary attachment figure (Quinn & Mageo, 2013; Wallin, 2007).

Quinn and Mageo, in the introduction to their edited volume of cross-cultural research challenging attachment theory's western bias, state: '... all of these authors agree... the universal fact that primary attachment is to mother or a single mother substitute. This is so even in cases where the mother is not the infant's or child's routine caregiver' (2013: 19).

It may be the case that the infant will internalise relationships with a wider range of carers than those considered in classic attachment theory, and that this can lead to positive adaptation, and the ability to seek comfort from more than one 'safe haven' in times of stress or danger. It is also true that some young people will have another figure as a primary attachment bond, such as an older sibling, grandmother or father. Research also indicates that, whoever their primary caregiver is, the child's fundamental patterns of attachment will have developed within a wide network of family and community caregivers where they grew up (Quinn &, Mageo, 2013). It is important to be aware of this in the therapeutic process.

However, it is also the case that the figure to whom the infant and developing child will automatically turn for comfort in times of stress is likely to be the mother.

This is reflected in my experience of therapy with young survivors of torture who have been separated from their family. For many of these young people (but not all), it is their mother for whom they have yearned as a primary source of comfort. This is most evident in societies where there is a clear division of gender roles.

The experiences of many young people who were tortured as children or adolescents and have fled to the UK show how important their primary attachment still is while they are under acute and severe stress.

Francois fled captivity in the Cameroon when he was 16 years old. His father was involved in anti-government politics, which led to the whole family being targeted by government forces. Francois was 14 when his father was arrested; the family never found out where the father was taken. Francois began to have nightmares, and would cry out during the night. His mother would come to him, to offer reassurance and comfort.

Six months after the arrest of his father, both Francois and his mother were arrested and detained. Francois witnessed the rape of his mother, before they were taken to separate areas in the detention facility. He was kept in a small cell with many other male prisoners, and was regularly beaten. There were no toilet facilities in the cell, and Francois was forced to clean up excrement (his own and that of other prisoners). He was able to escape when his uncle bribed the guards. His uncle then arranged false documents and a flight to the UK for him. He did not know what had happened to his mother.

On arrival, Francois was interviewed by the Home Office. The officials accepted his age, so he was taken into the care of the local authority as a 'looked-after child'. He was placed in foster care, and attended the local school. He already spoke good English, and he did well in exams at 16 and 18.

On leaving foster care at the age of 18, Francois was housed in a flat at the top of a high-rise building. He sometimes found himself standing at the window, feeling on the verge of jumping. At these times, he could hear two voices: the voice of the guard from the prison, ridiculing him and telling him to jump, and the voice of his mother, telling him how well he was doing, and that he had come such a long way. Francois said that hearing his mother's voice prevented him from jumping out of the window.

Attachment and trauma

Francois was 15 when he was held captive and tortured. He had a strong need to return to the secure base of his mother. The fact that he could not turn to her for comfort, and that he was forced to witness her rape, greatly added to the trauma of his own experience of imprisonment and torture.

Francois's attachment need for his mother would have added an extra layer of horror to his being made to witness her rape. His powerlessness to do anything to protect her, combined with his underlying need to be cared for by her, would have caused an unbearable dilemma.

> Worry about the safety of a family member or friend, whether in the next room or at a different location, adds an additional source of extreme stress... Witnessing the death of an attachment figure or peer evokes concurrent acute reactions to

the loss, even while the life threat continues. (Pynoos, Steinberg & Goenjian, 2006: 339)

This illustrates a clear connection between attachment and trauma for a young person: the disrupted attachment adds to and is part of the experience of trauma. This will influence the traumatic response, both in the short and long term.

Sinason writes of the connection between attachment and trauma in relation to child and adolescent refugees. While some early infant or childhood trauma can occur through difficulties in the primary attachment relationship(s), this is not always the case:

> Where the trauma is external but the parent is unable to mediate the experience because of her own traumatized experience... children experience more physiological and emotional anxiety whereas a parent remains calm and appears in control, the child's anxiety before and after is lessened. (Sinason, 2002: 131)

Francois had nobody to turn to for 'mediation of the experience of trauma'. Children and young people rely on their caregivers to be able to process and make sense of traumatic experiences. They need the opportunity to create, with a trusted adult, the narrative of what has happened, including how the child felt and still feels about the events:

> Children's traumatic narratives typically rely on co-construction with parents or other adult caretakers. Co-construction can assist a child in clarifying details of the traumatic experience, understanding its context and meaning, and addressing cognitive confusions. (Pynoos, Steinberg & Goenjian, 2006: 349)

This was not possible for Francois. He was left to cope on his own with overwhelming trauma and loss.

Francois lived through and survived layers of trauma over a relatively short period of time. This time coincided with early/mid adolescence. There is considerable research about the effects of early relational and developmental trauma on babies and young children (Schore, 2003; van der Kolk, 2014). Less has been written about what happens to children who have had a relatively secure early childhood, with good-enough attachment, who are suddenly faced with multiple and catastrophic loss and trauma. The young person in this situation often feels as if all familiar aspects of their life have been taken away.

'I have lost my self' is a phrase I often hear. That part of the self they feel they have lost may be their close family, and the internal and external coherence provided by that relationship (Steele & van der Hart, 2014). The long-term impact of this degree of loss and trauma can be devastating for them.

Adolescence is a time of immense developmental change. The rate and scale of changes occurring during this time means that a young person is extremely vulnerable to the impact of traumatic events. Music states: 'The teenage brain is fast reconfiguring but also vulnerable [and] easily damaged' (2011: 189). He writes of some of the ways that the brain is developing: 'Adolescence is marked by massive brain development and hormonal upheaval... These changes almost rival those of early childhood.' The changes in the brain include 'a major process of pruning, the loss of grey matter and an increase in myelination, the white wrapping around neurons leading to brain signals travelling around 100 times faster' (2011: 188).

This process is part of an adolescent's progression to an adult level of cognitive functioning. There are other processes in the developing brain that mean that a young person is vulnerable in other areas of function:

> The frontal lobes, central to what is often called executive functioning, are one of the last areas to fully develop, often not until the early 20s... the limbic system, where risk and emotionally driven behaviour is rooted, is definitely 'online'... whereas the parts which are involved with more 'top-down' control and executive functioning are at a level more like a child (Music, 2011: 188).

This suggests that, when considering a child's reactions to events that are experienced as highly traumatic, we need to do so in the light not only of the range of traumatic responses that we might normally see (van der Kolk, 2014; Schore, 2003; Herman, 1992), but also the particular stage of their brain development. Some reactions to events might not appear logical when viewed from an adult's perspective, but may be much more understandable when considered in terms of adolescent development.

It has been clearly demonstrated that the development of an infant's brain is adversely affected by prolonged exposure to stress hormones, such as cortisol (van der Kolk, 2014; Schore, 2013). However, as shown above, it is also true that the adolescent brain is vulnerable to the effects of trauma and prolonged stress, which have the potential to affect brain development, and so have an impact on future ability and functioning.

Francois experienced many layers of traumatic events. He felt frightened because of his father's political activity, and absorbed his parents' fear of being caught. He experienced terror and sudden loss when his father was arrested. These experiences, however, were mediated by his mother, who was able to provide some comfort to Francois, even while dealing with her own distress. At the point of Francois' arrest and detention, however, and his witnessing of his mother's rape, he was forced to confront his terror alone, with nobody to whom he could turn for comfort.

Pynoos and colleagues write that:

> Adolescents may acutely experience an 'existential dilemma' over the conflict of intervening on behalf of others or taking self-protective action... In violent circumstances, children may also feel compelled to inhibit wishes to intervene, or to suppress retaliatory impulses, out of fear of provoking counter-retaliatory behaviour (Pynoos, Steinberg & Goenjian, 2006: 338–339).

Francois experienced simultaneously a high degree of powerlessness while witnessing the rape and an urgent need to intervene to protect his mother. This would have placed an intolerable strain on a young person.

Trauma and dissociation

I had been seeing Bejana for psychotherapy for six weeks when she told me that she had been to see her friends the previous night. I asked Bejana who her friends were, and where she had met them. I was unable to understand her answer, and felt confused. I wondered whether Bejana was being exploited, or what she was finding difficult to disclose. Bejana finally told me that she had been 'to the sky', where her friends were. The journey started in her room, where she heard her friends calling, and then she went 'to the sky'. She felt happy there, and her friends were kind to her. She didn't know any of their names, or where she had initially met them.

> Derealization and depersonalization reactions allow the victim to avoid the reality of his or her situation, or watch it as a detached observer. These processes can create an experience of leaving the body, travelling to other worlds, or immersing oneself into other objects in the environment... If it is too painful to experience the world from inside one's body, even one's

> self-identity can become organized outside the physical self.
> (Cozolino, 2010: 269–270)

Bejana had experienced many painful events, including witnessing the killing of her family. Dissociation was a way to escape, at least temporarily, from experiencing the horror.

Dissociation is a common response to trauma. It has been described as 'the escape where there is no escape', which clearly alludes to the need to find some kind of release from extreme and unbearable psychological threat. Dissociation at the time of a traumatic event involves a psychological distancing or absence from the event. It may feel as if the person is not there at all, or is watching 'from the sidelines' (Levine, 1997: 138). There may be complete absences, or a person may feel that they are merging into an object in the room – for example, 'becoming part' of the pattern in the wallpaper. Dissociation as a response to trauma may enable a young person to survive physically, and may help them avoid total psychological fragmentation.

> Dissociation allows the traumatized individual to escape trauma via a number of biological and psychological processes. Increased levels of endogenous opioids create a sense of well-being and a decrease in explicit processing of overwhelming traumatic situations. (Cozolino, 2010: 269)

Thus, dissociation can be seen as an adaptive response to traumatic events. In the longer term, however, dissociative responses can become distressing. Dissociation involves a rupture in an individual's sense of a continuous self, and a disconnection from the body (Cozolino, 2010; Levine, 1997). This can lead to problems such as confusion and disorientation; difficulties in cognitive processing and forming memories, and a sense of being 'cut off' from the world. These responses may in turn inhibit recovery and rehabilitation from the trauma.

Mukhtar was a 17-year-old young man from Libya. He was held captive and tortured by a local militia group for two weeks when he was 16. When he was released, his older cousin helped him to flee by booking a flight and providing Mukhtar with false documents. When the plane landed in London, Mukhtar was confused and disorientated. His documents were identified as false, so he was taken for questioning by immigration officials from the Home Office.

Mukhtar was 17 on arrival in the UK. However, the Home Office stated they believed him to be older than this. He was therefore referred to social services for an age assessment. The social worker assessed him to be 18, so he was placed in adult accommodation, with minimal support. Mukhtar spent most of his time alone in his room, where he experienced frequent flashbacks to the torture. He missed his family, and did not know how to contact them.

Mukhtar was referred for therapy by his GP, who was concerned about his high level of distress and post-traumatic symptoms. In the second session of therapy, Mukhtar said that he had spent the previous night on a bench in the city centre. He did not know how he had arrived there. It was already dark and cold when he found himself there, and he was too frightened to move or to try to go home. Somebody tried to sell him drugs. When it became light, Mukhtar was able to find his bus stop and make his way home.

This level of dissociation, as well as causing distress and confusion, can lead to a high level of risk. Some young people self-harm while in a dissociated state, and then do not know how they were hurt. Some may walk in front of traffic, unaware of their surroundings. Young people may become at risk of assault or exploitation if they become lost and disorientated.

This can make it difficult for the therapist to work with a young person on strategies to stay safe. It is important to work closely with mental health professionals and the GP to manage the risk.

I saw Mukhtar for therapy for three years. During the first year, I became increasingly concerned by Mukhtar's high level of risk of self-harm. He would tell me that he would suddenly 'find' himself late at night in the city centre or in a local park, with no memory of how he had arrived there. At other times, he would wake up in the morning with cuts on his arms, and did not know how these injuries had been caused. My assessment was that Mukhtar had acted while in a dissociative state, and was then unable to recall what had happened. This lack of awareness and control of his actions meant that Mukhtar was sometimes unable to keep himself safe.

I helped Mukhtar develop strategies to find support while he was distressed, before he became dissociated. For example, visiting or talking to his friend would help him to become calmer. We also worked on plans of what to do when he 'came round' from a dissociative state, such as walking to the nearest bus stop, if he was in an unfamiliar place.

Throughout, I was in frequent contact with Mukhtar's GP and community mental health team. This meant that we were able collectively to manage the risk for Mukhtar. The mental health team was able to make home visits to Mukhtar and assess his mental health at times when he displayed a high level of vulnerability, dissociation and distress.

As the therapy progressed, Mukhtar had enough safety in place to begin to start processing his memories of the torture. His dissociative episodes eventually decreased in frequency and intensity.

Trauma-related voices

I first met Farhad when he was 20 years old. He had been in the UK for three years, having fled the Taliban in Afghanistan. The Taliban had forced his family to give him to a training camp, with the threat that all his younger siblings would be killed if they did not. Farhad had been forced to witness executions, and was expected to become a suicide bomber. A few days before his planned mission, a camp guard smuggled him out. Farhad managed to contact his father, who arranged for him to flee to Iran. From there, he travelled with a people smuggler across the Mediterranean and Europe. The people smuggler put him and a group of others into a refrigerated lorry in France that was destined for the UK. Farhad was found at a motorway service station in the north of England. He did not know where he was, or which country he was in.

Farhad was not able to see his mother or younger brothers and sisters before he left Afghanistan. His father had told him that they would all follow him out of Afghanistan. He had not had any news of them since then.

Farhad was referred to therapy by his legal representative as he became highly distressed and frightened when asked to recount his experiences.

When I first met Farhad for therapy, he appeared with a bag containing all of his belongings. He told me that he was too frightened to leave them in his house, as he believed they would be stolen by the Taliban. As I enquired more about this, Farhad told me that he heard the Taliban speaking to him at night. One time, the man from the Taliban had told him to kill himself, so Farhad went to find a knife from the kitchen drawer. One of the other men in the house stopped him from hurting himself by pulling the knife out of his hand.

Farhad believed that his life was at risk. He was terrified that the Taliban would be able to find him. Hearing the voice from the Taliban confirmed Farhad in his belief that this was the case.

Farhad also sometimes heard his mother speaking to him, especially during the night. At times, he found this comforting; at other times, he worried that she was angry with him. The telephone number that he had for his family did not work. Farhad was terrified that they were dead, particularly his mother: 'If I find out that she is dead, then I will kill myself.'

Both Farhad and Francois heard the voice of their mother, which enabled them to experience some comfort. They also both heard the voices of their persecutors. This caused terror and made them fear for their lives. Francois had psychological insight into his experience; he understood that the voice he heard from the prison guard came from the memories of what had happened to him. Farhad did not have this understanding. He felt consistently terrified of what the Taliban fighters would do to him when they entered his room at night.

This level of dissociative re-experiencing of events from the past might be experienced by young people who have been exposed to layers of traumatic events. This is particularly the case when the young person does not have a loved or trusted adult to help them process what has happened. The young person is therefore unable to assimilate their experiences or create a coherent narrative.

Following the period of captivity and torture, Farhad experienced multiple life-threatening events on his journey to the UK. He was frightened and uncertain for much of the time, and was beaten and threatened by the people smuggler. This is a common experience for young people who make this journey. On arrival in the UK, Farhad had to start to adjust to life in exile, while still uncertain about whether he would be accepted as a refugee. While still traumatised by all of these events, Farhad was longing for the comfort of his family. Farhad found not knowing the fate of his family, to whom he would otherwise turn for care and reassurance, almost too much to bear. This is the context in which he started to hear his mother talk to him in the night.

Young people who hear trauma-related voices may have had a straightforward development and attachment pattern until the time of the trauma. Other young people may have experienced conflict in their home country from a young age, and may therefore have absorbed the fear of the adults around them. Some of the family members may have been able to 'mediate' the frightening experiences for their children, and some not. The difference may be due to a range of factors, including temperament, family situation and surrounding levels of threat.

While there may be a link with the experience of psychosis, many young people who hear trauma-related voices and see visual hallucinations of those involved in their torture do not have more generalised symptoms. Their disturbing hallucinations are often directly connected with the traumatic events. These hallucinations are different from the flashbacks in that they are experienced as happening in the present, in the young person's 'here and now', and not as if the young person were back in the terrifying situation in which the torture occurred. I have been with a young person who has seen his torturer in the room, sitting behind me. He retained awareness of where he was and who he was with, and was clearly in the present, but he was convinced that the torturer was there.

These traumatic hallucinations are related to unprocessed traumatic memories (van der Kolk, 2014). For children and adolescents, it also suggests a developmental rupture, where there is no possibility of receiving support from someone with whom they have a close attachment.

Pynoos and colleagues state:

> ... intrusive images constitute memory markers that often capture moments of traumatic helplessness, terror, horror, and utter ineffectiveness – for example, at the occurrence of an irreversible injury to a parent. Of special importance is the fact that these memory markers may also indicate 'injury' to a developmental expectation... that may have serious developmental consequences. (2006: 345).

Resilience

Resilience has been described as the 'capacity to bend and bounce back after adversity' (Jones, 2013: 195). It is a word that is often used in relation to young people who have experienced many layers of traumatic events, including the loss of family and home. The fact that a young person has survived many life-threatening situations and is managing to build a life in the UK, even though it may be difficult and uncertain, can be seen to demonstrate 'resilience'.

However, resilience is a complex phenomenon. It is not something you either have or lack. It has been shown to be a mixture of factors, some neurobiological, some depending on circumstances and experience, which constantly interact with one another (Jones, 2013).

Young people who have survived torture, endured forced separation from their family and community and are living in exile will usually display a mixture of vulnerability and resilience. A young person's ability to survive a hazardous and life-threatening journey and to start learning a new language and navigate unfamiliar support, education and legal systems demonstrates a high level of resilience. The therapist needs to recognise this, and that the young person should be able to find emotional and practical support when they need it.

A young person's ability to make friends is an important part of developing resilience. Nadim lived on his own, and was frequently in a high level of distress. He said that he often thought of ending his life, and acted impulsively in ways which exposed him to risk of harm. For example, he would purposefully leave his house in the early hours of the morning to walk round his local park. At other times, he would walk to a motorway bridge near his house and consider jumping from it.

During a therapy session, Nadim disclosed that he had been having thoughts of ending his life. I asked Nadim how he might be able to keep himself safe. Nadim had the idea of asking his friend to stay with him overnight. By so doing, he was able to use his own capacity to build and maintain relationships, and to be creative at a time of intense distress. Nadim also managed to find the part of himself that wanted to live.

Lynne Jones, a child psychiatrist, interviewed more than 40 Serb and Muslim children in the immediate aftermath of the Bosnian War, and then returned 20 years later to find out about 'the adults they had become' (Jones, 2013). She found that they almost all described their lives as happy and meaningful. This was despite the fact that many still faced considerable challenges:

> How had they coped so well? The most obvious thing was that none of them felt isolated. They all had supportive families and communities with shared values... They were all still closely connected to their parents. (2013: 286)

An important part of a child's capacity to develop resilience might therefore be a supportive relationship with an attachment figure who is 'older and wiser' and who can help to 'mediate the trauma'. This is clearly not possible for young survivors of torture who have no contact with their family. However, if a young person has had a good-enough experience of early relationships with family and community members, he or she may have an 'internal working model' of relationships (Bowlby, 1969). This can be a great support in developing a new life with new relationships.

'My family would be proud of me'

The experience of torture for a child or young person is an experience of isolation and the devastating absence of adult protection; those who were responsible for keeping the child safe were unable to do so. A child or adolescent's view of the world, and of their place in it, has been radically altered. A young person's ability to trust may have been shaken to the extent that anybody might now be seen as likely to inflict harm.

Lynne Jones has written about research into the incidence of PTSD in children who have lived through conflict:

In conflicts studied around the world, 60 to 80 percent of children showed no psychological ill effects... their well-being was not necessarily related to the amount of violence they had suffered, but it was related to the way they made sense of their experiences, their subjective view of events. (2013: 20)

Young people need to receive therapeutic, social and legal support to enable them to develop trust and to feel safe. A young person is then able to use his or her own resilience to develop new friendships and relationships. These new attachments will inevitably be influenced by a young person's earliest experiences of being cared for as part of a community. With support from all of these relationships, young people are able to start to make sense of their experiences, and to find meaning in their lives. This is the start of recovery.

References

Adam H, van Essen J (2004). In between: adolescent refugees in exile. In: Wilson JP, Drožđek B (eds). *Broken Spirits: the treatment of traumatized asylum seekers, refugees, war and torture victims*. Hove: Brunner-Routledge (pp521–546).

Berry K, Danquah AH, Wallin D (eds) (2016). Introduction. In: Danquah A, Berry K (eds). *Attachment Theory in Adult Mental Health: a guide to clinical practice*. Abingdon: Routledge (pp3–15)

Bowlby J (1969). *Attachment, volume 1*. London: Pimlico.

Cozolino L (2010). *The Neuroscience of Psychotherapy: healing the social brain* (2nd edition). New York, NY: WW Norton & Company.

Herman JL (1992). *Trauma and recovery: the aftermath of violence – from domestic abuse to political terror*. New York, NY: Basic Books.

ISTSS Complex Trauma Taskforce (2012). *The ISTSS Expert Consensus Treatment Guidelines for Complex PTSD in Adults*. [Online.] www.istss.org/ISTSS_Main/media/Documents/ISTSS-Expert-Consensus-Guidelines-for-Complex-PTSD-Updated-060315.pdf (accessed July 2017).

Jones L (2013). *Then They Started Shooting: children of the Bosnian War and the adults they become*. New York, NY: Belle Vue Literary Press.

Levine PA (1997). *Waking the Tiger: healing trauma*. Berkeley, CA: North Atlantic Books.

Meehan CL, Hawks S (2013). Cooperative breeding and attachment among the Aka Foragers. In: Quinn N, Mageo JM. *Attachment Reconsidered: cultural perspectives on a Western theory*. New York, NY: Palgrave Macmillan (pp85–114).

Morelli GA, Henry PI (2013). Afterward: cross-cultural challenges to attachment theory. In:

Quinn N, Mageo JM (eds). *Attachment Reconsidered: cultural perspectives on a Western theory.* New York, NY: Palgrave Macmillan (pp241–250).

Music G (2011). *Nurturing Natures: attachment and children's emotional, sociocultural and brain development.* Hove: Psychology Press.

OHCHR (2016). *How Can Children Survive Torture? Report on the expert workshop on redress and rehabilitation of child and adolescent victims of torture and the intergenerational transmission of trauma.* Geneva: OHCHR.

OHCHR (1999). *Istanbul Protocol: manual on the effective investigation and documentation of torture and other cruel, inhuman or degrading treatment or punishment.* Geneva: OHCHR.

Pynoos R, Steinberg A, Goenjian A (2006). Traumatic stress in childhood and adolescence: recent developments and current controversies. In: van der Kolk B, McFarlane AC, Weisaeth L (eds). *Traumatic Stress: the overwhelming experience on mind, body, and society.* New York, NY: Guilford Press.

Quinn N, Mageo JM (eds) (2013). *Attachment Reconsidered: cultural perspectives on a Western theory.* New York, NY: Palgrave Macmillan.

Schore AN (2013). Relational trauma, brain development and dissociation. In: Ford J, Courtois C (eds). *Treating Complex Traumatic Stress Disorders in Children and Adolescents.* New York, NY: Guilford Press (pp3–23).

Schore AN (2003). *Affect Regulation and the Origin of the Self: the neurobiology of emotional development.* New York, NY: Psychology Press.

Sinason V (2002). Work with refugees. In: Papadopoulos R (ed). *Therapeutic Care for Refugees: no place like home.* London: Karnac Books (pp121–137).

Steele K, van der Hart O (2014). Understanding attachment, trauma and dissociation in complex developmental trauma disorders. In: Danquah A, Berry K (eds). *Attachment Theory in Adult Mental Health: a guide to clinical practice.* Abingdon: Routledge (pp78–94).

van der Kolk B (2014). *The Body Keeps the Score: mind, brain and body in the healing of trauma.* London: Penguin Books.

Wallin D (2007). *Attachment in Psychotherapy.* New York, NY: Guilford Press.

14. Be there but don't be there: working alongside interpreters with survivors of torture in exile

Jude Boyles, Desiré Kinané and Nathalie Talbot

In our experience, one of the barriers preventing survivors of torture from accessing therapy and mental health support is language and the resistance from therapists to working with interpreters. 'Language has been identified as a key barrier to accessing services and maintaining effective communication' (Smith, 2008: 21). The reluctance we have encountered has been driven not by a fear of working with people seeking asylum, or with survivors of torture and/or war, but by anxiety about having a third person in the therapy room.

Tribe and Thompson, in an article exploring the three-way relationship in therapeutic work with interpreters, argue that the use of interpreters in therapy and mental health work is viewed more negatively than is warranted: the 'inherent advantages of this way of engaging with the non-English-speaking client have been minimised or ignored' (2009: 13).

Individuals and families seeking asylum are part of the community to which therapists and mental health services deliver care. Whether or not a team includes bilingual therapists, there will always be a need for interpreters if services are going to be accessible to their whole community. The range of languages spoken now in migrant communities and those seeking asylum, and the fluctuations in global population movement, mean that therapists are unlikely to be able to avoid working with interpreters, despite their anxieties.

We are a therapist (Jude), an interpreter (Nathalie), and an African bilingual therapist and interpreter (Desiré). We have worked together for 14 years, and during that time we have delivered training to both therapists and interpreters, and have worked alongside each other to deliver therapy too. From our different positions in the triad, we have shared a commitment to ensure that the survivors we work with can freely express themselves in their chosen language and dialect.

Before we met in 2003, we had each worked for many years in our respective fields. When we began working together, we were establishing a new service as human-rights practitioners, and aimed to build a therapeutic setting for survivors where the presence of the interpreter enhances therapy, and where the interpreter bears witness alongside the therapist. We worked towards creating a dynamic where the interpreter is experienced as a reassuring and gentle presence by both the survivor and therapist, rather than an obstacle to be tolerated or endured. Our shared commitment is to challenge what Van Parijs (2004) refers to as linguistic injustice – the denial of the right to understand and influence of those who do not speak English as a first language.

> **The right to understand and receive appropriate communication support is a civil right and fundamental to an inclusive and democratic society that seeks to ensure that it provides for the needs of all its citizens.** (Scottish Translation, Interpreting and Communication Forum, 2004: 6)

In our experience, the therapist's ambivalence towards interpreter-mediated therapy leads to an underlying message: 'Be there, but don't be there,' and, we believe, this is often due to a lack of understanding and training on the part of the therapist. As interpreters, we have seen therapists arrive at a training workshop full of concern and doubt about working in a triad. However, by the end of the session, these therapists are open to a new sense of possibility and have developed a new-found empathy and understanding about the complexity and validity of an interpreter's role in therapy. They leave equipped with a fresh confidence, and even eagerness, to begin working in this way, to enable survivors to gain access to therapy.

In a profession where the relationship between a client and therapist is fundamental to the task, having a third person in the room, on whom both the client and therapist rely to communicate, can be anxiety provoking for the therapist. Helen Claire Smith states: 'One of the principal features of mental health practice is the therapeutic alliance that exists between client and therapist, which can be unique, special and curative in its own right' (2008: 21). She argues that, because most therapeutic approaches rely on aspects of interpersonal communication, it is understandable that 'introducing another individual into the relationship dynamic' can change it significantly.

It is widely acknowledged in the refugee sector that, whenever there is an interpreter present, there is a three-way relationship (Baker & Briggs,

1975). The interpreter is there and their presence is felt by both the client and therapist. Most writers in our field describe a triangular relationship, with the same distance between the three people. What we know from our work together, however, is that the distance between the three people can shift throughout therapy: 'The distance between the three participants is always in motion, shifting depending on the material being addressed' (Tribe & Thompson, 2009: 15).

Language is complex, and the process of interpretation is a challenging task. 'Interpreting requires more than just word-for-word translation, and advances meaning in the fullest linguistic and cultural sense, so that two people can understand each other beyond their words' (Raval, 2003: 16). Meanings may be coded, or there may not be a word for a concept that is part of the cultural landscape of a survivor's country. Social constructionist Mudarikiri writes that 'relationships between people can be thought about as existing within the web of meanings that are created by language' (2003: 183).

In this chapter, we aim to share what we have learnt, emphasising the importance of preparation of both interpreter and therapist for interpreter-mediated therapy, and clarity over the roles of both. Often, we have trained or supervised therapists who have struggled along without a framework or code of practice for joint working, over many years. We have frequently heard from both therapists and therapy service managers: 'I wish I could start again, knowing what I know now about what should be in place when we first start working with an interpreting agency, and what good practice looks like.'

The case studies used are fictional and based on amalgamated examples from our practice.

Preparation to work with interpreters

There are interpreting and translation agencies in most towns and cities with refugee communities. It is important to check whether the agency employs qualified interpreters: that is, they have a Diploma in Public Services Interpreting (DPSI), or equivalent, such as the Chartered Institute of Linguists (CIOL) Diploma, or the Ascentis Level 3 in Community Interpreting. Ask for the agency's code of conduct, ensure background checks and references are provided, and that the interpreters have been language-tested in all the languages they offer.

There are several published guidelines for therapists on best practice when working with interpreters, which services can adapt for their own use. It can be helpful to give an interpreter who is new to your service a copy of your code of practice before the first session. The British Psychological Society has produced a helpful set of guidelines, *Working with Interpreters in Health Settings* (Tribe & Thompson, 2008). The third-sector charity Mothertongue has published a *Code of Practice and Ethics for Interpreters and Practitioners in Joint Work* (Costa, undated). Nathalie and Jude have written a short-form guide on good practice, *Working with Interpreters in Psychological Therapy: the right to be understood* (Boyles & Talbot, 2017).

If the therapy team is new to using interpreters, setting up an in-house training course on good practice is helpful, to ensure therapists are fully engaged and prepared for the challenges it brings. Consider the training and support needs of the interpreting team, so they can be inducted into the work of the therapy service and support and supervision can be put in place. A lot of the learning will happen within the triad, but having some training in best practice can help the therapist and interpreter avoid some of the more common pitfalls.

Most agencies will have some interpreters on their books who have experience of working in mental health and therapy settings, but it is a good idea to ask the agency to identify those who want to work in a therapy setting, as interpreting in therapy is not suited to every interpreter's skillset. It is important that interpreters choose to take on this type of work and want to discover more about it.

The aim will be for the therapy team to have access to a small pool of interpreters who are committed to developing their practice in this specialised area. Meeting the training and supervision needs of interpreters is covered elsewhere in this book (see Chapter 15).

Once an interpreting agency has been engaged, it is crucial to outline some ground rules with its administration staff. The therapist must be able to request a specific interpreter, if they wish, and to specify the language/dialect and gender of the interpreter when making the booking. On some occasions, at the request of the client, the therapist may also need to specify a country of origin/region. It is important to agree that, if the requested interpreter is not available, the agency does not just send another interpreter, but informs the therapy service as soon as possible that the usual interpreter is not able to attend.

Organisational considerations before starting work with interpreters

Think about where the interpreter will sit while waiting for the session to start. If they sit in the same waiting area as the client, the client is likely to talk to them, or may ask them to translate documents or letters. They may ask them for their mobile number or for help to make a telephone call. This is understandable, given how rarely survivors have access to qualified interpreters; also, the professional boundaries of the interpreter's role are likely to be unfamiliar to most survivors when they first come to the UK: 'By using what they know and asking for help, they are not relinquishing autonomy but acting with autonomy' (West, 2006: 12).

If a relationship begins to form between the interpreter and survivor in the waiting area, the survivor may begin to align themselves more closely with the interpreter than with the therapist. Also, if a chatty and warm exchange between the client and the interpreter occurs before every session, it can be harder for clients to make the transition to the intensity of therapy and use the therapeutic space effectively.

It is best if the interpreters have somewhere separate where they can wait, so they can prepare themselves for the session, and recover afterwards. If this isn't possible – many therapy agencies lack space, and sessions can run back-to-back – talk to the interpreter about how to manage sharing the waiting area with clients and how they could respond to their questions and requests. Discuss with interpreters how these brief conversations, if they occur, can be brought into the therapeutic space. In a shared space, a skilled interpreter will take a book to read while they wait, to establish a comfortable separation from the client, and just offer a warm greeting when they arrive. If the interpreter is consistently being approached by a client in the waiting area, the therapist can address this directly in the session and explain the boundaries of the interpreting role.

This sense of separation and quiet before a triad meets is familiar in Desiré's culture. In West Africa, the third person, who may be a family member, and the person seeking counsel will sit in separate areas while waiting for their appointment with the Elder, to whom they are coming for advice. It is considered beneficial to have this space and silence before counsel, so that the focus is totally on the matter in hand and the energy of all participants is not scattered and focused on other issues or conversations.

There have been times, in our interpreter role, when we have been sitting in a shared waiting area and a client has approached us for advice or tried to instigate a personal friendship. It is a difficult position to manage as we do not want to create distrust or offence, or say or do something that will be experienced as rejection by the client, which could impact negatively on the therapy.

When the interpreter has been made aware of the necessary boundaries, we can be trusted to manage them, and will use debriefing to discuss any concerns and dilemmas we may be struggling with. The interpreter can operate within these boundaries in shared spaces, while still showing warmth and having appropriate social interaction with survivors. If the interpreter feels too tightly managed, or senses that they are not trusted, this may be detected by clients and affect the quality of the therapy relationship.

The other consideration for any therapy service is how to manage a situation where the interpreter is already known to the survivor, or has interpreted for them in a different setting. In our experience, it is better if the interpreter does not interpret in other settings for the same client, such as with the GP or their legal representative. This will not always be possible, if the client speaks an uncommon language or has asked for a particular, trusted interpreter.

When there is an established relationship between the client and interpreter, it can be challenging for interpreters to be completely present and not affected by knowledge of past disclosures that have not been shared with the therapist. When this dynamic occurs, there may be an unintentional non-verbal channel of communication between client and interpreter. This may put pressure on the client to disclose what has been said elsewhere, or the client may assume that the therapist already knows, as they are unaccustomed to confidentiality within services, or they expect the interpreter to share with the therapist things they have said outside the session.

Interpreters should always tell the therapist if the client is already known to them, whether it is in a professional or personal context. But they must protect the survivor's confidentiality, and should not disclose the details of the organisation where they have previously worked together.

Therapists should discuss within their agency whether they are prepared to work with interpreters who are also employed by the Home Office or the Asylum Tribunal. Therapists practising from a human-rights framework may feel that using interpreters who work with the Home Office decision-makers compromises their personal ethics, as the interpreter may not share their human-rights commitment. More importantly, the client may not feel safe in therapy if the interpreter also works for the organisation that is assessing their claim for asylum.

Briefing the interpreter

If you are working with an interpreter for the first time, arrange to meet them for a half-hour briefing session before the client arrives. This will be helpful in developing a good working relationship with them, as you can establish how you will work collaboratively, as colleagues with distinct roles, before the therapy starts. It helps to avoid confusion about working practices or unhelpful power dynamics, and is an opportunity for the interpreter to raise any anxieties they may have and get a better understanding of the context in which they are to be working. It is also important for the therapist to prepare the interpreter for the likely emotional content of the session, so they can manage their own responses to what they are hearing and translating.

At a practical level, the therapist can also check that the interpreter is willing and able to work at the same time each week in the weeks/months ahead, so the same interpreter can be used throughout the course of therapy.

Negotiate who will explain the interpretation process to the client. There is no right or wrong way to do this, but, in our experience, it works best if the therapist starts the session by introducing the interpreter to the survivor, and asks the interpreter to explain their confidentiality code to the client in the survivor's first language, before translating it back to the therapist.

We are now so used to working together that we don't always need to have these conversations at the pre-session stage, and almost instinctively know how we will manage introductions. After so many years of undertaking this often distressing and challenging work together, we now have a tacit understanding of the other's role. We can hear a break in a voice, or sense a shift in movement or tone that alerts us to a significant disclosure by the client or hints at a change in the therapist's pace. Our respect, trust and knowledge of each other's approach ensures that we are working towards offering survivors a partnership and a frame that can be experienced as containing.

It has taken many years of working together to arrive in this place, but even in established partnerships, it is important not to underestimate the interpreter's need for preparation, given the complexity of the task. Interpreters describe a full briefing as both reassuring and containing.

We have found that it is best not to make assumptions about a new interpreter's practice and to be explicit about what is required. Interpreters should reflect the therapist's tone and speak in the first person. They should be felt as a discreet and gentle presence, and their interpretation should reflect the hesitations, emphasis and pauses in the client's narrative. Interpreters can seek clarification, but they should not volunteer any knowledge from other professional fields. They should not touch clients, and should maintain an appropriate physical distance. When expectations are defined, it enables the interpreter to fully immerse themselves in the session, knowing that the therapist will trust them to fulfil their role.

When working with high levels of distress, arousal and shame, the therapist should explain to the interpreter how they would normally respond to distress in-session. They may find it helpful to explain a bit about trauma, and the principles of undertaking a suicide risk assessment. In some cultures, talking about suicide is taboo, and the interpreter will need to understand that the therapist may ask the client direct questions about self-harm or suicidal thoughts, and that they need to mirror their normalising tone of voice. It can be tempting for interpreters to soften the edges of these dialogues, because of their own cultural assumptions about what can be tolerated by a survivor, or what they can bear to say. If these issues are addressed openly and honestly, a new interpreter is more likely to trust the therapist's approach, even if it seems counter-intuitive at the time. This trust must be earned, of course, but a transparent conversation about these issues can help.

The briefing can also be an opportunity to explain to the interpreter that they shouldn't pass the tissues to the client, and should stay seated if the client jumps to their feet or appears dissociated and disturbed. The therapist should also tell the interpreter that they can request a break if they feel overwhelmed, at any stage. The more the interpreter knows about the therapist's approach to supporting a survivor in distress, the calmer they will be. Reassure interpreters that they will never be left alone in a room with a client.

Some interpreters are very experienced in a range of settings, and will have worked with GPs, legal representatives and support workers, who may have regarded them as advocates or cultural experts, and they may have held considerable power. The shift in power dynamic that is required in the therapy setting may feel disconcerting to some. Explore together how you will resolve misunderstandings in a session or how the interpreter will check with a survivor if they have not understood what they are saying. At no time should the therapist feel left out of an exchange.

If a client responds to a therapist's reflection or question by asking them to repeat it, the interpreter should leave it to the therapist to respond, rather than repeat their own translation; it might be a cue for the therapist to rephrase or slow the pace of the session. There can be some tricky moments in early sessions together, while the therapist and the interpreter establish a working alliance. Each challenge is an opportunity to explore how the partnership is developing.

In the briefing, therapists working from a human-rights framework often state their commitment to human rights and explain that the interpreter and therapist are both bearing witness to a survivor's testimony. Interpreters who do not recognise their role in witnessing, or fail to acknowledge the seriousness of the therapeutic endeavour, can significantly affect the safety of therapy and create a barrier to the survivor's ability to fully disclose. To assume that it is enough for the therapist's approach to be rights based and that the triad will be safe undermines the potential impact of the interpreter's presence and feeds into the notion that the interpreter is an invisible conduit of language – there, but not there.

If an interpreter expresses a prejudice towards a particular social group, or expresses values that cause the therapist concern, it is essential to explore this in the preparation stage. Interpreters need to be able and willing to reflect on their own values in refugee work. 'It is important to be mindful of the way in which power differentials originating in the country of origin may affect the relationship between psychologist, interpreter and client, particularly in the light of political and social conflict' (Tribe & Thompson, 2008: 3). In our experience, interpreters readily discard such preconceptions when they are confronted with the reality of a survivor's experiences in the torturing state and in the host country.

For a survivor who has experienced oppression, persecution and abuse, sensing disapproval or judgment from an interpreter is not only painful but is likely to inhibit the development of a therapeutic alliance. If the therapist senses ambivalence in the demeanour of an interpreter, then the client is likely to feel it too. If the therapist isn't comfortable, or the interpreter is inattentive in the briefing or interrupts the therapist, it may be an indicator of challenges to come. 'We cannot talk if we do not feel free' (Boyles, Talbot & Pahlevan, 2015: 17). This is especially the case if the interpreter is from the dominant social group in the survivor's country of origin and the survivor is from a persecuted minority or tribe. 'It becomes imperative that the therapeutic context does not recreate and reinforce the experience of being marginalised, disempowered and silenced' (Patel, 2003: 222).

Interpreters may hold strong feelings about a country or the atrocities committed there. There is a risk that an interpreter will over-identify with a survivor, or that their own emotions will dominate the therapeutic encounter. Many interpreters are survivors of torture, conflict, and/or gender-based abuses, and have their own histories of loss, separation and exile. These experiences can mean that the interpreter is sensitive, thoughtful and committed to working effectively, but they may also mean that the interpreter will struggle to stay separate enough to be helpful to both the therapist and the client. If a therapist senses this dynamic, explore with the interpreter whether they will need additional supervision or longer debriefings to sustain the work. Many writers in this book have referred to their commitment to practising self-reflexively, but interpreters frequently have no supervisory setting in which to examine their responses to clients.

It can be disturbing and painful for an interpreter to listen to and then voice a survivor's descriptions of abuse when this experience is similar to their own. The therapist should reassure the interpreter that there will be opportunity in the debriefing session to talk about the impact on them of the session, and that they should say if they have felt overwhelmed or are worried about the future direction of the work.

Interpreters may find managing silences challenging, and feel confused and anxious when they occur. It may take time for the interpreter to learn to sit comfortably with quiet periods in the session. The therapist should explain that silence is frequently part of the therapeutic process, and that the interpreter needs to remain calm and focused. Explain why there might be silences and ask the interpreter not to look expectantly at the therapist or client, and not to repeat or prompt the client. Most interpreters will dip their head slightly, but not so much that they come across to the client as embarrassed or uncomfortable. This is a subtle movement. When an interpreter makes efforts to give a discreet message that they are *sitting with*, it can be misunderstood as communicating that they are bored or irritated.

There have been many occasions in our work together when therapeutic engagement has been almost immediate, despite the presence of an interpreter. However, this is not always the case. A study by Miller and colleagues found that it was common for clients to initially form a stronger attachment to their interpreter (2005). Once trust has been established, a skilled and experienced interpreter facilitates the relationship between the client and therapist by keeping their eye contact with the client to a minimum. As therapy progresses, eye contact between the therapist and the client will develop organically. In some situations, there may be cultural or other reasons for limited eye contact, although often this too will change over time.

Sometimes a client can feel so drawn to the interpreter in early sessions that they wonder whether the therapist is a necessary presence. The experience of being understood, empathised with and attended to by the interpreter can leave many clients feeling almost as if the interpreter is speaking directly to them. The interpreter may be seen as a sister or brother, and they may have a shared history of persecution and oppression. Survivors may have expectations about shared experience or struggle that can lead to a quick and intense attachment, inevitably excluding the therapist.

If the therapist appears overly suspicious about a developing relationship between an interpreter and client, it can be challenging and destabilising for the interpreter. Interpreters may feel that the therapist is insecure and perhaps does not understand the cultural link that has been made. They may also feel they are not trusted, which is likely to lead to a closer alliance between the client and interpreter in the triadic relationship.

Survivors may want to know the country the interpreter is from or be keen to find out more about them, such as their tribe or faith. Survivors may not know what they can ask, or whether it is acceptable, but it is important to them. Be sensitive to this, as survivors may feel they need permission to ask questions or voice concerns without the interpreter present. Patel argues that 'the not-knowing can contribute to increased fear, suspicion and mistrust, which can be further compounded by the indifference or unwillingness on the part of the therapist and the interpreter to make explicit their roles and backgrounds' (2003: 232). Prepare for such questions as a partnership; think about how you will manage the situation if the client asks direct questions of the interpreter or if you sense a difficulty that is not named in the therapy room. Check first with the interpreter what they are comfortable with the client knowing.

Ask the interpreter simply to interpret a question, if one is asked. A colleague was working with a survivor who had fled the conflict in the Democratic Republic of the Congo (DRC). The survivor asked the Lingala interpreter: 'How long have you been here?' The interpreter interpreted the question back to the therapist. The therapist gently explained that the interpreter was not able to answer direct questions and was here to interpret, but also acknowledged the importance of the client's question, and opened up a conversation about what lay behind it. The survivor wanted to check whether the interpreter had lived through the conflict, as he felt so connected to him. Perhaps he could also feel a subtle but shared anguish about the continuing conflict.

The survivor, who had been tortured during the conflict, had said to the interpreter in the assessment, when describing his arrival in the UK, 'You know, don't you.' The interpreter and therapist had discussed this in the debriefing and wondered whether the client might be making assumptions about the interpreter's experience. The interpreter had his own story of persecution and exile, which at times could be felt by the therapist in the room. The survivor's question opened up an opportunity for further exploration in the session, and, as the issues were unpacked, it became apparent that what mattered to him wasn't that the interpreter had lived through the recent conflict, but that he felt comforted by his presence: it was familiar and knowing, in that he could sense a shared history and culture. He told them both that he felt 'recognised'.

The survivor was encouraged to explore how alien everything felt to him, including the act of seeking help at a crisis service. He described how reassuring it was to have an interpreter from his home country. His whole being shifted and softened whenever he looked at the interpreter or caught his eye. He was able to say that he knew that the therapist could not possibly understand the meaning of some of what he said, that it could never be completely understood by anyone who had not fled and survived conflict and who was from a different culture. 'Each different language makes particular meanings possible and allows us to experience certain aspects of ourselves' (Mudarikiri, 2003: 183).

The professionalism of the interpreter in just translating the question and the undefended approach and curiosity of the therapist meant that these exchanges became a process of developing understanding across cultures that deepened the relationships in the triad, rather than excluded the therapist, because *how could she really know*? Ortega (2011) argues that a rights-based approach to therapy requires us be grounded in cultural humility, rather than knowing. The therapist was able to make a space for dialogue about the strangeness of therapy, and the effects of the differences between client and therapist; how talking to a young, white woman about his distress was confusing and unfamiliar to him, and how the presence of the interpreter made it easier, because of their shared ethnic identity, culture and history. The interpreter's investment and confidence in the process gave the therapist some credibility in the eyes of the client, which itself encouraged openness and engagement. If the interpreter had simply answered the question and then continued interpreting, these dialogues might have been lost, and the therapist would have been excluded from the communication in that moment.

For some clients, it can be a relief that the interpreter is not associated with the atrocities they have been through. For others, the ache for home and search for connection mean that this distance presents a barrier to feeling safe in the triad. The therapist will need to balance the client's needs to connect with protecting the privacy of the interpreter. The impact of an interpreter's self-disclosures can be as great as when a therapist self-discloses. So, preparing for such questions is important, as it will reassure the interpreter that they will be protected. Most interpreters will give consent for their country of origin to be shared, but often that is all. This can change in long-term work as relationships in the triad deepen and the therapist and interpreter agree that self-disclosure around other aspects of an interpreter's identity or experience might be helpful.

Working together

> The experience of being unable to express oneself verbally can be a frightening and disempowering experience for anyone.
> (Tribe, 2007: 160)

At the first assessment session, it can help with engagement if the therapist goes alone to meet the client in the waiting area, leaving the interpreter in the therapy room following the pre-briefing. The chairs can be positioned so that the therapist is sitting opposite the client and the interpreter is to the left or right. This can encourage the survivor to look towards the therapist, if they are able to make some eye contact.

At assessment, the stability of the partnership between the therapist and interpreter can often determine how safe a survivor feels and lay the groundwork for developing a healthy, three-way dynamic. The first 10 minutes of dialogue will illustrate to the client how three-way communication can work. In some situations, particularly with newly arrived refugees, or with a survivor who has not had access to a qualified interpreter before, the therapist may need to describe how to use an interpreter. We always suggest that the survivor speaks just a couple of sentences at a time, as this allows the interpreter to capture everything that is said.

It is the therapist's responsibility to ask a client to pause if they are speaking for too long and not allowing time for interpretation. If the therapist does not pace the narrative, the interpreter can become anxious about not remembering the detail, and lose focus, or begin to summarise.

When the dynamic is working well, the therapist will have eye contact with the survivor as the interpreter translates the meaning of what has been said. Survivors may often still glance at the interpreter, or at both interpreter and therapist, but keep their key focus on the therapist. At turning points in the therapy, or where there is laughter or good news, we all have experience of survivors sharing eye contact with both professionals in the room, perhaps ensuring that the moment is shared.

Therapists can speak in their normal voice, tone and speed, and do not need to change what they say, other than to be culturally aware. It is the interpreter's role to translate the meaning of what has been said, so the therapist does not need to simplify or shorten what they say to take account of the interpreter. However, they may need to adapt what they say to the cultural framework of the client, remembering that 'the language of psychology and mental health has been largely based on a Western vocabulary' (Tribe & Morrissey, 2003: 207).

Try to limit the use of mental health jargon. Avoid using terms such as depression or anxiety on their own, and take care to explain what these diagnoses mean. Ask what meanings these concepts hold for clients. As Smith points out, there may not be 'words in their language for some of the commonest expressions in mental health practice' (Smith, 2008: 23).

In some approaches, such as Eye Movement Desensitisation and Reprocessing (EMDR), particular phrases are used when processing trauma, so precision in the language is vital for the model to be used effectively. Emphasise to interpreters the importance of tense in trauma work, where the therapist may revisit traumatic memories with the client in a managed way, aiming to ensure that the client remains connected to the present, and to separate what was felt at the time from what is felt in the present: 'It is vital that the interpreter understands what the therapist is doing and relays their questions and the client answers in the correct tense' (Boyles, Talbot & Pahlevan, 2015: 15).

Therapists can, of course, repeat themselves, pause or hesitate when they are unsure or curious. The interpreter needs to reflect the humanity and character of the therapist, as well as that of the client. The interpreter also needs to reflect the tone and volume of the words: it can be disconcerting when an observation is shared with a survivor in a gentle or quiet voice, only to hear it translated in a loud and firm manner.

Check a few minutes into the first session whether the client is understanding what has been said, and find time at the end to recheck that the survivor is comfortable with the interpreter, in terms of language/dialect and gender. If you sense a client is not understanding everything that is said, or they appear uneasy, anxious or watchful around the interpreter, check separately with your client whether the interpreter is the right fit.

Sometimes a client might not know that they can ask for an interpreter who can speak their preferred or first language, rather than the dominant language in their country. Ideally, a service should be able to offer a choice of languages. There are multiple and complex reasons why a survivor may choose to speak in a particular language. For example, it might have been assumed that a survivor will speak French if they are from the DRC, when Lingala or Swahili is their mother tongue. Be creative to ensure the interpretation is right for the client. If you think that a client isn't comfortable with the interpreter, telephone the client, using a different interpreter, and discuss it with them. A survivor from the DRC might ask for a French-speaking interpreter because they do not want an interpreter from their own community, but using a European French-speaking interpreter may also create communication challenges and inhibit a survivor. The French spoken in France is different from that spoken in DRC, which may have been 'enriched by words from one of the four native or indigenous languages' (Tribe & Morrissey, 2003: 207). Nathalie is a French speaker who has lived in Africa and grew up in a multicultural environment, so she is culturally aware of mannerisms, local sayings and coined phrases.

'For the multilingual person, it can sometimes be therapeutic to speak in a latterly acquired language. It may be that emotions are only accessible in one of their languages, depending on when and how they have learned' (Costa, 2011: 20). Ensure that time is taken to explore what language is appropriate in therapy, knowing that this might change over time in long-term work: '... many individuals are able to express their true feelings only in a first or second language. Particular words, phrases and emphases convey meaning within any cultural framework and are an intrinsic part of expression' (Boyles & Talbot, 2017: 7).

As therapy progresses, therapists will find that their relationship with the interpreter deepens too, and this connection may be witnessed by clients, and bring comfort to them. In the words of one client: 'It feels like you are one to me now.' As Bradford and Munoz state, when both therapist and interpreter have received training in how to work with each other, 'the translator becomes an extension of the therapist... the exercise of their respective roles entails momentary experiences of their sharing a single identity' (1993: 58).

Managing challenging dynamics

There will always be challenges for therapists in working with interpreters, and we often hear about the difficulties before we hear about the benefits. Certainly, interpreters face many challenges in working with therapists.

A common assumption is that the challenges in the triad relate to dynamics between the client and interpreter, but of course there are many occasions when the therapist is misreading the client's response, due to a lack of cultural or country awareness, or because issues of power and difference have not been explored and remain unspoken. This can place the interpreter in an uncomfortable position as they watch the therapy stall and can do nothing to prevent it.

If the inhibiting dynamic relates to a client's projections or their response to an interpreter, then it can be beneficial to explore this in the session. Jude was working with a Christian convert from Iran; the interpreter was a Muslim man. Jude noticed that the survivor never referred to his conversion, and only occasionally spoke about his new faith. She shared this with the interpreter in the debriefing, as she was worried that the client was avoiding talking about his conversion because he was afraid he would be judged by the interpreter. If this dynamic had been ignored, the client might have continued to censor what was brought to therapy, as he did during his calls home to Iran, where he could not admit to his Christian faith. When Jude shared in-session her curiosity about this avoidance, it enabled the client to say that he was worried about what the interpreter thought of him.

The positive, discreet and non-judgmental stance of the interpreter is often enough to resolve some clients' projections over time. However, if the therapist and the interpreter both sense that the dynamic is not changing, exploring the issues in a session may be helpful, even if it is uncomfortable. This curiosity gives permission for other concerns and complaints to be aired too.

It can be hard to decide when to stop working with an interpreter if their presence is inhibiting a client and progress is blocked by a survivor's struggle to trust. Persevering can be therapeutically helpful and deepen the relationships in the triad. However, sometimes introducing a new interpreter will be the only way forward. For example, a male survivor may be able to tolerate a female professional from the host country listening to their history of sexual violence, but to make such disclosures in front of a woman from his own culture may seem too inappropriate. No matter how confident the therapist is that the interpreter can sit comfortably with these disclosures, if the client feels embarrassed and ashamed and thinks that a change to a male interpreter would help, it is important to do this.

In our work with female survivors of torture, we have rarely found that a woman is comfortable working with a male interpreter. Women's experience of torture is different to men's, and usually involves sexual torture by men. 'Women suffer disproportionately from gender-specific torture, sexual violence and abuse, including rape, deliberate infection with HIV, enforced impregnation, sexual slavery, disfigurement, mutilation of sexual organs and enforced nakedness or sexual humiliation during questioning or detention' (Boyles & Smith, 2009: 4).

Survivors may have good enough English to know when the interpreter has made a mistake, and may become watchful if this happens, and correct them or clarify what they are saying. Survivors may also notice when the therapist pronounces a particular political group's name correctly but the interpreter asks for a repeat of a name, group or region. If the therapist is noticing mistakes or senses a lack of knowledge, it is likely the client will too. Asking the client for feedback on the interpreter shows respect and demonstrates commitment to finding the right fit for both the therapist and client.

The therapist needs to feel they can practise to the best of their ability, and they too have the right to decide not to use a particular interpreter, even if a client has requested them. The therapist might be concerned that the interpreter doesn't completely understand or respect their therapeutic approach. Whatever the reason, both client and therapist need to trust the interpreter.

Debriefing

A debriefing should follow every session. In most settings, therapists offer the interpreter 10 minutes. Interpreters should not be required to interpret for longer than an hour without a break. The debriefing provides the space for the therapist to offer support to the interpreter and provides an opportunity to clear up any misunderstandings or concerns about the interpreter's work, and to praise it, or talk about emerging dynamics or dilemmas. The interpreter may want to ask the therapist to clarify their approach to a particular difficulty, find out more about why a particular intervention was made, or ask why a therapist did not respond to a particular issue. It is also a time for the therapist to discuss their therapeutic approach and offer tools to the interpreter, such as relaxation or grounding techniques, to help minimise the risk of vicarious trauma.

Interpreters may find themselves disclosing personal details in the debriefing, as the partnership develops. Often these disclosures are not planned and are made in response to the highly charged and emotional session they have shared. The therapist should be aware that it may be uncomfortable if an interpreter feels as if they have become the client.

If a client has talked about suicide, it can be useful if the therapist shares with the interpreter their assessment of the risk. Interpreters will feel reassured to know there are measures in place to protect the client, and why the therapist believes these will protect the client from serious self-harm. Without this reassurance, interpreters may leave the session concerned that the client is more likely to harm themselves after talking about suicide.

Interpreters need to feel contained and informed by the therapist if they are to work at their best, especially with traumatised clients. It can be frightening or destabilising for an interpreter when a survivor has a dissociative episode or a flashback. Explaining to the interpreter what a flashback might look like and what the therapist's response will be helps them to remain calm.

Interpreters often share cultural observations or country knowledge in the debriefing, and this can help deepen the therapist's understanding. However, interpreters are not cultural experts or brokers, and, while their observations should be listened to, it is important that the therapist keeps in mind that survivors are the experts on their experience.

Therapists can feel inhibited by interpreters who believe they have expertise on a specific country or culture. It can be disconcerting when an interpreter has a very fixed set of expectations about people from a particular culture and views all the client's responses and the therapy dynamics through this lens. On the other hand, it can feel disempowering and frustrating for an interpreter when a therapist repeatedly misses cultural cues that are obvious to them.

In Jude's early work with an interpreter who knew that she was unfamiliar with her country and culture, the interpreter would share her cultural knowledge at every debriefing. Jude initially found her observations helpful but, as this continued and was repeated after every session, she began to feel inhibited by the interpreter's advice on what was or was not culturally acceptable. She struggled to remain congruent in the session and was blocked from expressing an open curiosity around meanings. She began to feel that the interpreter was softening the edges around her reflections and making judgments about what the survivor could tolerate.

The interpreter became all-powerful, and inhibited Jude from having an open dialogue with the client about his reluctance to talk about his experiences; issues of power and difference were not explored in the triad. The survivor's reluctance could have been cultural, but it might have been the interpreter's expectation that he could not disclose in front of her, an Arab woman, that was being transferred to him in some way. Jude certainly sensed this tension and was more tentative than usual, because she felt the weight of the interpreter's assumptions.

Interpreters will inevitably relate to some aspect of the experience of a survivor that has stirred their own emotions. They too will feel horror at hearing what one person can inflict on another. Their own anger at injustice may be ignited, leaving them feeling powerless or ashamed. Having the opportunity to express this in the debriefing will help them continue to work effectively, and will support their resilience.

As interpreters, we have left appointments in a daze after particularly distressing sessions, and have arrived home without remembering the journey. The debriefing is an essential way to assess how we might be affected by a session. Interpreters might not feel immediately aware of how they are feeling, and should be told they can ask for supervision at a later date if they want it, to help them process difficult therapeutic work.

Power in the three-way relationship

> Language is one of the ways by which we gain a sense of agency in the world. (Costa, 2016: 6)

The issue of power and the survivor's experience of oppression in the torturing state is a constant theme in the work, together with the survivor's experience of racism and exclusion in the racialised context of the host country, its institutions and the asylum process. The dynamics that can occur in the triad may reflect a client's experience of oppression or conflict, early family dynamics or their more recent experiences of interrogation and persecution. When reflecting on such dynamics in our work with interpreters, Tribe and Thompson advise the therapist to use a wide lens (2009).

It is good practice to explore cultural differences and the structural power of the therapist in therapeutic work with refugees. As human-rights activists, we may need to make clear that we are aware of the disparity between our position, as citizens of the host country, with all our rights, and that of the client, as someone seeking asylum, with no rights, in order to build a trusting and transparent working relationship: 'The fear of authority figures experienced by asylum seekers and refugees, in early and later phases, requires the counsellor to be particularly sensitive to the client's perception of power in the counselling relationship' (Griffiths, 2002: 211).

Exploring power in the three-way relationship and the power differentials between the individuals in the triad can feel unfamiliar for survivors and may provoke anxiety. 'The power differential and inequality between the therapist and the survivor becomes greater when there are differences in language and culture, and the service user is disadvantaged by not being able to speak the dominant language of the host country' (Raval, 2003: 10).

If these themes are not explored and acknowledged, it can be hard for a survivor to express or name how they feel about the therapist and the power and privileges they hold. For example, Desiré was interpreting for a therapist when the survivor, referring to an experience of racism, turned to him to seek his acknowledgement of the shared experience of living with everyday micro-assaults in the UK. Once the connection was opened up, the therapist and client explored the societal injury of racism, which became a frequent subject in the therapy. The therapist noticed the connections as they happened, and soon the survivor would openly include Desiré in his narrative about racism and xenophobia. Desiré felt his relationship with the survivor deepen, and the therapist could feel the strong sense of unity and shared experience between the survivor and Desiré. This connection strengthened the three-way dynamic. 'This means that anti-oppressive practices within therapy are required to explore the hatred, denigration and the internalisation of dominant oppressions, when racism and its effects breach the psyche' (Bains, 2010: 23).

It can be hard for clients to raise the issue of racism in exile with therapists who are not from an ethnic minority or refugee background. White therapists, too, can be reluctant to name and explore differences around race and culture (see also Chapter 4): '... many survivors of any form of persecution or abuse will carry a fear of racism, or harm, by the authorities into the therapy room' (Boyles & Talbot, 2017: 49). This is amplified when most of the therapists in the service are white and the therapy agency is not part of the refugee sector, and so may not be immediately recognised by survivors as refugee friendly.

Many of the institutions with which people seeking asylum are in contact, such as Border Control, the asylum and immigration authorities, immigration reporting centres and the police, may be overtly hostile. The culture of disbelief in the asylum system and the strong anti-migrant feeling in countries in the west mean that survivors will be careful about who they trust and who they talk to. This distrust is understandably going to surface in a setting where they do not know they will get a friendly and accepting reception.

It is vital that the interpreter understands the refugee context and the language of the asylum system. Survivors will notice if an interpreter is unfamiliar with the terminology of the asylum process, and may wonder if the interpreter has preconceptions about people seeking asylum or may be concerned about their ability to interpret accurately.

The interpreter as witness

As human-rights practitioners, we view all our therapeutic and interpreter work as coming from a rights-based framework. However, in the therapy and interpreting field, less is said in the literature about the ethos or frame of reference of interpreters and their role in bearing witness: 'Inevitably the interpreter is called upon to facilitate communication, not as a neutral linguist but as an active participant in the struggle against human rights abuses' (Patel, 2003: 222).

As interpreters, we have a commitment to human rights and oppose the use of torture under any circumstances. 'As such, the stance of non-neutrality can be interpreted as a political stance against human rights abuses' (Patel,

2003: 222). We would argue that this is important for the interpreter as well as the therapist. An interpreter is present in the room and alongside the therapist, bearing witness to the atrocities the client has experienced at home and in exile.

An interpreter is the voice for both the therapist and the client. They not only hear the client's painful and horrific stories; they also absorb the words, embody the story, internally translate it and speak it word for word. To be accurate and effective, the interpreter acts and speaks as the survivor, in the first person, so the story is transmitted as much as possible in the survivor's authentic voice. Interpreters speak the highly charged words, transmit their intensity, mirror the body language, and communicate the despair, powerlessness, grief and sadness. It requires a profound commitment to do this.

Sometimes, when the partnership between a therapist and an interpreter is well established, the therapist may use the word 'we', bringing the interpreter directly into the dialogue. Usually this has been agreed beforehand: for example, when there has been a bereavement, or good or bad news about a survivor's claim for asylum. At such times, to say 'I' would feel excluding of the interpreter. In our work together, it has been powerful when used and, we hope, not misjudged. It is usually the only time when the therapist refers to 'we', apart from at the closure of the three-way dynamic, or the ending of therapy.

Closure and ending

It is common, certainly in long-term therapy with survivors of torture, that the therapist and client end therapy with the interpreter before the end of therapy itself. This is usually because the survivor's proficiency in English is now so good that the survivor chooses to work in their second language.

As a client learns English, the interpreter may be in the room but only used when called upon. If the interpreter is rarely needed, the client and therapist will naturally consider the closure of the triad.

Whether all three participants are ending together, or the therapist and the client intend to continue without an interpreter, it is important to give attention to the ending between the interpreter and client.

In group supervision, interpreters often express concern that therapists transfer too early to working without an interpreter. Therapists may have noticed the client nodding and responding to the therapist's words before the interpreter translates. The client may have been replying instinctively in English to questions or reflections they have understood, or may have been managing in English during the interpreter's annual leave. Inevitably, the therapist wonders if it is time to proceed without the interpreter.

The invitation to work in English can be hard for clients to refuse, so it is important that the therapist explores with them the implications of working without the interpreter, and examines their own motivations for suggesting this to clients. Even if some of the session is in English, at times of distress, or when expressing complex feelings, our experience is that survivors tend to automatically revert to their mother tongue or the language they use to express distress. Therapists may make a judgment that their client is now fluent in English, but if the interpreter is withdrawn too soon, this fluency might elude survivors at times of distress, or they may lose the benefit of being able to express themselves freely and immediately in their own language. 'In therapy, clients should not have to search for words within a limited vocabulary or have to simplify sentences or lose tense and subtlety' (Boyles & Talbot, 2017: 68).

The final session is, we believe, one of the rare times when the interpreter is given space to say a few words about what the work has meant to them. If therapy is coming to an end, a three-way ending in the closing sessions is crucial. The therapist should give the interpreter some warning before the session that they will have the opportunity to speak directly to the survivor in their own words, as they may want to prepare themselves for this. Interpreters are used to speaking other people's words and may struggle to talk about themselves, using their own voice.

In this session, clients may also want, and can be encouraged, to talk directly to the interpreter and reflect on their relationship. This is more likely to happen if it has been a long-term relationship, with a well-established and trusting working alliance; it is unlikely in short-term therapy situations. However, making space for thanks and acknowledgements is important in any setting and will enable closure.

A skilled interpreter who has captured the meaning behind a survivor's words is bound to have personal significance for the client, and, like all endings, the closure of the relationship between the survivor and interpreter can be painful and complex. In our experience, this has been amplified when the interpreter and client are from the same community and/or country. In our combined years of practice in different settings, we have witnessed how often survivors have asked for continued contact with the interpreter and found it hard when the ethical framework to which interpreters adhere advises against this.

'You are one to me now'

The art of interpreting is moving and impressive to witness and can contribute to a survivor's rehabilitation. Working together as therapists and interpreters has been one of the most rewarding and interesting stages in our careers. We have learnt so much together about identity and culture, language, power and relationships. After so many years in this sector, Jude has found that she can feel alone in a therapy relationship without the familiar presence of an interpreting colleague. She finds herself missing the skilful and warm presence of another and the authentic partnership of mutual trust and respect.

When the three-way dynamic works well, the therapist welcomes the pacing that interpretation creates, where they can consider their responses to clients and reflect while a survivor's narrative is interpreted. These periods in which the therapist and the client have to *be* together, without talking, while they both listen to the interpreter, are meaningful.

As interpreters, this work has changed us and made us better human beings and more accomplished practitioners. Our depth of compassion, empathy and humanity has grown enormously through hearing and communicating these difficult stories and bearing witness to the therapeutic process.

Van der Kolk writes of the healing relationship: 'Being truly heard and seen by the people around us, feeling that we are held in someone's else's mind and heart. For our physiology to calm down, heal and grow we need a visceral feeling of safety' (2014: 79).

For us, the presence of the skilful and committed interpreter means the client is held in two people's hearts and minds for the length of therapy.

References

Bains S (2010). Racism as a trauma: reflective anti-racist practice in action. In: Lago C, Smith B (eds). *Anti-discriminatory Practice in Counselling and Psychotherapy.* London: Sage (pp23–32).

Baker R, Briggs J (1975). Working with interpreters in social work practice. *Australian Social Work* 28(4): 31–37.

Boyles J, Smith E (2009). *Justice Denied: the experiences of 100 torture surviving women of seeking justice and rehabilitation.* London: Medical Foundation for the Care of Victims of Torture.

Boyles J, Talbot N (2017). *Working with Interpreters in Psychological Therapy: a right to be Understood*. London: Routledge.

Boyles J, Talbot N, Pahlevan B (2015). We cannot talk if we do not feel free. *Therapy Today* 26(8): 12–17.

Bradford DT, Munoz A (1993). Translation in bilingual therapy. *Professional Psychology: Research and Practice* 24(1): 52–61.

Costa B (2016). Language matters to a refugee child. *Therapy Today* 27(8): 6–7.

Costa B (2011). When three is not a crowd: professional preparation for interpreters working with therapists. *ITI Bulletin January–February*: 20–21.

Costa B (undated). *Code of Practice and Ethics for Interpreters and Practitioners in Joint Work*. Reading: Mothertongue. www.mothertongue.org.uk/downloads/MTcode.doc (accessed July 2017).

Griffiths P (2002). Two phases of the refugee experience: interviews with refugees and support organisations. In: Papadopoulos RK (ed). *Therapeutic Care for Refugees: no place like home*. London: Karnac (pp189–212).

Miller K, Martell Z, Pazdirek L, Caruth M, Lopez D (2005). The role of interpreters in psychological therapy with refugees: an exploratory study. *American Journal of Orthopsychiatry* 75(1): 27–39.

Mudarikiri MM (2003). Working with interpreters in adult mental health. In: Tribe R, Raval H (eds) *Working with Interpreters in Mental Health*. London/New York, NY: Routledge (pp182–197).

Ortega RM (2011). Training child welfare workers from an intersectional cultural humility perspective: a paradigm shift. *Child Welfare* 90(5): 27–49.

Patel N (2003). Speaking with the silent: addressing issues of disempowerment when working with refugee people. In: Tribe R, Raval H (eds). *Working with Interpreters in Mental Health*. London: Routledge (pp219–237).

Raval H (2003). An overview of the issues in the work with interpreters. In: Tribe R, Raval H (eds). *Working with Interpreters in Mental Health*. London: Routledge (pp8–29).

Smith HC (2008). Bridging the gap: therapy through interpreters. *Therapy Today* 19(6): 21–23.

The Scottish Translation, Interpreting and Communication Forum (2004). *Good Practice Guidelines*. Edinburgh: Scottish Executive.

Tribe R (2007). Working with interpreters. *The Psychologist* 20(3): 159–161.

Tribe R, Morrissey J (2003). The refugee context and the role of interpreters. In: Tribe R, Raval H (eds). *Working with Interpreters in Mental Health*. New York, NY: Routledge (pp198–218).

Tribe R, Thompson K (2009). Exploring the three-way relationship in therapeutic work with interpreters. *International Journal of Migration, Health and Social Care* 5(2): 13–21.

Tribe R, Thompson K (2008). *Working with interpreters in health settings: guidelines for psychologists*. Leicester: British Psychological Society.

van der Kolk B (2014). *The Body Keeps the Score: mind, brain and body in the healing of trauma*. London: Penguin Books.

Van Parijs P (2004). Europe's linguistic challenge. *European Journal of Sociology* 45(01): 113–154.

West A (2006). To do or not to do – is that the question? *Therapy Today* 17(6): 10–13.

15. The strength and stress of triangles: training and supervision for interpreters and therapists
Beverley Costa

Triangular relationships are common in all our lives. Structurally, triangles are strong, but inflexible. They can withstand a lot of pressure, but they lose their inherent strength when you change the length of any one of their sides.

Triangular relationships provide the opportunity for collusions, alliances, inclusions, exclusions, oppression and competition. Triangles also offer opportunities for collaboration and support. This is particularly visible in the context of helping relationships. When therapists work with interpreters and clients in a triangular relationship, unhelpful dynamics can be magnified. Frequently, one member of the helping triangle is vulnerable and the other two members can be drawn into the roles of saviour or rescuer. When the vulnerable member is a survivor of torture, the pushes and pulls inherent in this triangular helping relationship can be stretched even further.

Many interpreters are working with survivors of torture in the triangular helping relationship of interpreter-mediated therapy, with scant training and even less clinical or reflexive supervision. Reflexive supervision allows practitioners to reflect on their work and to consider the dynamic processes involved in working relationships. Interpreters may have had excellent technical training and preparation for their role, but most will have had very little training in the practice of interpreter-mediated psychotherapy and very little preparation for the intensity of the material they will be required to interpret in this context. Interpreters seldom have the same professional and personal preparation as therapists, and rarely have access to professional support or supervision.

Interpreters who work in settings that require them to listen to clients' traumatic stories and where there are safeguarding and risk issues may be unaware of the impact this may have on them personally. They may themselves come from a refugee background. They may be survivors of torture and may be retraumatised by interpreting material that resonates with their own histories. Interpreters have their own codes of conduct, which emphasise neutrality and impartiality. Interpreting relationships with survivors of torture take place in emotionally powerful contexts. Although neutrality may be aspired to, the interpreter may become invested with feelings, albeit at an unconscious level, driven by the intense emotionality of the context in which the interpreting takes place (Costa & Briggs, 2014).

Reflexive supervision and training give a space and an opportunity for our unconscious processes to be explored safely so that we can act with awareness. They are essential components in our preparation for working in this context as therapist or interpreter, if we are to provide the best possible environments for our clients to access the help they need to heal and thrive.

This chapter will consider the dynamics of the client-therapist-interpreter triangle in the context of working with survivors of torture. It will make a case for the need to provide interpreters in mental health settings with supervision and training. It will offer examples of reparative, reflective, responsive supervision and dynamic training that can help prepare interpreters and therapists to work productively as a team in the context of working with survivors of torture. Without this preparation, interpreter-mediated therapy runs a constant risk of being a tool for linguistic injustice, where non-native English speakers have unequal capacity to be understood and to influence (Van Parijs, 2004)). Linguistic justice refers to the way in which some languages (such as English, which is the lingua franca of Europe) are dominant in discourses and have disproportionate power to influence. The lack of status of some non-native speakers' languages, compared with English, and unequal respect for the associated identities, intersects with racialisation processes (Burck, 2005: 326) and the legacy of colonisation. The possibility for clients to express themselves fully in their own language (not a lingua franca), often through an interpreter, means that their own narratives, infused with their own values, will be expressed, heard and acted upon.

The examples of supervision and training in this chapter are drawn from the work of Mothertongue multi-ethnic counselling service.[1] The case studies are fictional and based on amalgamated examples from our work. Mothertongue is a small NGO, based in the UK, that provides culturally and linguistically sensitive counselling and psychotherapy in a range of

---

1. www.mothertongue.org.uk

languages to people from black and minority ethnic communities. Since 2009, Mothertongue has had its own small pool of interpreters trained in working in a psychotherapy context. We provide training for interpreters and therapists in how to work effectively together, nationally and internationally to other NGOs, and to university training programmes, the NHS and social services in England. We also provide clinical supervision for all our interpreters who work in a mental health context, and train others in supervision skills for interpreters.

The stresses

Triangular relationships and unconscious processes

Anxieties are elicited when working in any mental health context, and they are magnified when working in the context of torture. The therapeutic frame refers to the micro and macro levels of structures and boundaries that enable anxieties to be contained and worked with productively in clinical practice (Milner, 1952). These structures and boundaries enable a client to feel psychologically safe, to experience an empathic relationship, and for the anxieties in the room to be sufficiently contained so that clients can reflect on and become active agents in resolving their problems. With the presence of a third person (the interpreter from the external world), the therapist will need to think carefully about how to incorporate them into the therapeutic frame so that it remains intact.

Building trust with the client is a crucial initial task for the therapist. Attribution of blame and the formation of inclusive and exclusive alliances, if left unexplored, impact on the dynamics and power relations of the triangular relationship in the room and are almost always counter-therapeutic (Tribe & Thompson, 2009).

In our training, one of the concerns about working with interpreters frequently reported by therapists is that they may not be able to form a rapport/relationship with the client, or they may lose control of the session. They mention a lack of confidence in their ability to ensure a psychologically safe environment for the client if they do not trust that what is being expressed in the room is being conveyed accurately. Therapists also report feeling excluded from the interpreter–client dyad. A creative way of attending to these dynamics is the formation of 'mini-equipes', described in Salaets and Balogh (2015: 63), which incorporate the interpreter into the professional team.

Professional triangular relationships can remind the participants of earlier triangular relationships, both personal and professional. Within these relationships, there may have been experiences of power and oppression, alliances, collusions and exclusions. Each person's personal history of such relationships, and the coping strategies they developed over time to deal with them, will be layered onto current triangular relationships, unless they are brought into awareness and reflected on.

The psychodynamic concepts of transference and countertransference take into consideration the unconscious stimulation of feelings towards a person in the present that have their origins in earlier, more significant relationships. Once the interpreter enters the mix, they become part of the transference, and therefore contribute to the ways in which the therapist and the client will be trying to make meaning of the experience together. The therapist can well-meaningly try to protect the interpreter from the transference, but it may be more helpful to acknowledge that the unconscious will not ignore the fact that there is a third person in the room.

In supervision sessions, we have considered the pressures on the interpreter, which can come from any side of the triangle. One example of this is when a client does not want to work with the interpreter because she thinks the interpreter is judging her. This may be very upsetting for the interpreter, who may feel this is an attack on her integrity. A therapist may want to protect the interpreter, or may feel annoyed that the interpreter's needs are getting in the way of the client's therapeutic needs. The therapist will have to assess this situation very carefully before they decide if they need to find a new interpreter or if the current interpreter can hold the transference with their help, without taking the client's objection personally. Working collaboratively with the interpreter as part of the team can provide a way of working constructively with the transference, wherever it shifts about in the room.

Therapists can find that they lose confidence in the face of the tensions in the triangle. A therapist needs to be able to tolerate uncertainty; therapeutic work, by its nature, requires an ability to hold assumptions at bay. However, if they do not share a language with the client, the therapist needs to have an even greater capacity to stay with not-knowing and not-understanding. This can stretch therapists to their limit and can be the cause of increased stress. Therapists may find it hard to hold their authority and containing function in the face of not understanding the client's language.

Feeling excluded may cause some therapists to try to hold on more tightly to the control and/or feel that they are losing their therapeutic footing. There are ways to maintain authority and control lightly in these situations, but it is difficult to make decisions when there are high levels of anxiety about not understanding. Supervision and training will help with these kinds of dilemmas and dynamics.

Karpman's drama triangle (1968) can help to frame some of the dynamics. The drama triangle draws on transactional analysis (Berne, 1961), and provides one explanation for human behaviour in relationships. It is particularly useful when considering helping relationships.

Figure 1: The Drama Triangle (Karpman, 1968)

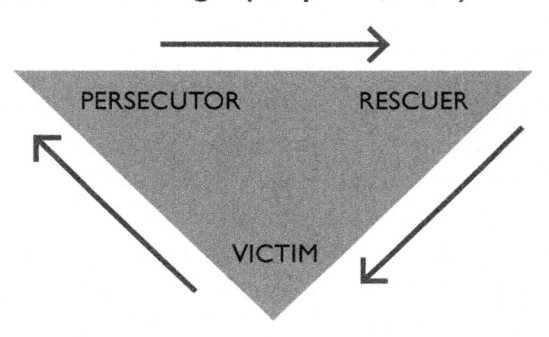

In the drama triangle, each person in the triad occupies a point on the triangle. They move between the positions of Persecutor, Victim or Rescuer. Although only one is called the Victim, all three originate out of and end up back at the victim position. If the therapist and the interpreter are not aware and do not pay attention to the way in which they move into and occupy these different positions, the dynamics will probably have a negative impact on the therapy. Alison Hetherington's research into interpreters' attitudes towards supervision revealed that interpreters often felt dismissed when they tried to offer advice and were ignored:

> You are seen to interfere, where really, I've often tried to offer some very polite advice but it's when that gets ignored and then they still do it, it's really quite painful. (Hetherington, 2012: 143)

The interpreter can align themselves with the client (as the Rescuer) in a cultural alignment if they perceive an interpersonal clash with the therapist, and this can lead them to ignore professional boundaries (Zimányi, 2012). The therapist and interpreter relationship is not immune to the powerful parallel processes that can occur when working with torture survivors, where both can feel a strong pull to be the Rescuer. A torture survivor's most recent experience of intensive questioning may have taken place in an interrogation room with two interrogators. Although the therapy room is a benign environment, it may remind the client of a previous experience of torture, and the therapist and the interpreter may find it almost impossible to bear the client reacting to them as if they were the torturers.

The following example from research examines the often neglected area of clients' own experiences of interpreter-mediated therapy and illustrates the client's point of view (Costa & Briggs, 2014: 238). The study explored patients' experiences of interpreter-mediated therapy in an NHS therapy service. This example focuses on a client's complaint about the behaviour of the interpreter, who laughed when the client described a painful experience. She was asked if the therapist addressed this in the room: 'No, he didn't say anything to her. Neither he, nor I. I only looked [at her] and that was it. I didn't tell her anything, because maybe I lacked courage.'

The behaviour of the interpreter and the therapist's lack of response left the participant isolated and unsure if she should have taken the responsibility for addressing the behaviour of the interpreter.

These unhelpful dynamics could have been avoided if the therapist had explained clearly the delineation of their role and responsibilities and those of the interpreter. But, as Zimányi observes (2012: 221): 'All three participants learn during an interpreted communicative encounter,' and this learning can be enhanced through external facilitation. Exploring conflicting dynamics is one of the functions of clinical supervision and dynamic training for both therapists and interpreters (Hetherington, 2012; Costa, 2016a, 2016b). With this type of support, participants can find ways to move out of the triangle and away from the reactive behaviour it evokes. They can move to a more reflective position, where they can carefully evaluate their options and their preferred way of behaving. Dynamic training can be particularly helpful for gaining perspective and moving out of stuck, repetitive positions (Kadrić, 2014).

Personal impact

Listening to and interpreting intense pain can cause vicarious trauma. Laurie Anne Pearlman and Karen Saakvitne (1995) define vicarious traumatisation as a transformation of the helper's inner experience, resulting from empathic engagement with a client's trauma material.

The interpreter who has the task of conveying traumatic stories through their own voice and body can feel this impact profoundly. Doherty and colleagues (2010) interviewed 18 interpreters, just over half of whom reported being emotionally affected by interpreting in a mental health setting. In total, 12 of the 18 (67%) said that they could find it hard to stop thinking about what had been said, and six (33%) reported that the work had an impact on their personal lives. This resonates with the experiences of Mothertongue interpreters, who say about supervision: 'You can get home and it can impact on the relationship you have with friends and family. Because if you don't offload here it's going to come out. And sometimes in the wrong situations.' Some interpreters said that a debrief straight after a session may not be enough: 'The clinicians, most will offer some support at the end of the session. You can't always remember, you can't always think, because during the session you're there 100 per cent trying to be professional, you don't let your emotions get in the way, you keep them buckled down.'

Dr Teodora Manea Hauskeller acknowledges the importance of these types of spaces in Mothertongue's creative writing project for interpreters, *In Other Words* (2015): '... where the ones used as voices are empowered to speak up and to express themselves in their own voice.'

Interpreters may attempt to protect themselves from excessive alignment that may lead to vicarious traumatisation. Without adequate self-care, they may erect a protective shell to numb them from the pain of compassion (Harvey, 2003). They – and some may share a similar history of torture – also report that they feel challenged to maintain boundaries when they hear these powerful stories, and when clients have expectations of them beyond their role (Sande, 1997; Tribe, 1998).

In our supervision sessions, we hear about situations where interpreters have been left alone with the client. This can occur when a therapist has had to leave the room quickly to fetch something for the session. In one example, while the therapist was out of the clinical room, the client made a disclosure to the interpreter that they did not want the therapist to know. The client said they did not trust the therapist. This put a great deal of pressure on the interpreter, who had to make an ethical decision about what to do with the information. In our supervision sessions, we often discuss the need for the interpreter to feel confident to make their professional needs known to the therapist and ensure the therapist is aware that an interpreter must never be left alone with a client.

The interpreter cannot be treated by the therapist as a bystander, a fly on the wall, simply translating words. As a Mothertongue interpreter says: 'Sometimes professionals and agencies see us like Google Translate – that we work only with words. But they are not only words or languages, they are also emotions and thoughts... our cultures.' Another commented: 'We're not add-ons. We are the link.' Therapists and therapy agencies will need to reflect on the impact of vicarious trauma on interpreters and consider what support can be made available to them. Therapists will often have some idea of the nature of the material to be discussed in the session, and can prepare themselves to hear very difficult material. The interpreter does not have this same preparation. It would help if the therapist were to brief them on what they can expect in the session, so they too can prepare themselves emotionally for what they are going to be hearing and voicing. Without this opportunity, the interpreter enters the therapy room emotionally naked and may find the material overwhelming. Without support, interpreters can experience burn-out and other negative impacts on their personal lives (Salaets & Balogh, 2015; Hetherington, 2012; Doherty, MacIntyre & Wyne, 2010).

The personal impact on interpreters of working with victims of torture is compounded by other factors. One significant factor that can impact and create additional stress for an interpreter is the clash between an interpreter's working methods and those of the therapist.

The stress created by differences in working practices

Counsellors and psychotherapists have their own codes of conduct, practice and ethics, as do interpreters. Although these professions may have contrasting professional models of interaction and professional values, it is essential that both professions find a way to work together as a professional team. They need to negotiate their respective team positions in order to work collaboratively, as professional colleagues. To find these positions, professionals will need to share their thinking about boundaries, empathy and agency, and share their anxieties about working in this collaborative way.

When working methods are not shared, interpreters can feel excluded from understanding the practice of the therapist, such as why the therapist has asked a particular question, or focused on one aspect in a survivor's narrative. In supervision sessions, interpreters have reported that therapists can disempower them by not sharing information. Interpreters have also said that they are frequently given too much power. Interpreters may be left to manage clients' distress or unexpected reactions (Maatta & Simo, 2014). Therapists may not understand the limits of the interpreter's role and may ask interpreters to share information they have gathered from other interpreting assignments in different settings. An interpreter in one of our supervision sessions described how a psychiatrist had asked her to share information she already knew about the client. The interpreter was aware of her personal temptation to do so, but did not breach confidentiality as she had become skilled at reflecting on her own motivations during supervision. She understood that her temptation arose from a desire to increase her own sense of importance in the professional relationship. With that awareness (and personal honesty!) she felt confident to inform the psychiatrist about her professional boundaries.

In the supervision sessions offered by Mothertongue, interpreters report that the support from group supervision has been invaluable in helping them make the right ethical decisions in the moment, with the knowledge that they will have an opportunity to process it later: 'Sometimes we're not certain that we approach some problems in the right way or not. This space gives us the opportunity to find out what other people think.'

The following example illustrates the problems that can occur when interpreters and therapists do not share their working methods with each other.

In a therapy session, a client had just begun to express themselves with some freedom and the therapist felt it was useful for the client to continue, even though the therapist did not understand what was being said. The therapist therefore decided not to pace the client's flow, trusting that something useful was emerging from the uninterrupted narrative. The interpreter, assessing this situation with no guidance, attempted to follow their code of conduct, which requires them to interpret everything. The interpreter may even have felt that the therapist had frozen and that they were rescuing the situation. Research shows that interpreters can take the initiative in managing the session, because they think they are 'trying to keep a peace that the interviewer (practitioner) was not aware he was constantly disturbing' (Zanen & Gillogley-Mari, 2014). This unhelpful tension could have been avoided if, before the session began, the therapist had discussed with the interpreter what to do in such a situation. In our training at Mothertongue, we refer to this as 'talking about the talking'. The discussion could also cover the delineation of roles and responsibilities. An exploration of the fears brought by both the therapist and interpreter is extremely useful and can form the basis of an approach to working supportively together. Through dialogue, the therapist and interpreter can establish a joint code of conduct, practice and ethics to underpin their work together.

The strengths

Supervision

Training, ongoing professional development and mentoring are all ways to help interpreters to become and remain fit to practise. Supervision for interpreters working in sensitive settings is an additional and necessary form of support. The use of the word supervision, in a clinical context, differs from its usage in other contexts, where it may include the functions of line management and assessment. The British Association for Counselling and Psychotherapy (BACP) describes supervision in this way (2015):

> Supervision is a specialised form of professional mentoring provided for practitioners responsible for undertaking challenging work with people. Supervision is provided to:

ensure standards; enhance quality and creativity; and enable the sustainability and resilience of the work being undertaken.

Supervision can also be described as a protected, reflective, shame-free space to think about the work and the unconscious processes in the therapeutic frame. It is an opportunity for transformative learning that otherwise may be lost in the repetitive cycle of acting out familiar dynamics.

Interpreters can find it helpful when the therapist spends time offering support after an emotionally difficult session. However, given that the therapist is also a part of the triangle, there is sometimes a danger that the interpreter can begin to feel like another client in the room. For this reason, it can be more productive for both to discuss the situation with someone outside the triangle, in a more systematic way.

The examples from supervision that will be described here occur mainly with interpreters and therapists in separate supervision groups. This is clearly not ideal; however, it is realistic, and represents the reality of the organisation described. Joint supervision is a relatively new idea in interpreter-mediated therapy, and these are early initiatives. Hopefully, in the future, when its significance is realised, it will be possible to resource joint supervision for therapists and interpreters.

Michael Carroll's description of one of the functions of supervision is to help us to take a 'perspective outside ourselves' (2010: 13). In interpreter-mediated therapy, interpreters and therapists need to be able to consider the perspectives of two, rather than one other person. A new model of supervision does not need to be created from a vacuum. The model described here derives inspiration from other models: for example, Page & Wosket's (2001) cyclical model of reflection and learning; Inskipp and Proctor's (1995) normative, formative and restorative stages of supervision, and Hawkins and Shohet's (2006) seventh eye of the meta-organisational perspective, in their seven-eyed model of supervision.

It is beyond the scope of this chapter to address the supervision of therapists as a separate entity, but some of the examples given in this chapter illustrate how thinking about interpreter-mediated therapy can be incorporated into ongoing clinical supervision of therapists. A model of supervision for mental health interpreters follows, together with a section on dynamic training, which focuses on therapists' needs.

A proposed model of reflexive supervision

A three-stage model of reflexive supervision for mental health interpreters focuses on three purposes of supervision (Costa, 2011, 2016a). The model is drawn from the research (see below) (Doherty, MacIntyre & Wyne, 2010; Miller et al, 2005; Hetherington, 2012; Costa & Briggs, 2014) and the experience of supervision of mental health interpreters from Mothertongue. The supervision is provided to the group monthly. (New interpreters are offered more frequent one-to-one supervision with trained, senior interpreters.) Group supervision is valued by the interpreters, who welcome the peer learning, the sharing of experiences and feeling part of a team.

Supervision model for interpreter-mediated therapy

The supervision model for interpreter-mediated therapy incorporates key learning and recommendations from research (Doherty, MacIntyre & Wyne, 2010; Miller et al, 2005; Hetherington, 2012; Costa & Briggs, 2014).

To summarise, these include recognition:

- that all three people in the room are subject to their own anxieties elicited by the triadic relationship
- that the interpreter may experience vicarious trauma and may have no space where they can explore the emotional overload they experience in a safe and confidential space
- that the interpreter is subject to the same dynamic processes as the therapist: that the interpreter becomes invested during therapy sessions with the client's hopes, fears and wishes (transference) and can have powerful emotional reactions and experiences in the therapy (countertransference)
- that the inclusion of the interpreter is an essential part of the therapeutic process
- of the importance of training and reflexive supervision for interpreter and therapist in working with therapeutic dynamics
- of the importance for the therapist to develop a form of collaborative and reflective co-working with the interpreter as a colleague – (although we would not go so far as to suggest the interpreter becomes a co-therapist, a new collegiate status could be established, such as 'co-communicator').

The supervision serves three purposes:

1. Reparative – to provide personal and pastoral support for interpreters and build on their self-care strategies; to discuss how outside factors may be affecting the work; to help interpreters process distressing and traumatic material they might hear that may affect them emotionally and personally, so they stay fit for work because they can manage stress before it becomes critical.

2. Reflective – to provide case management and mentoring to deal with ethical issues; to ensure that guidelines are followed; to identify gaps in skills, training and development; to provide reflexive/clinical supervision; to explore and reflect on the client work and the interpersonal dynamics of the helping relationship, including risk issues, transference, countertransference and alliances.

3. Responsive – to provide managerial supervision. Contextual supervision plays a vital function if there is going to be a systemic change. If there is no mechanism or process for feedback to the therapists, their managers and/or commissioners, it can leave interpreters feeling disempowered and unsupported, with no hope for the possibility of change. Interpreters from Mothertongue say that they find the inclusion of this managerial function empowering.

The following are examples of the ways in which interpreters can make use of supervision. These examples are generic and do not represent any individual piece of work or person and illustrate each of the purposes of supervision, as described above.

1. Reparative purpose: personal and pastoral support

An interpreter shared in supervision that she had been interpreting for a woman whose husband had recently revealed to her that he was raped while he was a political prisoner. The client was very distressed and was suffering from depression. The interpreter was finding it very hard to stop thinking about her after the sessions.

When the interpreter talked about this in supervision, she revealed that her brother was also raped in prison, and she was worried about his mental health. As a result of the supervision, she decided that she could use coping strategies to manage her own anxieties, but decided that she would not take on working with more than one survivor of torture at a time.

2. Reflective purpose

a) Case management and mentoring

In one of our supervision sessions, we discussed what interpreters would do in a therapy session if the therapist kept falling asleep. We considered several suggestions: for example, the interpreter could suggest opening the window, as it was quite hot and offer to go out of the room to get glasses of water for everyone. This would give everyone a chance to move around and re-energise without anyone having to lose face. Supporting interpreters to be assertive without undermining anyone in the triangle is a frequent theme in the supervision sessions.

b) Reflexive supervision

In one supervision session, we discussed the fact that some clients will feel disempowered by having to use an interpreter, regardless of the interpreter's competence. In Julie Telvi's research about mental health patients' experiences of interpretation, a participant reported that speaking through someone else about pain and intimate internal struggles can feel as if the interpreter '... enters you as the second arrow. It makes you upset, of course it makes you upset' (Telvi, 2006). Group members explored how clients come with different anxieties and that all kinds of dynamics are at work in the triadic relationship, which can make each member feel disempowered.

Some issues of power differentials can be resolved on a practical level, such as a client's choice of the gender of the interpreter. Some situations are more complex and benefit from the reflective space, such as racist or elitist attitudes from the client to the interpreter, and vice versa. It is hoped that supervision will not have to focus on challenging these kinds of attitudes from the interpreter, as interpreters selected to work with an organisation with a human rights-based approach should hold the same values as the organisation and therefore have an awareness of oppression and anti-oppressive practice.

3. Responsive purpose: managerial supervision

One Mothertongue interpreter has noted: 'We have the supervisor who runs the group and who's in charge and we can talk to her. She is sometimes in a better position to go back to a clinician and say, "These things have come up and what can we do about those?"'

Unlike therapists, interpreters are not afforded the relief of intervening in a therapy session. They can feel quite powerless. An interpreter commented that our supervision sessions gave her the space where 'we can share our doubts' and talk about their issues with practitioners: 'When we work with professionals, it doesn't mean that every relationship with professionals goes very smoothly.'

In our supervision sessions, interpreters share that they believe that the confidence of all the team members is the key element to successful interpreter-mediated therapy. As one interpreter said: 'As therapists become more confident to work with us, so it becomes easier for us to do our job and for us, together, to provide an effective service for the clients.'

These examples illustrate the subtlety and sensitivity of the work of an interpreter working with survivors of torture and the resilience it requires. Interpreters may need help to deal with the feelings that arise when their own histories of trauma are retriggered or on occasions when an interpreter is vicariously traumatised by the material. Supervision can help interpreters to become aware of how to contain their emotions and recognise when they are overwhelmed and unable to manage strong emotions in a session. It is important for interpreters to have a supportive space where they can accept that knowing one's limitations is a strength and crucial to ethical work with the client.

Dynamic training for therapists in collaborative team-working

We have already considered that, if the therapist and the interpreter do not pay attention to the way in which they move into and occupy their respective positions, repetitive cycles of relationships will be played out. The following example demonstrates a training intervention for therapists and interpreters that explores these repetitive cycles using action training methods inspired by psychodrama techniques (Moreno, 1946). For the purpose of showing different perspectives, we will use an example from a supervision session for interpreters, but from the therapist's perspective, which is helpful for exposing underlying dynamics in relationships (Costa, 2016b, 2016c).

An interpreter is worried because the therapist seems to be annoyed with her. The client keeps looking at the interpreter and not at the therapist. The therapist wants the interpreter to stop looking at the client, as it is disrupting his ability to achieve a rapport with her (the client). The interpreter is worried about the impact it might have on the client if she avoids her gaze.

Miller describes situations where therapists, initially excluded from the eye contact, experience feelings of 'exclusion and uncertainty and even competitive feelings... towards the interpreter' (2005: 32). In training, this situation is role-played with trainees occupying different chairs in a triangle, representing the roles of client, therapist and interpreter. The re-running of a scene in several different ways can provide the space for a creative solution to a difficult situation.

The above scene is one that is frequently presented in supervision by therapists. Supervisees often report feeling anxious about addressing the communication flow in the room and drawing attention to the inclusions, exclusions and alliances that are occurring. Role play has also been used successfully in supervision to help therapists build their confidence in addressing these dynamics.

The feedback we have received from therapists is that, after the role plays, they have felt more able to manage their own anxiety and the anxieties in the room, at the same time as addressing the pushes and pulls they are noticing. This has resulted in a more transparent and equal sharing of power in the communication by all three participants.

An evaluation of this training, and other trainings developed by Mothertongue and delivered to therapists, was conducted in 2017 (Bager-Charleson et al, 2017). All 88 participants who completed an online questionnaire, and seven who participated in further in-depth interviews, reported improvements in their practice as a result of the training, with scores of at least four on a rating scale of nought to five. One participant commented on her new understanding: 'They (interpreters) have that same power as I do, as well as the knowledge of the language, which is also a power factor in the relationship.'

Three elements of the training were highlighted: reflectiveness on the relationship with the interpreter; collaborative working with the interpreter, and maintaining clinical control of the session: 'Thinking in terms of triangular relationships and the therapeutic frame dynamics enables therapists to remain in control without losing the patient-centred approach/rapport.'

Participants reported that the use of action training methods helped them maintain perspective, clarified roles and enabled them to feel safe to practise: 'Having the training has given me safety into my work with interpreters and clients and the relationship, and to learn from mistakes.' Most participants commented on the fact that they had never considered the interpreting triangle from the interpreter's perspective before.

One participant mentioned that she now had 'a clearer understanding of the impact on the interpreter if I don't take control of the session'. Another reflected: 'I think the most significant impact of the training was recognising that we work as an equal threesome, that the interpreter isn't just there as a tool to be used, but that we need to open the work as a triangle.'

Practicalities, motivation and professional development

Should responsibility for supervision and support for the interpreter rest with the individual therapist, or should it be held at organisational level? Certainly, organisations should ensure that pre-briefing time with the interpreter is added to any client appointment. There should always be a debriefing at the end of the session too, so that therapists and interpreters can reflect on their collaboration together. Clients should be informed about the debriefing and its purpose, as this will emphasise the importance of the working partnership between the interpreter and therapist. In the UK, only a handful of third-sector clinical organisations budget for and provide supervision for their interpreters, as they regard this as best practice. However, many interpreters are contracted by agencies and there are limited ways of influencing these services. If the organisations that commission these agencies were to insist on the interpreters being trained to work in a mental health context and supervised appropriately, this would lead to a dramatic improvement in their conditions and the quality of their work.

It can be difficult for interpreters to prioritise attending supervision over paid work. Some organisations pay interpreters to attend supervision. Another way of increasing interpreters' motivation to attend supervision (and of providing professional development) is to offer senior interpreters free training in supervision skills. At Mothertongue, interpreters who have undertaken this training are paid to provide one-to-one supervision for newly qualified interpreters. This adds to the status of supervision and provides the opportunity for progression for this new professional role within the team.

We are not like 'Google Translate'

Triangles can hold large loads without collapsing. Triangles are also excellent containers. So perhaps we can conclude that the triangular relationship of client, interpreter and therapist, where the containing structure is reflected on and attended to, can be a positive asset in working therapeutically with the effects of trauma and torture. Certainly, therapists interviewed by Miller and colleagues (2005: 33) valued working collaboratively with an interpreter when they were working with very intense experiences: '[It] made the intensity of the client's reaction easier to sit with, and I was glad to have someone with whom to process the experience after the session.'

In order to work collaboratively as a team, interpreters and therapists need to be trained in working together, and receive ongoing supervision.

Preparation, in the form of training and supervision, can increase the confidence of the interpreter and the therapist in their professional roles. A confident interpreter can make an honest appraisal of their own capacity and their limitations. A confident interpreter will feel able to challenge therapists non-defensively, to improve the quality of the client's experience.

A therapist who feels confident to work with an interpreter will be able to work collaboratively, incorporating the interpreter into their working triangular 'team', and they will not abdicate their authority to the interpreter. Therapists are used to helping clients to find a way to form a bridge between their cognitions and affect. Interpreters are frequently referred to as a 'bridge' to aid the communication flow. When an interpreter joins in the therapy relationship, they share in this co-creation of meaning across and within the triangle, and across and within languages. This does not happen by chance.

Supervision and training are tools for applying the strength of the triangle. A strengthened triangular team can witness and work therapeutically with survivors of torture without fragmenting under stress.

Acknowledgements

With gratitude to all our interpreters at Mothertongue, who care and learn and teach, in equal measures.

References

Bager-Charleson S, Costa B, Dewaele J-M, Kasap Z (2017). Can awareness-raising about multilingualism affect therapists' practice? A mixed-method evaluation. [Online.] *Language and Psychoanalysis* 6(2). www.language-and-psychoanalysis.com/article/view/1900 (accessed June 2017).

BACP (2015). *Ethical Framework for the Counselling Professions*. Lutterworth: BACP.

Berne E (1961). *Transactional Analysis in Psychotherapy: a systematic individual and social psychiatry*. New York: Grove Press.

Burck C (2005). *Multilingual Living: explorations of language and subjectivity*. London: Palgrave Macmillan.

Carroll M (2010). Supervision: critical reflection for transformational learning (Part 2). *The Clinical Supervisor* 29: 119.

Costa B (2016a). The importance of training and clinical supervision of interpreters and practitioners for best teamwork in gender violence contexts. In: del Pozo Triviño M, Toledano

Buendía C, Casado Neira D, Fernandes del Pozo D (eds). *Construir Puentes de Comunicación en el Ámbito de la Violencia de Genero/Building Communication Bridges in Gender Violence*. Granada: Comares (pp61–71).

Costa B (2016b). Team effort: training therapists to work with interpreters as a collaborative team. *International Journal for the Advancement of Counselling* 39(1): 56–69.

Costa B (2016c). Roles in triangles: the interpreter, the client and the therapist. *The Psychotherapist* 64: 18–19.

Costa B, Briggs S (2014). Service-users' experiences of interpreters in psychological therapy: a pilot study. *International Journal of Migration, Health and Social Care* 10(4): 231–44. Costa B (2011). Managing the demands of mental health interpreting: why training, supervision and support are not luxuries. *ITI Bulletin*, March.

Doherty SM, MacIntyre AM, Wyne T (2010). How does it feel for you? The emotional impact and specific challenges of mental health interpreting. *Mental Health Review Journal* 15(3): 31–44.

Harvey MA (2003). Shielding yourself from the perils of empathy: the case of sign language interpreters. *Journal of Deaf Studies and Deaf Education* 8(2): 207–213.

Hawkins P, Shohet R (2006). *Supervision in the Helping Professions* (3rd ed). Maidenhead: Open University Press.

Hetherington A (2012). Supervision and the interpreting profession: support and accountability through reflective practice. *International Journal of Interpreter Education* 4(1): 46–57.

Inskipp F, Proctor B (1995). *The Art, Craft and Tasks of Counselling Supervision. Part 2: Becoming a supervisor: professional development for counsellors, psychotherapists, supervisors and trainers*. Twickenham: Cascade.

Kadrić M (2014). Giving interpreters a voice: interpreting studies meets theatre studies. *The Interpreter and Translator Trainer* 8(3): 452–468.

Karpman SB (1968). Fairy tales and script drama analysis. *Transactional Analysis Bulletin* 7(26): 39–43.

Maatta, Simo K (2014). Public Service Interpreting with Male Survivors and Alleged Perpetrators of Sexual Offences. Madrid: Universidad de Alcala Publicaciones.

Miller KE, Martell ZL, Pazdirek L, Caruth M, Lopez, D (2005). The role of interpreters in psychotherapy with refugees: an explanatory study. *The American Journal of Orthopsychiatry* 75(1): 27–39.

Milner M (1952). Aspects of symbolism and comprehension of the not-self. *International Journal of Psychoanalysis* 33: 181–195.

Moreno JL (1946). *Psychodrama. Vol. 1*. New York, NY: Beacon House.

Mothertongue (2015). *In Other Words: the interpreter's story*. Reading: Mothertongue

Page S, Wosket V (2001). *Supervising the Counsellor: a cyclical model* (2nd ed). Hove: Brunner-Routledge.

Pearlman LA, Saakvitne KW (1995). *Trauma and the Therapist: countertransference and vicarious traumatization in psychotherapy with incest survivors*. New York, NY: WW Norton & Company.

Salaets H, Balogh K (2015). Co-Minor-IN/QUEST research findings. In: Balogh K, Salaets H (eds). *Children and Justice: overcoming language barriers. Cooperation in interpreter-mediated questioning of minors*. Cambridge-Antwerp-Portland: Intersentia (pp175–226).

Sande H (1997). Supervision of refugee interpreters: five years of experience from northern Norway. *Nordic Journal of Psychiatry* 53(5): 403–409.

Telvi J (2006). *Living in Translation: experiences of Turkish-speaking clients when they use interpreters.* Unpublished MA dissertation. London: Birkbeck, University of London.

Tribe R (1998). A critical analysis of a support and clinical supervision group for interpreters working with refugees located in Britain. *Group work Journal 10*(3): 196–214.

Tribe R, Thompson K (2009). Exploring the three-way relationship in therapeutic work with interpreters. *International Journal of Migration, Health and Social Care 5*(2): 13–21.

Van Parijs P (2004). Europe's linguistic challenge. *European Journal of Sociology 45*(01): 113–154.

Zanen DE, Gillogley-Mari E (2014). *Ethical Conduct of Interpreters on Mission: survey findings.* Unpublished presentation given to the Round Table on Ethical Requirements for Interpreters on Mission for the International Criminal Court, 18–19 September, The Hague.

Zimányi K (2012). Conflict recognition, prevention and resolution in mental health interpreting: exploring Kim's cross-cultural adaptation model. *Journal of Language and Politics 11*(2): 207–228.

16. Holding hope: the challenge for therapists working with survivors of torture

Jess Michaelson

> The nature of torture makes it difficult for us to acknowledge its existence, let alone respond humanely, realistically, and effectively.
> (Pope & Garcia-Peltoniemi, 1991: 269)

It is no wonder that psychological therapists can sometimes feel overwhelmed and deskilled when working with clients who have experienced torture and other human-rights abuses. They may be listening for the first time to horrific details of torture that are unlike any experiences they have encountered before. They may be affected by the immense and intense distress the survivor continues to experience, and the multitude of urgent needs, many of which are not usually presented in therapy.

Working with people who have been devastated by torture, are under threat of return to the country they fled, and are dealing with the challenges of seeking asylum and living in exile, presents the therapist with a huge emotional, psychological and human challenge. Holding hope for clients until they are able to hold it for themselves is at the heart of all therapeutic practice. This can be a particular challenge for the therapist working with survivors of torture, who are likely to be living with high levels of hopelessness, both in their day-to-day lives and in their search for safety through the asylum process.

In this chapter, I am drawing from relevant literature on working with survivors of torture as well as from my experience in this field over the last 15 years as a psychotherapist, supervisor and trainer. I currently work for a human-rights non-governmental agency in the UK that provides rehabilitation to survivors of torture. My role also involves supervising and training psychological therapists working with survivors in other services.

I describe myself as a human-rights therapist. I have consciously chosen to work in settings where I can offer free psychotherapy to clients who would not otherwise easily access it. I am not impartial; I have opinions about what happens in the world and will express these to clients. I will also at times use my power and privilege to act on behalf of clients when they are unable to act for themselves. I previously worked in a small, community-based therapy service in a deprived part of Manchester, and began to work with people seeking asylum in 2003. I did not directly choose the refugee sector, but, on reflection, it now seems an inevitable path that I would follow and it has provided me with a personal and professional challenge that has enhanced my life and work.

People seeking asylum are often discussed as though they are different from the rest of us. A history of migration or fleeing from one country to another for economic reasons or to seek safety is found in many of our family histories and the history of the countries we live in. I am a British citizen because members of my family fled persecution in Eastern Europe in early 1900s, and in Austria and Germany before the Second World War.

My hope is that this chapter will help normalise the feelings therapists are likely to experience when working with survivors of torture and to offer reflection on when these may arise. I hope to increase awareness of the risks of vicarious traumatisation and to explore ways to keep healthy and work effectively. Finally, I will explore how the impact of working with survivors can also be positive and even life-changing for therapists.

The clients' stories used in this chapter are fictional and based on amalgamated examples from my practice.

My experience as a therapist new to working with survivors – Alain

Alain is from the Democratic Republic of the Congo (DRC) and was one of the first refugee clients referred to the small NGO therapy service where I worked. It was also the first time I had worked with a survivor of torture, let alone one who was traumatised and destitute. I had previously worked with a diverse group of both short- and long-term clients, many of whom were survivors of childhood abuse, domestic violence and other historical traumas. However, I found sitting with Alain an entirely different experience. I had always shied away from working with recent trauma; there was something about the freshness of the trauma that I found disturbing. I did not identify as a trauma therapist. This was also my first experience of working with an interpreter. I did not understand what Alain was saying, and I was not used to having another professional sitting in the therapy room.

I remember the overwhelming feelings I experienced throughout those early sessions. I sat opposite a man in profound distress, who did not seem capable of psychological contact. He did not appear to know why he was there, but he was desperate for help. I struggled against feeling overwhelmed by the enormity of the therapeutic task. 'What can I do? What difference can I make in these 50 minutes in the face of the atrocity that Alain has survived? How can I help someone whose daily life is so harsh?'

Alain had been tortured and had witnessed the brutal killing of his family. He had fled his village and his country, and then sought safety in the UK. His story was not believed by the authorities and his asylum claim had been refused. By the time Alain was referred to our service, he had no money, nowhere to live and was suicidal. He had no hope for a future. I remember reeling after these early sessions. On one occasion, I sighed out loud after a session, and said to my interpreter: 'That was hard.' My interpreter nodded: 'I'm glad you said that.' We were both feeling overwhelmed. My role was to hold and contain the client and the interpreter, but I was struggling to keep myself usefully present in the therapy room.

I shared my work with Alain in every supervision session, and cried as I talked about him. I struggled to know what to do with my huge feelings of anger. Having been brought up in a Jewish community, my childhood was full of stories, films and images of the Holocaust, from a very young age. The words 'Never again' were often spoken in my community, and the importance of not forgetting, to ensure such atrocities do not happen again. In the words of Primo Levi, from *If This is a Man*:

> Never forget that this has happened.
> Remember these words.
> Engrave them in your hearts,
> When at home or in the street,
> When lying down, when getting up.
> Repeat them to your children. (1979: 7)

I knew about human rights abuses in the past and was aware of what was happening in the present. However, listening to survivors' testimonies and witnessing the effects of torture had a very different impact on me. As I began work with survivors of torture, the enormity and prevalence of human-rights abuses in the world overwhelmed me to the extent that I found myself questioning the nature of humanity.

If I was asked about my work in social settings, I would launch into an angry tirade about torture and violence. I felt guilty, as a privileged, white, middle-class woman. With such overwhelming feelings to contain and my anxieties about whether therapy could make a difference for Alain, I realised that, if I wanted to continue in the field, I needed to find another way to be with my clients. I was not sure if this was possible, and so began a personal and professional journey that has been life-changing for me.

The challenges for therapists working with survivors of torture

Working with complex trauma and experiences of torture

> Trauma therapy profoundly changes the therapist. We give up our familiar ways of being and beliefs about the world when we embark on this work with survivors of traumatic life events. These changes are both inspiring and disturbing, involving gains and losses. Rarely do therapists enter the field of trauma therapy with full understanding of the implications of their choice.
> (Pearlman & Saakvitne, 1995: 279)

Trauma therapists working with survivors of childhood abuse, road accidents, domestic violence and sexual assault can find themselves questioning their ability to work with survivors of torture. Despite having therapeutic skills that are transferable to this client group, the impact on the therapist can be unexpected and disturbing. What makes the difference?

Working with survivors who have been tortured physically, psychologically and sexually as part of a systematic abuse of their human rights is often outside the therapist's experience. To think that men collectively design methods of torture to cause the most harm and leave the fewest scars is to consider aspects of humanity that most of us understandably wish to avoid. Therapists are also confronted by the realisation that this is systematic and deliberate harm perpetrated by states that face no consequences for their actions. There is usually no justice for the victim and no punishment for the perpetrator. In addition, survivors seeking asylum live under the constant threat of being returned to the countries from which they fled in fear of further torture or even death.

Torture is designed to overwhelm the person, to 'kill a person without his or her actually dying... [it is] a reminder of the omnipotent destructive power of the state' (Bamber, cited in Korzinski, 2003: 194). It is therefore not surprising that therapists find themselves feeling overwhelmed at times too. Many writers in this field talk about the contagion of trauma. Herman, in writing about traumatic countertransference with survivors of atrocity, describes how 'the therapist at times is emotionally overwhelmed. She experiences, to a lesser degree, the same terror, rage and despair as the patient' (1992: 140). At these times, therapists may forget or undervalue the therapeutic importance of their human presence, which forms the basis of all therapeutic approaches.

Jovic and Cvetkovic-Jovic differentiate between what could be described as 'universal reactions' of anyone reading a client's experience of torture and an unconscious traumatic countertransference reaction that leads a therapist to doubt their therapeutic effectiveness. They describe this as being 'an unconscious identification with feelings of hopelessness and helplessness that, although originating from the traumatic experience of the patient, could develop more easily if there is an unconscious conflict within the therapist related to the feeling of [their] own competence' (2004: 313).

Van der Veer and van Waning describe out-of-awareness approaches that therapists may use to manage their feelings, such as numbing, denying, avoiding, distancing, holding on too tightly to their professional role and reducing the therapeutic process to the application of method and theory. All of these will 'interfere with his or her ability to be completely "with" the client' (2004: 193).

Herman refers to feelings of helplessness that 'may lead the therapist to underestimate the value of her own knowledge and skill... to lose confidence in the power of the psychotherapy relationship' (1992: 14). If the therapist can retain their belief in the core principles of psychological therapy, then there is an opportunity for the client to restore their faith in humanity. Witnessing a survivor benefit from psychological therapy has helped restore my faith in humanity too.

The focus for therapists initially is to build a trusting therapeutic relationship, as well as stabilise a survivor's mental health and help them manage their trauma symptoms. Some survivors of torture may be reluctant to engage with trauma processing, but therapists too can avoid offering them the opportunity, even when it is clinically appropriate. Herman writes about 'bystander guilt' that may extend to therapists feeling guilty for 'causing the patient to re-experience the pain of the trauma in the course of treatment' (1992: 146). It takes courage for clients to explore and process traumatic experiences. It is understandable that the survivor may wish both to avoid and engage with trauma processing. The therapist's challenge is not to collude with the avoidance.

Ibrahim was a survivor from the Central African Republic. I had many discussions with him about what course he wanted therapy to take. When we began working together, he had recently been granted refugee status, was in the process of settling into his new flat and was keen to look for work. He had recently found out the whereabouts of his wife, whom he had been forced to leave behind, and his solicitor had applied for family reunion. Ibrahim was experiencing frequent disturbing nightmares and distressing memories of his prolonged period of torture. On the one hand, he wanted to process his trauma to reduce his distress, but he also felt an urgency to search for work so he could be a provider, and to focus on rebuilding his relationship with his wife after such a long separation. My role was to hold both possibilities and explore the choices available to him. Ibrahim made a choice to prioritise work, which made it difficult for him to attend weekly therapy, and so we agreed to end our work together. Ibrahim may choose to revisit his trauma in the future once his life is more settled.

One of the challenges for the therapist is to bear witness to survivors of torture. Cooper and Rendall describe bearing witness as 'the capacity to be able to bear to listen, to tolerate the grief, rage, helplessness... the clients' communication of their experiences evokes in oneself; but also to bear, in the sense of carry away, and be a bearer of some portion of this feeling; and finally, be capable of managing this pain rather than passing it on yet again for someone else to bear' (2002: 243).

Bearing witness is not only a therapeutic task; it is a human-rights task. 'The very act of bearing witness is a political act in itself and furthers human rights. What we witness must inform how we live our lives' (Boyles, 2006: 165).

Therapist as torturer

In my first assessment appointment with Zahra, I became aware that she was out of contact and had not heard what I or the interpreter had said. I said her name and she did not look at me, but seemed agitated and started looking around her nervously. I reminded her of my name and where she was, and spent time gently grounding her in the present. After this dissociative episode, we reflected together and she explained to me that she had suddenly found herself back in prison, where she was being interrogated. She had begun to see me as the torturer, when I asked too many assessment questions. Therapists may inadvertently trigger memories of torture by what they do or say. There may also be triggers from the environment, such as sudden noises, bars on windows or dark corners in a clinical room. Survivors whose experiences of past trauma and present experience are enmeshed in this way may experience everyone around them as potentially harmful, including the therapist. This can be painful for the therapist. Countertransference may be so strong that the therapist may feel as if they are the torturer and/or interrogator. I have had supervisees bring this to a session, and when I name this process and remind them that they are not the torturer, they describe a huge sense of relief as they became aware of how a part of them has identified with the survivor's transference.

The impact of the asylum process on the therapist

In my professional life, I have experienced little that is comparable with the impact of the asylum process on people who have sought protection in the UK. At the same time, I have never been alongside a person who was kept in poverty, treated like a criminal and was living under constant threat, with very little chance of influencing their position. The asylum process impacts significantly on the client, the therapy and the therapist.

Therapists may consider that it is not appropriate to offer therapy to a survivor still in the process of seeking asylum, and that they should wait until they are safe. They may cite Maslow's theory of human motivation (1943) to explain this view. Maslow describes a hierarchy of human needs, where basic needs must be fulfilled before higher needs can be met. These basic needs begin with physiological wellbeing and physical safety. Herman describes how '[s]urvivors feel unsafe in their bodies. Their emotions and their thinking feel out of control. They also feel unsafe in relation to other people' (1992: 160). Both of these needs are addressed during the stabilisation phase of trauma therapy. It is true that the precarious process of seeking asylum can impact on the therapy, the client's mental health and the therapist's struggle to create a safe therapeutic relationship. Survivors can, however, benefit from therapy, even though they have not yet been granted asylum. Therapy can help them better manage the challenges of the asylum process, develop insight into their trauma symptoms and learn tools for managing their responses. By helping to build their emotional resilience, therapy can improve a survivor's ability to reconnect with others.

The therapist may feel they are a powerless witness to the cumulative impact on clients of the asylum process. It is painful to see the deterioration in a survivor's mental health when there are delays, administrative mistakes and refusals that deny the truth of their account. A negative decision on a claim for asylum can dominate sessions and hijack other therapeutic work. There are times when the therapist finds themselves in the position of delivering bad news to a client, when the client receives a refusal of the claim from the Home Office, and gives the letter to the therapist to translate in a session.

On one occasion, I agreed with the legal representative that I would inform a client, Huguette, from the DRC, that her fresh claim had been refused, to ensure that immediate support was available to her and minimise any risk of serious self-harm. What shocked me was the impact I felt in delivering the negative decision. I knew intellectually that this was the most supportive way for her to receive the news, but when I witnessed her immediate distress and shock, I was left feeling responsible for her distress. I found it helpful to voice this out loud to a colleague and explore my feelings in supervision. The following session, I explored with Huguette how it had been for her to hear this news from me. She immediately replied that she was glad she had not been on her own. She said that my presence and support enabled her to stay connected in the face of the shocking news that I was telling her.

Many survivors have fled from the authorities and are fearful of being returned to further torture. Many believe that they will be killed if they are returned. Survivors live with a constant fear of being removed if their claim for asylum is not successful. In the UK, people seeking asylum are required to report regularly at their nearest immigration reporting centre, and their fear increases as the reporting dates approach, and they may be at risk of being detained.

Home Office interviews and Asylum Tribunal hearings are also frightening and anxiety provoking for survivors. Many survivors describe feeling as if they are on trial for committing a crime. Contact with the authorities can be particularly frightening if a survivor has no legal representation or current asylum claim. Therapists may fear for a client's safety and feel powerless to influence the outcome. It is important for therapists to understand the different stages of the asylum process so they know when survivors are at more risk of being removed. Awareness of the process will help them manage their client's risk, and provide containment. As therapists, we have to find a way to sit with the reality that both we and our client have limited power in the face of the asylum system. We need to find a way to bear this in order to continue to value what we can offer.

> The threat of detention and/or removal hangs over our clients from arrival and can last many years. It hangs over their therapist too. Managing this threat is part of the day to day work of psychological therapists working with people seeking asylum.
> (Boyles & Shaez, 2015: 11)

All therapists have experience of clients not turning up for therapy or failing to respond to attempts to contact them. However, the impact of a survivor of torture disappearing can be significant, as frequently it is not from choice. Survivors may just disappear (possibly to avoid detention) or be suddenly detained, pending removal, and this can be extremely stressful for the therapist. Some therapists may work in settings where they are able to keep in contact with clients by phone while they are in detention, to provide ongoing support. This can be an essential lifeline for a survivor, but enormously distressing for the therapist. At this time, the therapist will require support to manage the impact of working with someone who is facing return to a country where they are likely to experience further harm, and even death. The therapist is likely to witness a rapid deterioration in a client's mental health, and clients are often retraumatised when they are detained in the UK. 'The experience of being imprisoned and the conditions in the removal centre can trigger existing post-traumatic stress disorder (PTSD) symptoms and detention can be a traumatic experience in its own right' (Boyles & Shaez 2015: 12). Therapists and services working with people seeking asylum are in a better position to respond helpfully if they know about the support and legal representation available in the immigration removal centre. Knowing when and how to 'do something' for the client at these difficult times is not only important for the client, who may not have anyone else to turn to, but can also help the therapist manage the impact on them of their client facing the possibility of being returned to further torture.

Therapists expect to hear about human rights violations in the survivor's country of origin and on their journey to seek asylum. However, it can be a shock to hear about human rights violations in the host country. It is painful to watch survivors deteriorate during the long wait for refugee status and as their claims are refused. As a therapist working in the UK, I am outraged when I see a survivor's mental health affected by unsuitable accommodation, poverty or destitution.

It can be difficult for therapists to return to their warm, safe home, knowing a client is living precariously on other people's couches or on the street. It is anxiety-provoking knowing that a vulnerable, destitute survivor may be at risk of sexual exploitation. At such times, managing our own sense of powerlessness is crucial if we are to sustain the quality and integrity of our therapeutic work. I remember the pain of a colleague when her young, psychologically vulnerable client was forced to live on the streets for several months, despite great efforts to find alternative accommodation for him, when his claim was refused. It was important at that time to support the therapist to maintain her therapeutic work with him, despite the severity of his situation. Informal team support and debriefing was as important as clinical supervision, as well as the recognition by her manager of the challenges inherent in her work with this young man.

Immigration is frequently on the political agenda. Therapists and clients are both affected by xenophobic media reports about people seeking asylum, and by anti-immigration legislation that is intended to serve as a deterrent to people seeking refuge.

Boundaries

Working with survivors who are very isolated, living in poverty and experiencing severe psychological distress can present the therapist with a heavy emotional burden. Sometimes the urge to step over ethical or organisational boundaries can be great. However, these lines are the cornerstone of ethical therapeutic practice, and it is essential to stay within them. Survivors may ask for practical help – to read a letter or resolve a housing issue, for example. For most therapists, this is a huge departure from their usual remit. There are times when the therapist may choose to use their personal and professional power to resolve a practical issue for a survivor. However, responding to these requests requires careful consideration, both in terms of the therapist's motivation (conscious or otherwise), as well as empowerment-based practice (Freire, 1971; Alinsky, 1971). Freire and Alinsky's ideas on empowerment led to a change in community work that emphasised working *with* and *alongside* disadvantaged groups, rather than on behalf of them.

Esther was a destitute survivor. She had to walk 10 miles to attend each appointment. She was sleeping on various friends' couches, and had no money. She often had very little to eat. In my bag were some beans that a colleague had just given me from her allotment. I noticed my urge to offer them to Esther, and, as the session went on, I found myself reaching into my bag and giving them to her. My usual approach, when I feel a desire to do/say something in a session, is to reflect on whether this is from my need or from my client's, and consider my therapeutic choices. In that moment, it felt simple: here was a person with no money or food, and here I was, with extra food, and the ability to buy more.

I reflected on my struggle in supervision. I could have asked Esther how it felt to live with nothing to eat, and nowhere to live. We could have explored what she needed and what agencies could provide support, such as destitution projects and food banks. In this instance, by offering her beans and stepping outside of my role (and there certainly are times when it is right to do this), I denied Esther the space to share and reflect with me. This may not seem a huge transgression, but it is a struggle that is familiar to me in my supervisory work. Many experienced and ethical practitioners have been tempted to telephone a survivor from home, outside working hours, or to offer them items they need or even give them money. These impulses would be inconceivable in any other therapy setting, but for therapists working with destitute people, such breaches become a possibility in the face of such need. This incident was many years ago and I would make a different choice now, but I have learnt to carefully consider what is motivating me to act, whenever I feel this pull in sessions. Sometimes it can feel that there is not much time to reflect while with the client. Therapists will make their decision based on their assessment at that time. Honest self-reflection and the willingness to explore these instances in supervision are vital to ensure the therapist maintains appropriate therapeutic boundaries.

Survivors have often said to me, 'You and the interpreter are my family in this country.' The impact on the therapist of hearing these words can be significant and can create a sense that they are responsible for the survivor. This weight of responsibility can be amplified if a survivor is socially isolated and has no connections in the UK. We may also be frightened that the survivor may expect more from us than is in our role to offer. But it can be the survivor's way of telling us how important we are to them, how they trust us and are attached to us. It is an understandable way for survivors to make sense of the close, trusting relationship with the therapist and interpreter. It is vital that the therapist is not isolated in their work with the survivor, but shares this responsibility with and feels supported by colleagues, their manager and their supervisor.

The impact of working with prolonged risk

Many therapists work in settings where it is not unusual to see clients at risk of suicide. However, this can feel more intense when working with survivors of torture, who may feel suicidal over a long period, and have fewer resources and personal support networks. The risk of a suicide attempt can be ever-present, and this risk will increase at times of bad news.

At the core of this work is instilling hope, and monitoring the client when hope has been lost. At such times, we may need to act in order to keep the person safe, sometimes against their wishes. It can be shocking to hear a survivor say that they plan to kill themselves and their family if they are removed from the UK. This is likely to have a greater impact on therapists who work in isolated settings, without the support of a team. Therapists working with high levels of risk should have access to adequate line management and clinical supervision to support them in holding this risk.

Power and powerlessness on the therapist

The dynamics of power within the therapeutic relationship with survivors of torture are too complex to explore fully in this chapter. Therapists may experience profound feelings of powerlessness when working with survivors. These, in my experience, can have a greater impact on the therapist than similar feelings evoked by other client groups. Survivors may ask for practical help. While the therapist has more power than the survivor (in terms of their role, access to information in a language they understand, and their status as a professional, to name but a few), they may not have the power that the survivor thinks they can wield. Therapists want to help and cannot always help in the way the survivor wants or needs. On the occasions when a therapist chooses to use their power to advocate on behalf of a vulnerable survivor and is successful, it may increase a client's expectations of the therapist's ability to assist and influence in the future.

The complex dynamics that can occur when practical assistance is provided require ongoing self-reflection and access to regular clinical supervision.

I remember working with Yasmin, a traumatised Iranian woman who was feeling powerless in the asylum process and overwhelmed by her symptoms of trauma. I found myself feeling compelled to 'do something' to avoid the sense of helplessness I was experiencing and wanted to avoid. I could have offered to make a phone call to her legal representative in order to feel that I was *doing* something. However, instead, I chose to allow myself to experience this sense of powerlessness and share my responses with my client. What ensued was a therapeutic dialogue and exploration of how she felt, which also included the choices and power she did have in her situation, however insignificant they felt to her at the time.

Following this exploration, the client decided to ring her legal representative herself. The risk of viewing our clients as helpless can further disempower them. It is important to be aware of each person's resources and resilience, and remind clients where they can make choices and where they do have some influence.

Vicarious trauma and compassion fatigue

Vicarious traumatisation is defined by Pearlman and Saakvitne (1995: 31) as the 'negative effects of caring about and caring for others... the cumulative transformation in the inner experience of the therapist that comes about as a result of empathic engagement with the client's traumatic material.' Working empathically with a traumatised survivor, whether hearing or reading details of their experiences of torture, will have an effect on the therapist.

> **The expectation that we can be immersed in suffering and loss daily and not be touched by it is as unrealistic as expecting to walk through water without getting wet. (Remen, 1996: 52)**

There is considerable literature about vicarious trauma and compassion fatigue in psychological therapists (Meichenbaum (undated); Figley, 1995, 2002; Pross, 2006; Hernández-Wolfe et al, 2014; Figley & Abendroth, 2013). The symptoms of vicarious trauma include the following:

- feeling overwhelmed
- feeling exhausted
- increased illness
- persistent feelings of anger and sadness
- feeling hopeless that things can improve for the client
- feeling isolated as a therapist
- bystander guilt
- questioning competence as a therapist
- similar symptoms to the client: eg. intrusive images, body sensations, difficulty falling or staying asleep
- struggling with boundaries with clients
- more negative view of the world, the world feeling less safe
- nightmares
- thinking about clients outside of work
- easily startled
- feeling overly emotionally involved with clients
- less reflective about your client work
- feeling less in control of your work and life
- negative effects on relationships with colleagues/friends and family.

Our understanding of the impact of vicarious trauma on therapists is evolving, and we use a variety of terms to describe how we respond to the demands placed on us by trauma work, including compassion fatigue and secondary traumatic stress. The literature emphasises the importance of therapists being aware that it is a normal consequence of empathy with traumatised clients, and encourages good self-care. We cannot meet our clients' therapeutic needs if we do not take care of our own.

Maintaining therapeutic effectiveness and self-care

> Therapists who work with traumatized people require an ongoing support system to deal with these intense reactions. Just as no survivor can recover alone, no therapist can work with trauma alone. (Herman, 1992: 141)

Herman stresses the importance of not working in isolation when working with survivors. All therapists need a good work/life balance, supportive networks around them, and an eye on self-care. However, in my personal and supervisory experience, support alone may not be enough to sustain therapeutic work with survivors of torture.

Training and reading can be a source of support and information in understanding what survivors of torture have experienced in their country, during flight and in exile. It can be helpful to understand the asylum process, as well as the rights to benefits, accommodation and healthcare of people seeking asylum. Understanding how to work with interpreters in therapeutic settings is vital for those new to working with refugees.

Therapists can feel deskilled when their therapeutic approach or trauma model does not easily transfer to working with such a diverse population. It is vital to have a clear, flexible theoretical framework, as well as an understanding of complex trauma. Over the years, many therapists have expressed uncertainty about how to adapt their therapeutic approach to working with survivors of torture. Most trauma models involve a three-phase approach (Herman, 1992). Phase one (stabilisation and relationship building) can be considered an appropriate therapeutic approach in and of itself for therapists who do not have the flexibility to offer long-term therapy.

'Window of tolerance' is a concept introduced by Dan Siegel (1999: 281). It is the area of arousal within which the individual can function well. With our traumatised clients, we are working to increase their tolerance of sensations, feelings and thoughts so that they can experience and process them. Taylor considers the therapist's window of tolerance in her chapter 'The well-resourced therapist' (2014: 180). Therapists need a sufficient window of tolerance to stay emotionally regulated when working with complex trauma. The therapist may experience symptoms of hyper-arousal, a racing heart, or feel overwhelmed and breathless.

Therapists working with trauma will be familiar with the use of grounding tools with clients who are highly aroused or dissociative. Being able to attend to one's own breathing and bodily sensations with curiosity, not judgment, and an ability to regain an equilibrium during or after a session with a survivor, is important. Neuroscience, through the theory of mirror neurons, describes how we can experience what we observe in another person, as it can activate part of our brain *as if* it were happening to us. Cozolino describes how that 'facial expressions, gestures, and posture of another will activate circuits in the observer similar to those which underlie empathy' (2010: 188). This theory not only explains how we can empathically experience what our clients may be experiencing, but also how survivors can benefit from our ability to stay self-regulated within our window of tolerance (Taylor, 2014: 210).

Life events in the past or present, such as experiences of trauma, bereavement and physical health issues, may decrease a therapist's window of tolerance for working with survivors. This needs attending to in supervision and/or in therapy. Therapists who are refugees may have their own experiences of torture and racism, which can be a resource but can also be triggered when working with clients with similar experiences.

In my early days of working with Alain, I was fortunate to have a Jewish supervisor who encouraged me to explore what was being triggered from my Jewish family experiences. I joined a Jewish co-counselling peer support group in the US, and together we began to share and explore the impact from our families' histories of persecution. It is still hard to put this into words as I have no narrative of the immense emotions that this provoked in me. However, giving myself space to experience these emotions fully, with the support of others, began to lessen their intensity. I started feeling less overwhelmed with clients and found a deeper place within myself from which to bear to hear and work with Alain's experiences. I have no doubt that, without having undertaken this personal work, I would have chosen to withdraw from working with torture survivors. I still feel angry at the human-rights abuses in the world, including in my country. However, I no longer feel so engulfed by feelings of anger, sadness and hopelessness that I cannot be effective as a therapist.

Van der Kolk, reflecting on neuroscience research, states: 'The only way we can change the way we feel is by becoming aware of our *inner* experience and learning to befriend what is going on inside ourselves' (2014: 206).

Clinical supervision

It is important for therapists to have a containing supervisory space to identify and explore the impact of this work. This process involves separating out what is being evoked *in them* that belongs to the survivor (feelings they may not be able to experience or express) from what belongs to their own experiences or reactions. Supervisors can also support the therapist to transfer existing skills to their work with survivors and to further develop their therapeutic approach.

Van der Kolk writes that, 'Feeling listened to and understood changes our physiology; being able to articulate a complex feeling, and having our feelings recognised, lights up our limbic brain and creates an "aha moment"' (2014: 232). Although he is referring to his work with clients, this is equally true for the therapist. It has been vital for me to have a supervision space to articulate what I experience in my work, gain deeper understanding and feel supported as well as appropriately challenged by my supervisor.

Shame is present in the therapy room; it is a common experience for survivors of torture who may feel as if they are 'going mad' and not understand why they cannot cope with day-to-day life. Many survivors have also experienced humiliation as part of the torture and/or have been sexually violated. Supervision is vital to help therapists explore the impact of the client's shame on them, as well as how their own experiences of shame may affect the therapy. Therapists new to working with survivors may feel ashamed of their inadequacy or disconnected from the 'well-resourced therapist' that they usually are (Taylor, 2014: 186).

Organisational support

The organisations we work for have a duty of care for therapists working with traumatised survivors of torture. The organisation can support resilience in therapists working with survivors of torture in the following ways:

- **Commitment to provide therapy to survivors of torture**. This will ensure the responsibility for working with survivors is being held by the wider organisation and not just by a small number of interested therapists. Organisations can review the accessibility of the service to refugees and address barriers to access.
- **Commitment to specialist training**. Organisations can support therapists to develop their approach to survivors by encouraging specialist training on themes such as working with interpreters in therapy, working with complex trauma and increasing knowledge of the asylum process and asylum support arrangements.

- **Peer or facilitated supervision groups.** These groups provide opportunity to share experiences and explore impact of the work, as well as increase therapeutic skills and confidence. They may also reduce professional isolation and minimise the risk of vicarious trauma.
- **Mixed caseloads.** In generic counselling services, it may be possible to mix therapists' caseloads, to reduce the risk of vicarious trauma. Therapists may choose to avoid working with this client group, which can lead to one therapist becoming the 'expert' on working with refugees. Ensuring traumatised survivors are shared across a team can enhance the development of new skills and increase peer support opportunities.
- **Recognising and normalising the potential for vicarious trauma.** Organisations have a responsibility for the welfare of staff who are working with complex trauma. Acknowledging the impact on both the individual and the organisation is important.

After 15 years of working with survivors of torture – Mahmoud

Mahmoud is a new client who looks uncomfortable in his chair, uncomfortable in his body and uncomfortable with me. We have not yet built a trusting relationship; he has not discovered the possibility for psychotherapy to help him, and I have not yet found a way to connect with him. Mahmoud is used to finding his own solutions in life, something he is currently unable to do now, due to the impact of torture. Mahmoud wants to die; he has lost all hope for his future. As we explore this together, I notice my heart rate speed up; I feel anxious and tearful in his presence; I can sense a desperate need to reach out to him from my heart, wanting to keep him alive long enough to see that there is hope, that therapy can make a difference, and that he is not alone. I finish the session feeling exhausted and worried that he might kill himself. Mahmoud is overwhelmed by what he is experiencing and I am managing to stay in my window of tolerance, despite experiencing a range of sensations and emotions.

What has helped me stay in my window of tolerance? I have confidence in my therapeutic approach and my model of working with trauma. I have good support from colleagues, my manager and clinical supervisor. I know when I need to reach out for more support if I am particularly affected. I also know it is normal to be affected and that I do not want to become numb to the atrocities our clients have survived. I do not become overwhelmed by anger, as I know I am contributing to the wider struggle for human rights. I pay attention to what I am experiencing with a client and know how to keep myself grounded. I am curious about what is happening for my client, for me and between us. I do not judge what I am aware of, whether it is from my history or a countertransference reaction.

Vicarious resilience and the positive impact on the therapist

Vicarious resilience is a concept described first by Hernández, Gangsei, and Engstrom (2007). Vicarious resilience is referred to as a process that 'transforms the therapist's inner experience, resulting from empathic engagement with the client's trauma material' (2007: 237). Their work has shown how therapists working with survivors of torture can learn about coping with adversity from their clients. They reflect that working with survivors of torture can have 'a positive effect on the therapist, and that this effect can be strengthened by bringing conscious attention to it' (2007: 237).

It is also important to consider the resilience of survivors and its positive impact on therapists. I am often in awe of their strength of human spirit and their drive to recover and overcome. This therapeutic work is life changing for the therapist, as it is for the client, and can be profoundly rewarding. Seeing Alain smile at me for the first time and begin to have a sense of the person he was before the torture touched me greatly, and felt like a huge therapeutic step forward. So too did the first time he was able to talk about his country and remember the good times, without the traumatic events swamping him. Focusing on the small, yet hugely significant changes in our clients can sustain us.

This work can increase the therapist's awareness of global issues and galvanise human rights activism (Herman, 1992). Contributing to the wider fight against torture and human rights abuses has enabled me to manage overwhelming feelings of powerlessness.

Honouring those who have survived and remembering those who did not

> The reward of engagement (with survivors) is the sense of an enriched life. (Herman, 1992: 153)

It takes courage for therapists to engage therapeutically with survivors of torture. It is normal, and I would say necessary, for therapists to experience some of the myriad reactions I have described in this chapter. Therapists cannot avoid being affected by what survivors have experienced and the challenges they continue to face in exile. It takes commitment from therapists to develop their existing therapeutic skills, gain specialist knowledge and seek out appropriate support in order to ensure they offer the psychological therapy so badly needed by survivors. I also see it as a chance to stand up for human rights as a therapist and to choose to offer our skills, support and human caring to people who are desperately in need.

While I will never stop feeling overwhelmed and hopeless at times, I know that I can manage my feelings. *Seeing* someone who has been so nearly totally destroyed recover, find new ways to cope and begin to live their life and have real choices is the most humbling therapeutic work I have ever embarked on. The resilience I see in my clients inspires me and gives me hope for humanity once more.

References

Alinsky S (1971). *Rules for Radicals: a pragmatic primer for realistic radicals*. New York, NY: Random House.

Boyles J (2006). Not just naming the injustice: counselling asylum seekers and refugees. In: Proctor G, Cooper M, Sanders P, Malcolm B (eds). *Politicizing the Person-Centred Approach: an agenda for social change*. Ross-on-Wye: PCCS Books (pp156–166).

Boyles J, Shaez M (2015). In the shadow of detention. *Therapy Today 26*(4): 10-14.

Cooper A, Rendall S (2002). Strangers to ourselves. In: Papadopoulos, R (ed). *Therapeutic Care for Refugees: no place like home* London: Karnac Books (pp239–252).

Cozolino L (2010). *The Neuroscience of Psychotherapy: building and rebuilding the human brain*. New York, NY: WW Norton & Company.

Figley CR (ed) (2002). *Treating Compassion Fatigue*. New York, NY: Brunner-Routledge.

Figley CR (ed) (1995). *Compassion Fatigue: coping with secondary traumatic stress disorder in those who treat the traumatized*. New York, NY: Taylor & Francis.

Figley C, Abendroth M (2013). Vicarious trauma and the therapeutic relationship. In: Murphy D, Joseph S (eds). *Trauma and the Therapeutic Relationship: approaches to process and practice*. New York, NY: Palgrave Macmillan (pp111–125).

Freire P (1971). *Pedagogy of the Oppressed*. New York, NY: Herder & Herder.

Herman JL (1992). *Trauma and Recovery: the aftermath of violence – from domestic abuse to political terror*. New Yor, NY: Basic Books.

Hernández P, Gangsei D, Engstrom D (2007). A new concept in work with those who survive trauma. *Family Process 46*: 229–241.

Hernández-Wolfe P, Killian K, Engstrom D, Gangsei D (2014). Vicarious resilience, vicarious trauma, and awareness of equity in trauma work. [Online.] *Journal of Humanistic Psychology* 55(2): *153–172. http://journals.sagepub.com/doi/abs/10.1177/0022167814534322* (accessed November 2016).

Jovic V, Cvetkovic-Jovic N (2004) (trans A Krstic). Torture in the therapy environment: countertransference in working with victims of organised violence. In: Špiric Z, Kneževic G, Jovic V, Opacic G. *Torture in War: consequences and rehabilitation of victims – Yugoslav experience.* Belgrade: International Aid Network (pp309–327).

Korzinski M (2003). Somato-psychotherapy at the Medical Foundation in London. In: Krippner S, McIntyre T (eds). *The Psychological Impact of War Trauma on Civilians: an international perspective.* Westport, CT: Praeger (p193–202).

Levi P (1979). *If This is a Man/The Truce* (trans S Woolf). London: Penguin Books.

Maslow A H (1943). A theory of human motivation. *Psychological Review 50*(4): 370–396.

Meichenbaum D (undated). *Self-Care for Trauma Psychotherapists and Caregivers: individual, social and organisational interventions.* [Online.] www.melissainstitute.org (accessed November 2016).

Pearlman LA, Saakvitne K (1995). *Trauma and the Therapist: countertransference and vicarious traumatization in psychotherapy with incest survivors.* New York, NY: WW Norton & Company.

Pope K, Garcia-Peltoniemi E (1991). Responding to victims of torture: clinical issues, professional responsibilities, and useful resources. *American Psychological Association Professional Psychology: Research and Practice 22*(4): 269-276. www.kspope.com/torvic/torture1.php (accessed November 2016).

Pross C (2006). Burnout, vicarious traumatisation and its prevention. *Torture 16*(1): 1–9.

Remen RN (1996). *Kitchen Table Wisdom: stories that heal.* New York, NY: Penguin Group.

Siegel D (1999). *The Developing Mind: how relationships and the brain interact to shape who we are.* New York, NY: Guilford Press.

Taylor M (2014). *Trauma Therapy and Clinical Practice: neuroscience, gestalt and the body.* Maidenhead: Open University Press.

van der Kolk B (2014). *The Body Keeps the Score: mind, brain and body in the transformation of trauma.* London: Penguin Books.

van der Veer G, van Waning A (2004). Creating a safe therapeutic sanctuary. In: Wilson JP, Drožđek B (eds). *Broken Spirits: the treatment of traumatized asylum seekers, refugees, war and torture victims.* New York, NY: Brunner-Routledge (pp33–52).

17. Walking a journey alongside a survivor: therapeutic social work with survivors of torture

Anna Turner

This chapter offers practical guidance on therapeutic social work approaches to working with torture survivors in exile. I will draw on my knowledge as a qualified social worker with 10 years' experience of working with refugee adults and families. I hope to demystify social work with survivors of torture, which is frequently seen as a specialised area of work. My intention here is to raise awareness of therapeutic interventions and encourage confidence among fellow social workers in applying these approaches. I will reflect on various models of social work practice and attempt to recapture the essence of social work as a human rights-based profession by exploring the political, societal, personal and inter-relational challenges for professionals and clients.

The three case studies are based on an amalgamation of my work with torture survivors, and are used here to illustrate key themes and effective methods of working. These case studies are drawn from my work at a charity offering a range of holistic services to refugees and people seeking sanctuary. In my role as a social work co-ordinator, I developed several projects, including a complex case work service, a weekly drop-in and a duty and short-term crisis service. I also supported the development of user-led campaigning and action groups.

My passion for working with refugees stems from my deep-rooted commitment to humanity, equality and social justice, which is embedded in the traditions of social work values and practice. While the work is challenging, it is also deeply rewarding.

I draw strength from the resilience of refugees and people seeking asylum and enjoy being part of a rich fusion of culture and diversity. There is also a unique sense of solidarity among colleagues, partners and clients that motivates and binds a drive for change in this sector.

Defining social work

The following Global Definition of the Social Work Profession was approved by the International Association of Schools of Social Work (IASSW) General Assembly and IFSW General Meeting in July 2014:

> Social work is a practice-based profession and an academic discipline that promotes social change and development, social cohesion, and the empowerment and liberation of people. Principles of social justice, human rights, collective responsibility and respect for diversities are central to social work. Underpinned by theories of social work, social sciences, humanities and indigenous knowledge, social work engages people and structures to address life challenges and enhance wellbeing.

Thus, social work focuses on the interconnections between:

- the micro – understanding the individual(s) internal psyche, behavioural functioning, and the processes and systems within families
- the mezzo – their position and relationship within their community, including spiritual, religious and cultural connections, friendship groups, the wider family, social networks, local services and policies
- the macro – their position and relationship within the social-political sphere that includes national and international legislation, government operations, wider public opinion and popular social discourse.

In practice, among many other things, this involves holistic assessment, advocacy, crisis and risk management, and therapeutic psychoeducational interventions such as understanding symptoms, developing coping strategies and goal setting. Effective social workers need to be acutely attuned to the interplay of power and oppression and committed to working with individuals, families, services and governing bodies to alleviate injustice and disadvantage.

This has significance when working with refugees because of the systematic abuses of power that they experience on multiple levels, both within their home countries and in the host country where they seek protection. It raises two important questions: what might be a good framework for social work with torture survivors seeking asylum in exile, and what are the knowledge and skills required to aid the therapeutic relationship?

Creating a framework

The role of the social worker is multi-faceted and, if given the time and space to reach its full potential, offers real opportunities for creativity and flexibility when working with torture survivors, particularly in the voluntary sector. However, this broad scope can also make it hard for social workers to balance working therapeutically with the practical/political tasks of advocacy, safeguarding and crisis intervention. In the organisation where I previously worked, this regularly arose in discussions about how we developed service provision. In group supervision, it has been argued that it is not possible to separate therapeutic work from the practical aspects of the role, as they are intrinsically linked. Clients value help with dealing with their practical needs, such as support in accessing services and liaising with legal representatives, which are important in helping them establish stability in their lives. They also value the planned therapeutic sessions where they can explore symptoms of trauma and develop personal resilience. Social workers combine an ability to influence and make changes in the external social and political environment, while encouraging the client to connect with their internal self. This complements the role of the therapist, whose primary focus is on the internal experiences of trauma. It can be difficult to undertake this work when a client's external environment is so unstable.

Social workers often first meet a client when they are in crisis or where there are safeguarding concerns. There may not be time to build a relationship. Therefore, each task, whether practical or therapeutic, needs to have a purpose. Without this, it is easy to lose direction in the complexities of the work. My social work colleagues and I developed the following simple framework of objectives to anchor our work with clients: to promote access to rights, choice, stability, safety and improved wellbeing. Each social work action or interaction links into one or more of the objectives, and the framework ensures that the client remains central to the work.

We visualise our work as 'walking a journey', accompanying survivors in exile, and we use a fluid process, incorporating relationship building, assessment, collaborative working and applying knowledge-based practice.

Building a relationship

In my experience, it is the quality and consistency of the relationship that is the most important aspect of work with torture survivors. This requires the practitioner to be a containing presence, who listens and encourages the survivor when the system has rendered them powerless, and takes practical steps to ensure their rights are recognised.

I have found that taking time to build a relationship with a client can enrich the assessment process and the subsequent interventions. Clients are then more likely to engage actively in assessing their own strengths and needs by exploring their past and present, which acts to empower them, and their family.

In building a relationship, I incorporate several informal sessions into the process of engagement. For example, when I can, I will take a client to the vast, open space of the local country park. This has proved powerful with clients who struggle to feel at home in their new environment. One client at risk of removal told me: 'Since being in the UK, this is the first time I have felt free.' Undertaking creative sessions that are led by client's needs breaks down barriers to relationship building and enables freer conversations to take place, as the sessions are less intimidating than formal assessment processes, and can be enjoyable.

I once worked with a young male torture survivor who wanted to be an engineer. He liked to work out how mechanisms function. Following his traumatic experiences, he believed he had lost his skills and ability to concentrate. I suggested that we try some basic engineering tasks in one of our sessions. Together we built a (semi-successful) water filter, and, in another session, we made paperclips float in water. Through this process, I was not only building a relationship with him; I was also tuning into his skills and inner strengths. To our amusement, we found that he was much more patient with the exercises than I was, and he still had a strong attention to detail. I reflected this back to him, and from here we began to explore his resilience and personal qualities. He told me that the quality of patience was held in high regard in his culture and community. At the time, he was waiting for a Home Office decision, and so we then looked at how he could use his personal qualities and cultural beliefs to help him cope with the here-and-now.

Building trust

Building trust is pivotal; it cannot be taken for granted. For a survivor of torture, their ability to trust is often severely damaged, which may influence their response to a practitioner. For example, they may regard the process of assessment with suspicion; they may feel as though they are being interrogated, and may withdraw or disengage. Often there are overwhelming feelings of shame as a result of torture, particularly for those who have suffered rape.

Trust is developed when a practitioner is able to bear witness to the disclosure of rape and torture. Maintaining the dignity of a survivor is paramount.

Social workers also need to be aware of the potential for traumatic transference in the therapeutic relationship, and that their trustworthiness may be tested by survivors. Alternatively, the survivor may idealise the practitioner as the rescuer, and place high expectations on them that cannot be met. Then, when the practitioner fails, it reinforces the survivor's belief that others cannot be trusted.

Social workers may feel drawn to rescue the client and lose sight of what they can realistically achieve. Therefore, it is important for the social worker and client to discuss and identify a collaborative means of working in which the limitations on the practitioner's role are clearly understood.

A collaborative approach

The first principle of establishing a therapeutic relationship is to listen to the survivor. Use active listening and enquiry to encourage them to talk. Consider using the exchange model (Smale, Tuson & Statham, 2000) as a process of communication. The exchange model is based on the sharing of information between client and social worker. It pays attention to the client's expertise and draws on the expertise of the practitioner and wider networks in a collaborative, solution-focused approach.

I strongly advocate multi-agency working. Working in isolation leaves less space to develop a therapeutic relationship, which can lead to the disempowerment of clients. A practitioner who is managing multiple cases, with high volumes of crisis intervention and multiple demands on their time, is likely to focus more on advocacy work and on delivering practical interventions on behalf of a survivor, rather than alongside them.

A holistic approach

It is important for social workers to have some knowledge of the client's life before, during and after the traumatic events. This is to ensure that their identity and that of their family are not lost in the problems of the here-and-now. It is also important to identify the survivor's strengths, resilience and resources, alongside the challenges facing them, in order to gather a fully rounded sense of the person.

I usually explore early childhood experiences and childhood development. I ask about the survivor's work and family life and their education pre-torture, and about their culture. I explore emotions and characteristics by asking them to assess how they were before torture and how they are now, after torture and relocation. I ask what led to the torture, the subsequent migration process, such as being trafficked to the UK, and how this has added to their traumatic experiences. With children, I explore their likes, dislikes, fears and wishes.

This holistic approach helps me put myself in their shoes, which is essential in this work. However, the timing of these dialogues is crucial. If a client is displaying acute symptoms of trauma, or is in crisis, it may be too distressing for them to delve into their past, and counterproductive rather than therapeutic. The purpose is to enhance their wellbeing, safety and stability. Only ask a survivor to share their life experiences when necessary and if there is a clear purpose, and explain why you are seeking this information.

Internal and external barriers to recovery, settlement and improved quality of life

There are many barriers to helping survivors build a new life and move forward, and they are often directly related to the external environment. For example, if survivors are refused asylum, they are no longer entitled to housing, and become homeless. Having lost the right to stay in the country where they have sought protection, and unable to return to their home country, they become stuck. The instability of their immigration status and the punitive asylum and immigration systems have a detrimental impact on recovery. A survivor I worked with described the system as 'killing him slowly'. He was a survivor of rape and prolonged torture. He was homeless for several years after his initial claim for asylum was turned down. He disengaged from services as he was so ashamed of what his life had become. He could not comprehend that a country he thought would protect him could leave him living 'like a dog'. He was eventually granted refugee status, but his experiences of abandonment, with no safety, stability or therapeutic help, resulted in significant damage to his emotional psyche. If the system had given him protection sooner, his recovery process would have been very different.

Women are particularly vulnerable if their asylum claim is refused. Many are forced into exploitative relationships and withdraw from services through fear of being removed to their country of origin.

Processing the physiological and psychological impacts of torture can be extremely difficult. Family systems may break down, trust in others may be ruptured and the survivor often experiences overwhelming grief, loss and a sense of powerlessness.

Some people may have pre-existing trauma or attachment difficulties because of early childhood experiences, which may hamper the process of recovery. Additional barriers to recovery include cultural shock, loss of cultural identity, disconnection from other people, systemic oppression and language barriers. Transition to refugee status can also be problematic, as survivors then face the pressures of finding employment and housing and accessing higher education.

Social work values and ethics

Social work values and ethics are central to working therapeutically with torture survivors. They are based on human rights and access to justice and involve a commitment to an ethical framework of practice that promotes respect, dignity, a right to self-determination and protection from harm. As a social worker, I grapple with the concepts of modern social work practice, including the core values and ethics that appear at times to have lost their original meanings in the UK. Systemic layers of power and oppression are entrenched into political and organisational frameworks and filter directly into the social worker and client relationship. This presents a number of ethical dilemmas for social workers, and in particular for those working in statutory services, which are centred around care and control. In the UK, there has been a gradual shift in the delivery and cultural attitudes of local authority social services in response to government agendas and austerity measures. Tighter guidelines have been drawn in relation to eligibility for services, and social workers' caseloads have increased significantly. There can be time for little more than risk and resource management. A woman survivor and her child, with no recourse to public funds (NRPF) and in need of shelter, will be assessed against her immigration status and how much it will cost services to care for them.

The constraints on social workers in local authority services should not detract from the good work that some services and individual social workers are doing to protect vulnerable adults, young people, children and families. However, there is a need for social workers and their employers to recognise and, where possible, address the conflicts between the political, organisational and social work frameworks. It is these conflicts that impact negatively on the core values and ethics of the profession. I encourage social workers to be mindful of their approaches to working with torture survivors seeking asylum, particularly when they are assessing or declining access to statutory service provision.

Understanding of power and oppression

There are many theories and volumes of literature on power and oppression in social work, yet they remain among the most challenging and complex of challenges. Power and oppression take place on multiple levels and are intrinsically linked to fear, discrimination and alienation. Bourke argues: 'Emotions such as fear do not belong only to individuals or social groups, they mediate between the individual and the social. They are power relations... fear sorts people into positions of social hierarchy' (2005: 354).

Where there is social hierarchy, there is privilege. Social workers should reflect on their own social position and that of their clients in relation to personal, professional and political privilege. Hays (2001) created a theoretical framework known as 'ADDRESSING', as a tool to promote the recognition of the cross-cultural influences that form identity. Brown (2009) and Wilkin & Hillock (2014) discuss its use in social work practice. The tool encourages practitioners to assess how each of the domains below inter-relates and how each is connected with the others:

A = Age-related factors, including chronological age and age cohort
D = Disability status, developmental and acquired, visible and invisible
R = Religion and spiritual issues
E = Ethnicity, race and culture
S = Social status (current and former)
S = Sexual orientation
I = Indigenous heritage, colonisation, coloniser history
N = National origin, immigration or refugee status
G = Gender, biological sex or gender identity.
(From Brown, 2009: 177–178 and Wilkin & Hillock, 2014: 197–198)

Treating each domain separately risks overlooking the unique experiences of marginalised groups and fails to acknowledge how power and oppression are experienced differently in each realm. Civil rights activist and professor of law Kimberly Crenshaw argues that we must adopt this intersectional perspective to understand how identity can impact on an individual's experience of loss of power through oppression (1989). For example, an African woman who has been raped and has been refused asylum will experience multiple burdens of oppression, based on her ethnicity, gender, legal status, culture, national origin, economic status and health.

Western countries are bound by bureaucracy and complex systems, which can lead to survivors of torture and their families feeling paralysed.

I frequently work with adults and families who are overwhelmed by the bureaucratic systems that serve to reinforce internal persecutory messages that the state is deliberately taking away their freedom. This can be challenging for the practitioner when trying to build a professional relationship with clients, as they may think that the worker holds some power in this system and is doing nothing to help them.

Social workers are restricted as to what they can achieve, but they must always keep in mind the privileges and power they hold and acknowledge the disparities between them and their clients and the loss of power and choice that refugees experience.

Culturally sensitive practice

Culture is very influential in forming both our collective and our individual identity. Holding onto one's cultural and spiritual identity is, for many, a way of holding onto a sense of self, which can be significantly damaged by traumatic experiences. Settling successfully in a new environment requires being able to adapt to a new system while maintaining a sense of self and cultural community.

Maintaining cultural identity and adapting to a new environment are complex, as there are challenges from all angles: pressure from a societal construct to 'adapt' and 'integrate'; pressure from one's community to meet certain cultural expectations, and the individual need to retain a sense of self and belonging. Practitioners can make efforts to learn about and understand other cultures and must avoid making assumptions in their work with refugee survivors and imposing their own cultural norms and expectations on those with whom they work. Social workers should work flexibly, and be prepared to adapt their practice and invite an open relationship that welcomes discussion and understanding.

Most refugees have experienced multiple losses, including loss of family members and friendships, so it is not uncommon for the practitioner to be seen as a substitute family and emblematic of hope. The significance of this is not to be ignored or dismissed. While we do not want to create dependency and a false sense of attachment, culturally, for many refugees, the concepts of family and collective identity are very symbolic, and it is important that the practitioner works with this notion, rather than against it. For example, the practitioner may be invited to participate in family or community life. However, as the relationship develops, there will be many opportunities to define roles and expectations, explore professional boundaries and encourage more authentic connections and relationships with people outside the service and beyond the professional relationship. This needs to be discussed honestly and openly with clients, and they should also be made aware that the relationship is professional and will, in time, come to an end.

Advocacy and a human rights approach

Advocacy can serve several therapeutic functions if used appropriately. The Latin word *advocatus* translates literally as 'one called to aid'. This kind of relationship is graphically illustrated by one of my clients, a woman survivor of torture, who told me her traumatic experience had affected her capacity to receive and interpret information. She described wanting to shut off, wanting people to stop talking and just 'do something'. What she was describing was a 'call to aid' – a handing over of responsibility; a request for someone to act on her behalf because she couldn't handle the situation herself. By taking on this advocacy role, I was forming an alliance of trust, and thereby supporting a connection that had been ruptured by her traumatic experience. Social workers should be mindful, however, that by taking on responsibility for negotiating systems and processes, our role can quickly and imperceptibly shift into that of rescuer, and the client becomes the victim. Thus, a contractual approach is useful in these cases, where together the practitioner and client define the goals, aims, expectations and responsibilities of the relationship.

Advocacy is about human rights and raising the voices of the voiceless and least heard. It takes place on several levels: through campaigning, influencing policy, developing services and supporting access to rights and justice. A human rights-based approach to social work is a belief that refugee survivors of torture have the right to be treated with respect and dignity, and are entitled to the rights and protections conferred by the international conventions and treaties to which many countries have signed up. Many people seeking asylum are unaware of their rights to access services under national and international laws, policies, conventions and treaties. Social workers can use and share their knowledge with clients, professionals and services. This requires practitioners to ensure they are up to date with and alert to these rights and how to support, advocate and inform their clients on how to exercise them.

I would also recommend that practitioners and services promote and develop opportunities for self-advocacy, both within their projects and externally. Through my work, I have been part of several grassroots initiatives led by refugees and people seeking asylum, such as awareness raising through drama and singing groups, education in schools, conferences, campaigning, and contributing to research to support political activism. The latter has involved being interviewed or providing case study material to be used for lobbying or campaigning. Promoting and supporting self-advocacy groups is important and richly beneficial. It gives individuals a more powerful, collective voice; they learn new skills; they form longstanding connections and friendships, and it can shift a person's identity from potential victim to activist. Survivors can be involved in raising awareness and contributing to changing local and national policy and, importantly, are seen as experts in their own right.

Understanding the context and refugee awareness

There are several reasons why a person or family may seek sanctuary in another country: war; terror; persecution because of their political beliefs, sexuality, ethnicity, gender or religion; family feuds; land feuds; trafficking and slavery; natural disaster and poverty. However, not all these reasons warrant recognition and refugee status, and many people have difficulties proving their need for asylum to the required standard.

Article 1 of the 1951 UN Refugee Convention, as amended by the 1967 Protocol, provides the definition of a refugee. Once recognised under the Convention, refugees are granted the same rights and access to services as citizens of the host state. In reality, in the UK, they are likely to experience further exclusion, discrimination and poverty. People going through the asylum process and awaiting a decision are commonly referred to as 'asylum seekers'. Those whose application for refugee status is not recognised are widely referred to as 'failed asylum seekers'. Popular discourse attaches suspicion, disbelief and dehumanisation to these terms. I use the terms 'people seeking asylum' and 'people refused asylum'. In both cases, their rights to access services are significantly fewer and their human rights are often breached and largely ignored.

The practitioner's role becomes complex when survivors become destitute following refusal. Their commitment to a human rights-based approach must be consistent, as far as this is possible. In practice, this involves the practitioner being persistent and seeking legal advice to push for action from agencies who have a duty to ensure human rights are met. In my experience, the most effective therapeutic approach is to uncover and bring to the fore the resilience and personal strengths of a survivor while also being committed to multi-agency working and safeguarding.

Popular social discourse has significant influence on political, civil and social frameworks, both internationally and in individual host countries. In the socio-political sphere, there is conflict, largely fueled by fear, between a humanitarian response to refugees and discourse about resources, public safety and entitlement. This includes fear of overpopulation, fear of difference, fear of terrorism and concerns about public safety, which are unfairly associated with refugees and those who seek asylum.

These messages filter down to mainstream services and local communities, giving a platform to Islamophobia and xenophobia and resulting in the further exclusion of people seeking asylum. Refugees and people seeking asylum are lumped together under the umbrella of 'migrants', and the humanitarian messages and understanding of the plight of people seeking asylum and our duties under the 1951 UN Refugee Convention and the European Convention on Human Rights (European Court of Human Rights, 2010) are forgotten.

Understanding the impact of torture and trauma

From my experience of working with survivors, how individuals respond to torture varies. Some may recover quite quickly and draw strength from their experiences, and others who have survived prolonged and severe ill-treatment, including sexual violence, have an acute reaction. For all, trauma is exacerbated by significant experiences of loss.

When I first began working with torture survivors, I worked with several young men from the Democratic Republic of the Congo (DRC). Many described unsettled lives as children. Their communities had for decades been disrupted and torn apart by war and persecution. There were similarities in their presentations, which included a deep suspicion of others, paranoid ideation and noticeable difficulties in remaining present in appointments. Intrusive images and thoughts would repeatedly trouble them, especially at night, when they experienced nightmares and flashbacks. One young man, who had been kidnapped as a child, was easily startled by loud noises and sudden movements, which triggered a return to his experiences of being attacked by soldiers. He would have long episodes of dissociation, resulting in paranoia, and would often misinterpret the intensions of others. On three occasions, he was admitted to a mental health ward.

These young men were completely fixated on the external factors, such as their immigration status, housing and health services, and were in constant conflict with service providers, professionals, partners and friends. They were repeatedly involved in risky or harmful behaviours that threatened their tenancies, which they would have lost if it had not been for my intervention.

As my experience has grown, I now recognise this as traumatic transference and countertransference. I had a strong pull to nurture, while they were unknowingly testing everything around them, and relying on me to rescue them. Their focus on the perceived flaws of others allowed them to avoid looking at themselves. Drinking alcohol distracted them and numbed their feelings. This resulted in self-loathing and hidden shame.

It is not uncommon for torture survivors to present with feelings of helplessness and persecution. These strong feelings often find expression in somatic and physiological symptoms, which are a primary complaint for most torture survivors. Survivors report stomach pains and burning sensations in the stomach and chest, pains in the body, sweating hands, difficulties in swallowing, racing heart, tension in the shoulders, pain in the eyes, blurred vision, dizziness and severe headaches. Difficulties with sexual intimacy may also arise, for both men and women. In addition, some survivors have long-term physical injuries from their experiences, which are constant reminders of the torture.

Babette Rothschild explains that, during life-threatening events, our autonomic nervous system (ANS) releases hormones that are telling our body to prepare for defensive action (2000: 8). The body mobilises for flight or fight, and produces a number of physical sensations, including freezing and numbing. Often people feel guilt after freezing, despite freezing being a natural reaction to a terrifying event. Thought processes and how one stores memories and recalls information can also become disorganised and confused. The amygdala (part of the threat system) alerts our body and brain to danger. During this process, the hippocampus (where we store memories) is suppressed, leading to difficulties in recalling and placing memories in time and place. It is not uncommon for the physiological sensations associated with fight, flight or freeze to remain long after the event, and thus some torture survivors may have difficulties in distinguishing past dangers from the present.

Social workers will find it helpful to learn about the effects of trauma, so they understand what is happening when clients behave in unusual or unexpected ways. I use the website http://psychology.tools, which has helpful diagrams of the body and brain that explain how they react during life-threatening events. Diagrams can be useful when explaining to survivors about the effects of trauma.

Children, depending on their level of exposure to torture and conflict, will also develop some of the above presentations. Children and young people are resilient; they are also vulnerable and often express high levels of anxiety and worry for their families. They may have experienced multiple losses and may feel abandoned, isolated and disconnected, especially if they have been separated from their family. Children who are living with a parent/s who has survived torture may take on a parenting role and caring responsibilities, and may absorb the emotional distress of their parents and become vulnerable to vicarious traumatisation.

Diagnosis and psychosocial factors

In western societies, someone displaying these presentations to the extent that they interfere with everyday life is likely to be given a diagnosis of post-traumatic stress disorder (PTSD). Masocha and Simpson (2011) and Wilkin and Hillock (2014) question the application of westernised constructs to the mental health of refugees. They criticise the medical model for its preoccupation with biological factors, symptoms and diagnoses, such as PTSD, and individual pathology, and the way it understates the significance of the wider social context and barriers to social inclusion.

To strengthen service provision, there needs to be an increased awareness of culturally appropriate interventions, and flexibility within frameworks of practice to incorporate an understanding of spiritual pain and loss and a much deeper analysis of biological and psychosocial causation (Masocha & Simpson, 2011).

Recovery models

There are several theories of trauma and recovery, notably those of Babette Rothschild (2000), Judith Herman (1992) and Ravi Kohli (2007). In Rothschild's theory, the phases of recovery include the following stages: stability and safety, processing the trauma, and integration. Similar to Rothschild, Herman identifies safety as the initial stage, followed by 'remembrance' and 'mourning', then 'reconnection'. Movement between these stages is fluid and does not necessarily occur in a straightforwardly linear direction.

Kohli (2007) explores social work practice with unaccompanied minors. He suggests three domains of trauma recovery, which are also transferable to working with adults and families: cohesion (bringing order to the outside world), connection (resettlement of inner worlds), and coherence (resettlement as feeling reconstructed). While the social worker's role is not to process trauma with a survivor, they are required to respond to disclosures of loss and trauma through emotional support, psychoeducation and validation.

All theories emphasise the importance of torture survivors being the authors of their own recovery. Herman discusses the healing relationship between therapist and client and defines recovery as based on 'the empowerment of the survivor and the creation of new connections' (1992: 133). Achieving a sense of safety can be challenging, particularly for people who are refused asylum, made homeless and destitute, and are at risk of removal. Bringing stability to the person's circumstances is often the first necessary step on the journey of recovery.

Social workers and care professionals who are not qualified therapists may find overwhelming the idea of working therapeutically with torture survivors. Given that the principles of human rights and social justice are embedded in the traditions of social work practice, workers may feel frustrated and angry at the injustice in how refugees and people seeking asylum are treated in the UK. They may feel powerless as they try to find solutions within a restrictive framework, which in turn may lead them to doubt their ability to do anything to help. Self-doubt and powerlessness can impact on the worker's relationship with clients, or can lead to 'empathy burnout', or compassion fatigue.

Professionals should pay attention to how they process their emotions and seek support at the end of each working day, and have a good self-care plan in place. It is also the responsibility of agencies to ensure they support their staff. In the refugee organisation where I previously worked, I set up reflection meetings where workers could bring these issues and explore challenging cases, as in a case conference. We paid attention to our own thoughts and feelings and shared what we knew with one another. I would strongly encourage this in all social work environments – the goal is not to work in isolation but to develop, learn and improve, both personally and collectively.

Social work theories, models and approaches

Practical approaches

Crisis intervention is a central component in this area of work, particularly when assessing risk to self and other, or risk of homelessness and detention and/or removal. I use a visual mapping sheet to highlight the key areas of crisis, followed by an action plan that clearly sets out the tasks for each person involved. It is important to review and monitor the crisis on a regular basis and identify when it has escalated, reduced or ended.

Task-centred practice is simple but effective. I find it useful when creating action plans with clients, as an inclusive model of working and one that promotes their participation and development of personal skills. It involves setting out the tasks for each person involved and creating a timeframe for completion. For example, tasks for a client may be to gather evidence for their asylum case, attend regular appointments, speak to their GP about their health problems, and so on. Tasks for the social worker include agreeing roles, co-ordinating access to services, setting up multi-agency meetings, and liaising with professionals. I encourage clients to write down their tasks in their own language. If a client is not literate in any language, diagrams and colour coding can be helpful.

Psychological perspectives and interventions

Cognitive behavioural techniques, compassion-focused practice, person-centred practice, psychoanalytical approaches and psychoeducation are all important and relevant to therapeutic social work practice. Psychoanalytic work, which usually involves exploring attachment and child development, is helpful with single adults and with families with children.

From my experience, cognitive behavioural techniques can be helpful in addressing negative thought patterns and raising awareness, which may complement the deeper therapy work a survivor may be undertaking with a qualified psychological therapist. However, this type of intervention is limited when used on its own, as trauma is often located and processed within the body, outside of conscious decision-making, and therefore not always in the control of the survivor (van der Kolk, 2005).

Family perspectives and approaches

Systems theory and the ecological perspective are particularly relevant to this work. Systems theory focuses on the internal functioning of a family. Within each family, there are open and closed systems and subsystems. The key is to identify the target system or subsystem requiring intervention that will bring about change (Teater, 2014: 16). The ecological perspective addresses the relationships and connections between the individual, their family and their environment. This perspective throws a wider spotlight on external barriers to recovery, such as access to the necessary recourses and adequacy of the environment to meet a family's needs (Teater, 2014: 27).

Each country will have its own guidelines and legislation for protecting children. In undertaking assessments, I use a nationally recognised UK government policy document, *Every Child Matters* (HM Government, 2003), which sets out five key outcomes for a child: being healthy, staying safe, enjoying and achieving, making a positive contribution and achieving economic wellbeing.

In the following three case studies, I demonstrate how the frameworks discussed in this chapter can be incorporated into practice.

'There my life is in danger, here I have no freedom'

These are the words of Ali, a survivor of ethnic and political persecution in Sudan. Ali fled his home country in search of freedom, but was met with complex systems, systemic racism and lack of opportunity. He is seeking to hold on to his individual and cultural identity as he tries to adapt to a new environment that competes and contradicts with his core sense of self and his understanding of how to be in the world. He asks if he can ever belong in this society and questions if he will ever recover. He misses his wife and children and worries about them constantly. He misses the warm sun and his community, sharing meals, social gatherings and religious responsibilities, and his work as a teacher. In the night, he sees violent images of the soldiers torturing him. He does not trust others. He is startled by loud noises and is easily irritated. He finds it difficult to separate his experiences in Sudan from where he is now. He has been granted refugee status, but finds himself homeless, with a limited choice of housing. He attempts to negotiate the dogmatic, bureaucratic systems in organisations such as the welfare benefits centre, where the staff refuse to use an interpreter and accuse him of not actively seeking employment. He convinces himself that he is 'going crazy'. He begins to feel helpless and angry.

With the above information, the first stage is to begin to map out the information I have for Ali, pre-and post-migration (see Figure 1).

With clients like Ali, the initial stage requires a crisis intervention, in which risks and safeguarding are paramount. An assessment is needed to address his immediate needs for housing and benefits, with targeted questioning about his health, his coping strategies, and the risks of psychological and physical deterioration. A risk assessment is required to explore risk to self and others, including risk of exploitation. The social worker needs to explore protective factors, and identify any other services involved with Ali, and include them in the crisis plan, with Ali's consent.

It is important to note that these types of assessment and subsequent interventions can easily lead to the pathologising of a survivor's responses to trauma and stress. It is an ethical dilemma for practitioners, but it is sometimes necessary to use a diagnosis to access services and establish safety. During this process, the social worker should not lose sight of the client's resilience and strengths and should feel confident that they are advocating from a rights-based approach and applying principles of recovery, which include establishing a sense of safety. Ali's immediate need is for shelter. Without this, his health is

Therapeutic social work with survivors of torture

Figure 1: Ali's pre- and post-migration maps

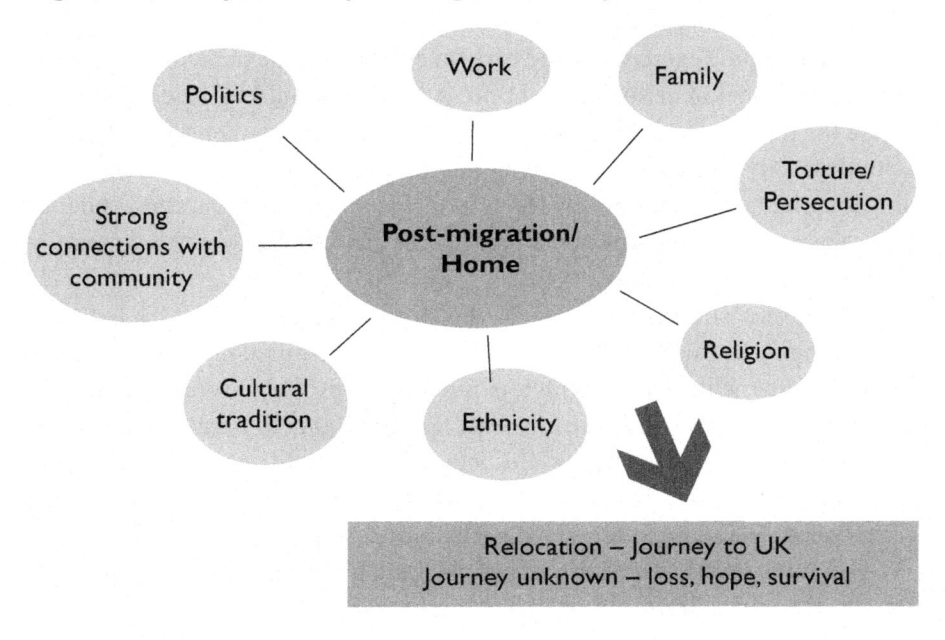

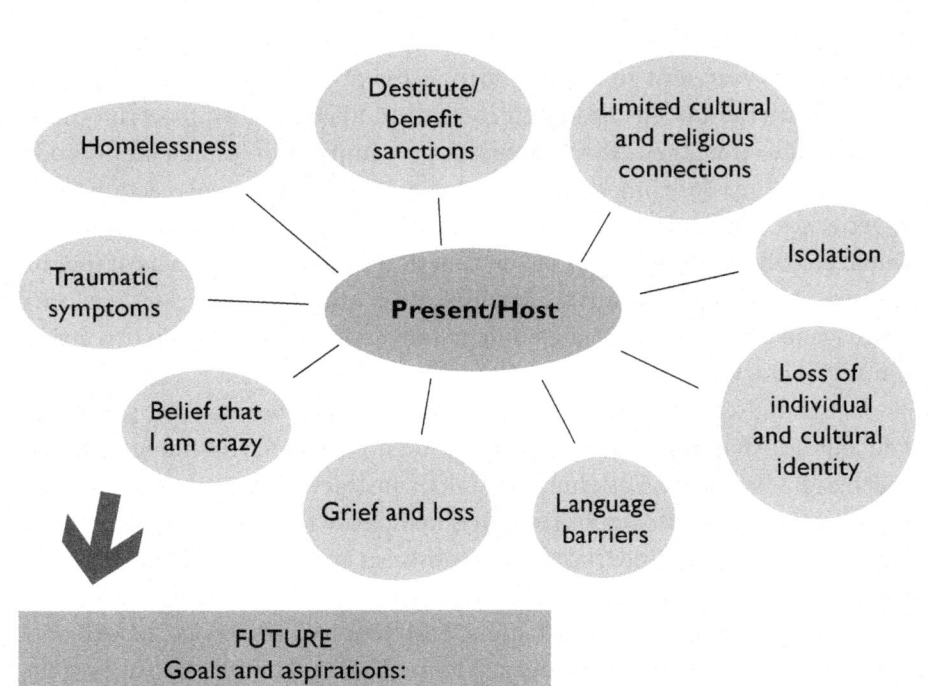

Post-migration/Home
- Politics
- Work
- Family
- Torture/Persecution
- Religion
- Ethnicity
- Cultural tradition
- Strong connections with community

Relocation – Journey to UK
Journey unknown – loss, hope, survival

Present/Host
- Homelessness
- Destitute/benefit sanctions
- Limited cultural and religious connections
- Isolation
- Loss of individual and cultural identity
- Language barriers
- Grief and loss
- Belief that I am crazy
- Traumatic symptoms

FUTURE
Goals and aspirations:
- to be reunited with family
- to be healthy

387

likely to deteriorate and his process of recovery may be significantly hindered, with potential lasting damage.

The mapping exercise is used early to ensure that the person does not get lost in the model of crisis intervention. Attention should be paid to Ali's life before the traumatic events: he had a profession; he was a father, a husband and a political activist. He had strong religious beliefs, and described a strong sense of belonging to his community. He used his personal strengths and resilience to escape persecution and embark on a journey to relocate to another country. He has a capacity for survival.

Attention should be given to the power dynamics in Ali's external environment. In this case, there is a distinct power imbalance in relation to the welfare benefits centre, which is refusing to provide an interpreter. My role is to use positive power to advocate for Ali's rights to have an interpreter. This is achieved by using equalities legislation to hold services to account. In this process of crisis intervention and advocacy, my approach remains compassionate and maintains a strengths-based perspective.

Ali has told me that he thinks people think he is crazy. He is experiencing flashbacks, feels irritable and has nightmares. In response to this, I acknowledge and validate his experiences and empathise with his emotional distress. Attuning to Ali's loss of a sense of self, I try to gain insight into his grief and his reactions to torture, such as his physiological, emotional and somatic experiences, his thought process and his relationships with others. My aim is to strengthen Ali's awareness of the impacts of trauma on his body and psyche. I reassure him that his current feelings are a normal reaction to his experiences. If he can take in information and engage with psychoeducation, I would consider using a diagram to explain the physiological impacts of trauma and ask Ali to identify any similarities. This empowers him to develop a language to explain what is happening to him and move away from perceiving himself as crazy.

I find it useful to introduce grounding techniques during these situations. I encourage Ali to regulate his breathing, and notice his surroundings through touch, sight and smell. I ask him to think of an object that might ground him, such as a stone or photograph. The aim is to increase his ability to remain in the here-and-now. When undertaking an assessment and planning an intervention with him, I use thinking questions and engage him as much as possible in the decision-making process. For example, I ask him to think about the personal strengths he used to make the journey to the UK. I undertake a positive traits exercise, and ask Ali to think about how he can apply it in the here-and-now. My role is to work alongside Ali to reconnect and strengthen his sense of self. By completing these simple exercises, the social worker is building a therapeutic alliance and setting a foundation for a trusting relationship.

Ali may need a referral for psychological therapy, and it may be necessary to collaborate with other services. This should be discussed further with him, and any referrals made only with his consent.

In line with the model of crisis intervention, I will explore the power dynamics between us and have regular reviews of progress, with continuous goal-setting, aiming to improve his wellbeing and emotional and functional stability.

Guita and Asif

Guita and Asif are from a rural region of Afghanistan. They live with their two children, Samia (12) and Mohammed (14). Asif's brother became affiliated with the Taliban and pressured Asif to join him. When he refused, he became a target for daily harassment. The children saw Asif being kidnapped and Guita being beaten by Asif's brother.

Guita is the main carer in the home. She has raised concerns about Asif's psychological wellbeing. She says his memory is poor, he cannot concentrate, he is irritable and withdrawn. She says he screams in the night. Samia is wetting her bed at night, and seems extremely anxious and depressed. Mohammed often accompanies his parents to medical and legal appointments and speaks on behalf of the family, who have limited English. Guita reports that Mohammed has been praised for good behaviour in school but has anger outbursts at home. Their asylum claim has been refused and their appeal rights are exhausted. They are frightened of removal and there are high levels of anxiety and high expressed emotion within the home.

I conduct my initial assessment over several visits. As the family has had a refusal of their asylum case and fear removal to Afghanistan, my priority is to attend to their need for protection. I ask for their consent to contact their legal representative to establish the status of their asylum claim. Good legal advice is vital in such cases. I ask to see a copy of their asylum interview and refusal, as this will provide a wealth of information about their claim. Practitioners who are more familiar with asylum and immigration law may be able to see whether adequate information about their case has been presented. A social worker should never provide immigration advice unless qualified to do so, but social workers do have a key role in updating the legal representative about the family's health concerns and risks, which are often associated with torture and trauma.

When families are under acute stress and desperate, such as when they are at risk of removal, it is not uncommon for parents and children to feel suicidal. A full risk assessment needs to be carried out, including an exploration of protective factors, and appropriate strategies can then be put in place. This could involve identifying support networks and who to contact in a crisis.

With permission from Guita and Asif, I make referrals to other services, such as the local children and families' service, and hold multi-agency meetings, with the family's involvement. Together, we identify a list of actions and desired outcomes. We use this list to gather information for the case, including medical reports, social work reports, risk assessments and recommendations for services and the family. Along with paying attention to any safeguarding concerns about the children, I assess how they are currently achieving against the *Every Child Matters* outcomes. I assess how the external environment, such as access to school, health, housing and legal services, is impacting on the family's internal world, and if it is adequate to meet their needs. I explore the systems within the family, which involves discussions with both parents and the children, together and separately.

There are many ways to engage children in conversation. My social work colleagues have been particularly creative, and have developed a worry-eater toy, a game with stones (looking at past, present and future) and a wish, hopes and fears game. In this case, there have been significant changes to the roles within the family home, and traumatic transference is also occurring, from Asif to the children. The children are very anxious about their asylum case and worried about their parents – particularly about their father, who they can see is not well. I explore with them the effects of witnessing so many traumatic events and make referrals to a child and adolescent therapy service for Samia, and to a young carers project for both. I identify school activity clubs and ensure the family can have an interpreter, so they are not reliant on Mohammed.

I use the early assessment meetings to collect information about their wider family and social networks, including close extended family and local community, cultural and religious links, friendships and any daily activities that the family undertakes. As part of establishing a therapeutic relationship, I build on the information from the initial assessments and interventions by finding out more about their internal family systems, their strengths and where there are challenges. I involve Asif and Guita in completing the pre/post migration mapping sheets and begin to explore their experiences. I explore individually with each of the parents how they have been affected by their experiences and current circumstances, and refer them to appropriate services.

I also ask Asif's GP to refer him to the local community mental health team.

Asif is convinced he is no longer a good father, so I hold six sessions with the family to identify and work on their functioning and systems of communication within the home.

I first complete a genogram with both parents to get an understanding of their family life before and after they fled Afghanistan. I ask them to think about their personal strengths and the resilience it took to come to the UK. I ask how they made decisions in the past and what their roles were and how these have changed. I also ask how they like to spend time with the children, and what they enjoy doing as a family. From this I establish that Asif and Guita had an arranged marriage, and that their way of communicating their affection is by acknowledging and appreciating each other's functional roles and contributions. It is important that I respect and work with the cultural dynamics of their relationship.

I can see that the children are their primary concern. I ask how they can reduce the anxiety within the home to protect the children. I ask them to think about how they spend their time, and what parenting tasks they can still manage. Asif is able to say that he is having flashbacks and that there are times when he completely shuts down during the day and can only sit and rock back and forth. I acknowledge his traumatic experiences and explore his sense of loss and how this affects him in the here-and-now. I work with him to identify triggers in the home that cause him distress. I encourage him to plan strategies to reduce the children's exposure to this distress. He suggests going out for a walk, attending the local mosque to pray and listening to music.

I ask Guita and Asif to think of fun activities they can do with the children, when Asif is able to engage. They say they like to go to a nearby town and to visit relatives. They also enjoy cooking and eating meals together. Asif suggests that, on a good day, he can collect Samia from school. Asif and Guita put some of these strategies into action, and report back that the children have enjoyed the time together. Following the sessions, I also link Guita into English classes, volunteering opportunities and access to family activities and community events.

The family continues to fight to secure asylum.

Yolanda

Yolanda is from the DRC. She was studying to become a nurse but experienced many problems because of her ethnicity. She was arrested during a political protest and taken to prison, where she was gang-raped. Her uncle paid money to an officer to help her escape. She was given a false passport and travelled to the UK seven years ago. Yolanda's asylum case has been refused and she has lost her right to accommodation and financial support, and is liable to be detained. Yolanda has a son aged 10, who is with an aunt in Burundi. She has not seen him since he was three years old.

In the UK, Yolanda has moved around, sofa-surfing, until she began a relationship with a much older man, Jonathan, who wants Yolanda to marry him. She says he emotionally abuses her, telling her that he is her only provider and no other man would want her. Yolanda has very low self-esteem and is disconnected from other people. She has severe migraines and cannot sleep because of nightmares. She says she has memory problems and feels trapped in the relationship.

Before undertaking interventions with Yolanda, I first explore her strengths and resilience. Yolanda has been resourceful in finding ways to support herself. She is scared to talk to services, particularly to people in authority. While she does need an assessment of safety and risks, she does not need immediate intervention. As her asylum claim has been refused and she has no right to financial support or housing, she has very few options in terms of alternative accommodation. I establish that Yolanda is not in any immediate danger. She explains that, when she has arguments with her partner, she stays at a friend's house, but this is her only friend and she cannot live there permanently.

My initial work is centred on building trust, paying attention to the exchange model to aid communication. Rather than enquire too deeply, I ask Yolanda to talk about feels comfortable to tell me. I ask how she feels about herself and she says she has low self-esteem. She also has pains in her stomach and severe headaches. Her reactions and responses are slow and she appears very distant. After a few appointments, I ask Yolanda if she has been raped, which she confirms. As my relationship develops with Yolanda, she describes her sense of deep shame and the cultural stigma attached to rape. She also talks about missing her son. She has had telephone contact with him, but can no longer afford the phone cards. I apply to a charity for some money towards a phone card each week. I also support her to request a copy of her file from the Home Office, as she has lost it. We agree that, when the file arrives, I will refer her to a legal representative for advice. I offer to refer Yolanda to a counselling organisation working with survivors of rape, but she initially refuses this, as she does not think it will help and blames herself for her circumstances.

Alongside compassion-focused work, I bring in some basic cognitive behavioural approaches to explore her patterns of destructive thinking, and help her redirect the blame from herself. I use a feminist perspective and focus on normalising Yolanda's responses to traumatic events. Yolanda feels unsafe going out of the home. I acknowledge some of the dangers and we discuss potential safe environments. I encourage her to use self-help techniques to give her somatic relief, such as stretching and grounding techniques. My aim is to reduce shame and disconnection and lift Yolanda's confidence so she feels able to make new connections. With this new confidence, Yolanda asks for a referral to a counselling service and to women-only peer support services. I help her register with a GP, who prescribes medication for her stomach pains and sleep problems.

Referring Yolanda into a project specifically for refugee women proves to be very therapeutically healing. Like Yolanda, many other women in the group have survived rape and have children from whom they have been separated by migration. Her contact with these other women is powerful and beneficial.

Yolanda's new legal representative asks for a medico-legal report. Once her case is reactivated in the asylum process, I can support her to find accommodation and financial support, so she can leave the abusive relationship. Following a review, we establish that Yolanda is successfully linked into services and does not need further support.

Summary

Therapeutic social work is based on working with both the internal and external worlds of a refugee survivor. In my experience, the successful outcomes of the work rely on establishing a therapeutic relationship, upholding the principles of dignity and respect for human life, attuning to clients' personal strengths and resilience, and acting to ensure the voices of the voiceless are heard.

It is for this reason that this chapter ends with the voice of a survivor, Abdelaziz Al Nour Mousa, who I am truly inspired by and grateful to have worked with.

> My name is Abdelaziz Mousa, I'm from Sudan. I came to the UK on 28 October 2013. During my journey, I passed through three cities in the UK: Dover, London, Liverpool, and then I arrived in Manchester, or, more accurately, Salford. I have been here since 28 February 2014.
>
> In that time, I was suffering a lot from different situations as a result of harsh conditions that passed by my life, including my

arrests in prisons, which I find too difficult to talk about.

When I arrived in Salford, I did not know anybody. I could not even be with any group of people because I was scared, and my circumstances were preventing me from that. One day I met a man in the road who guided me to go to the enlightened road [a voluntary sector social worker].

I remember carrying everything I had – my immigration papers, my letters and my medicine – and headed out to a local centre, as I was looking for rescue. I was immersed in what felt like a bottomless sea and I needed to be plucked from the crisis. I was suffering from severe depression and I cried bitterly every day. I chose to stay lonely as I did not trust anyone. I emptied all I had out of my bag on a table and I was very lucky to find a saviour who was Anna. It is possible we can call her 'Iron Woman', as a result of her role for helping each person who suffers as I suffered.

We have done a lot of work together. The relationship has been very important because before I did not have trust for anybody or hope for my life. Over time I developed trust in Anna, as I felt comfortable and safe in her presence, so I started to confide in her about my past. She has helped me grow my confidence and trust in others. Step by step, I have started to believe the words that I couldn't believe before: that life is not lost and I can regain my confidence.

Actually, with great conviction I want to say thank you, as she has helped me so much, fighting for my rights and also at times challenging me. She saved my life from being lost and she continues to help me regain even half my life I had before. Finally, I wish my God keeps her in good health and wellness and thank her forever. She became for me as mum and dad and sister and I am thankful for all staff and volunteers, in their great effort of helping others. I wish God to bless all of you.

References

Bourke J (2005). *Fear: a cultural history*. London: Virago Press.

Brown LS (2009). Cultural competence. In: Courtois CA, Ford JD (eds). *Treating Complex Traumatic Stress Disorders: scientific foundations and therapeutic models*. New York, NY: Guilford Press (pp166–182).

Crenshaw K (1989). Demarginalizing the intersection of race and sex: a black feminist critique of antidiscrimination doctrine, feminist theory and antiracist politics. *University of Chicago Legal Forum 1*: 139–167.

European Court of Human Rights/Council of Europe (2010). *European Convention on Human Rights*. Strasbourg: Council of Europe. www.echr.coe.int/Documents/Convention_ENG.pdf (accessed July 2017).

Hays PA (2001). *Addressing Cultural Complexities in Practice: a framework for clinicians and counsellors*. Washington, DC: American Psychological Association.

HM Government (2003). *Every Child Matters*. Cm 5869. Norwich: the Stationery Office.

Herman JL (1992). *Trauma and Recovery: the aftermath of violence – from domestic abuse to political terror*. New York, NY: Basic Books.

International Association of Schools of Social Work (IASSW)/ International Federation of Social Workers (2014). *Global Definition of the Social Work Profession*. Berne: IFSW. http://ifsw.org/get-involved/global-definition-of-social-work/ (accessed July 2017).

Kohli R (2007). *Social work with Unaccompanied Asylum-Seeking Children*. Basingstoke: Palgrave Macmillan.

Masocha S, Simpson M (2011). Developing mental health social work for asylum seekers: a proposed model of practice. *Journal of Social Work 12*(4): 423–443.

Rothschild B (2000). *The Body Remembers: the psychophysiology of trauma and trauma treatment*. New York, NY: WW Norton & Company.

Smale G, Tuson G, Statham D (2000). *Social work and Social Problems: working towards social inclusion and social change*. London: Palgrave.

Teater B (2014). *An Introduction to Applying Social Work Theory and Methods*. Maidenhead: Open University Press.

UNHCR (1951). *Convention and Protocol Relating to the Status of Refugees*. Geneva: UNHCR. www.unhcr.org/uk/3b66c2aa10 (accessed July 2017).

van der Kolk (2005). Developmental trauma disorder: towards a rationale diagnosis for chronically traumatized children. *Psychiatric Annals 33*(5): 401–408.

Wilkin L, Hillock S (2014). Enhancing MSW students' efficacy in working with trauma, violence, and oppression: an integrated feminist-trauma framework for social work education. *Feminist Teacher 24*(3): 184–206.

Postscript
Jude Boyles

The last two decades have seen the erosion of support services for all those in mental distress. The introduction in 2008, in England and Wales, of the Improving Access to Psychological Therapies (IAPT) service has not brought the benefits it promised. Rather, it has imposed a limited model, with a limited choice of therapies, tight restrictions on numbers of sessions, and inflexible expectations of progress through treatment. Alarmingly, we are also now witnessing the third sector beginning to adopt the manualised models of therapy offered in IAPT services, in order to win contracts for their services and ensure their financial survival. In the process, these services are abandoning the non-pathologising, accessible and flexible practices that meant their doors were open to the socially excluded.

I hope this book goes some way to demonstrate that, despite and within these organisational constraints, it is still possible to practise from a human-rights framework and to be flexible, holistic and, therefore, genuinely helpful in our work.

I will finish with Reza's words:

> I will always feel bad because what I lost cannot be given [back] to me. I lost my home and my life and family. But it has been good to talk about the hurt I never thought I would tell someone. It is good you know what happened to me there [in the cell], but everyone should know what happens to us.

Contributors

Colsom Bashir is a clinical psychologist with more than 10 years' experience of providing direct therapeutic services, training and supervision for practitioners and expert medical reports in relation to adult refugee and children/family survivors of torture. She has worked across the voluntary and statutory sectors.

Jude Boyles is a BACP-registered, senior accredited psychological therapist and feminist activist. She has been practising for the last 24 years. Before qualifying in 1994, Jude worked in the women's movement, in a rape crisis centre and in Women's Aid refuges for women fleeing domestic violence. She then worked as a counsellor in a non-medical mental health crisis service for 11 years, before establishing the Freedom from Torture North West Centre in Manchester in 2003, where she carried a caseload of torture survivors and managed the centre for 14 years. Jude currently works as a psychological therapist with Syrian refugees in the Syrian Vulnerable Persons Resettlement Programme. Jude has published several articles about therapy with refugees and has co-written a book for therapists: *Working with Interpreters in Psychological Therapy: a right to be understood.*

Beverley Costa is a UKCP registered psychotherapist. After training and working as a group and individual psychotherapist and psychodramatist, she founded Mothertongue multi-ethnic counselling service in 2000, and remains its director. The organisation has developed a model for working therapeutically with mental health interpreters and has a dedicated team of interpreters who work across Berkshire. Beverley has published several articles and peer-reviewed papers and chapters on the experience and impact of therapy conducted across languages. She holds an honorary research fellowship at Birkbeck, University of London.

Carl Dutton is a UKCP registered psychodrama psychotherapist and mental health nurse. He has worked in asylum and refugee mental health for the past 14 years. He was lead therapist for the Haven in Liverpool, which was a community-based service for asylum-seeking and refugee families. He is now based in a statutory setting and uses psychodrama, creative therapies, and horticultural therapy in his work to support children and young people affected by torture and trauma.

Ashley Fletcher has developed a speciality in working with sexual minorities, with over 30 years of practice in the NHS and the voluntary sector. He currently trains on sexuality and sexual minorities. Ashley is qualified to diploma level in counselling and supervision and is BACP accredited. Ashley has been Deputy Manager at Freedom from Torture North West since September 2008. He has spent 25 years working in mental health, trauma, bereavement and terminal care in the NHS and voluntary sector. He was Clinical Director of North West HIV Services for the George House Trust, working extensively with sexual minorities and refugee/asylum seeking communities.

Prossy Kakooza is a refugee from Uganda and has lived in the UK for nine years. In Uganda, before she was imprisoned, Prossy was a university student studying business administration while assisting with the family business. She now works as an outreach co-ordinator at the British Red Cross, with refugees and people seeking asylum who are newly arrived. Prossy is an activist and is involved in the Lesbian Immigration Support Group, which supports women seeking asylum on the basis of their sexuality.

Desiré Kinané worked as an interpreter and trainer at Freedom from Torture North West from 2003 to 2016. He is dedicated to teaching good practice when working with interpreters and has been training professionals to work effectively with interpreters in a therapeutic setting since 2006. He is now a qualified counsellor working in a primary care setting, as well as doing outreach work in the community with vulnerable adults and people seeking asylum

Kirsten Lamb is a clinical psychologist and a UKCP registered psychodynamic psychotherapist. From 2001 to 2016, Kirsten worked as the Tameside and Glossop Secondary Care Psychological Therapies Services Manager in Pennine Care NHS Foundation Trust. Kirsten started volunteering with Freedom from Torture North West at the end of 2003 and has since had a variety of roles at the centre. Kirsten is currently working as a psychological therapist running therapy groups for torture survivors. Throughout her career, Kirsten has offered longer-term individual therapy to survivors of childhood sexual abuse and over time has developed her interest in offering psychological therapy within a human-rights framework.

Norma McKinnon is a community worker, counsellor and psychotherapist registered with BACP and UKCP. She lives and works in the UK, and is based in Scotland. She has almost 20 years' experience of working with refugees in a variety of different roles. Her current clinical work is focused on working with survivors of torture. She works within a torture rehabilitation service, and in private practice.

Jess Michaelson is a UKCP registered Gestalt psychotherapist, supervisor and trainer, who has been working with survivors of torture for more than 15 years. Jess currently works at Freedom from Torture North West as training officer, psychotherapist and supervisor. Her work involves designing and delivering training on working with traumatised survivors of torture, and she also offers psychotherapy to survivors and supervision to therapists. Jess has recently completed training in EMDR, which she has begun to incorporate into her work. Jess has a longstanding interest in the therapist's journey when developing their work with survivors of torture.

Rajita Rajeshwar is a UKCP registered psychodrama psychotherapist and works as a freelance group therapist, trainer, researcher and associate senior lecturer. She has been working with asylum seeker and refugee children, adults and families for the past 15 years. Currently she co-facilitates a long-term therapy group for Tamil- and English-speaking male survivors of torture and offers long-term trauma therapy in a horticultural project to asylum seeking and refugee families. The thread that connects Rajita's work is commitment to a transcultural, creative, integrative and rights-based approach.

Emma Roberts is a systemic family therapist and psychological therapist who has worked with survivors of torture for the past 15 years. Emma currently works for Freedom from Torture as a family therapist, adult therapist, group worker, supervisor and trainer. She has a developing interest in family and group approaches to trauma therapy and rehabilitation.

Ann Salter has worked with separated young people who are survivors of torture for over 10 years, in a variety of settings. She is a UKCP registered Gestalt psychotherapist, and holds a postgraduate diploma in child and adolescent psychotherapy. She works at Freedom from Torture as a therapist, supervisor and trainer. She has an interest in attachment and complex trauma, and in developing this understanding to support children and young people who have experienced torture.

Nathalie Talbot was born in the Ivory Coast, where she began her education in a multicultural environment. After completing a Master's degree in Techniques of Translation (English and Russian), she moved to Moscow to work in international banking, and wrote her PhD on Russian literature. Nathalie has worked with the Stockport Ethnic Diversity Service as a bilingual assistant, helping refugee children who have fled from war zones to learn English in schools, and as an interpreter and tutor in community interpreting. Nathalie has worked as an interpreter and trainer at a torture rehabilitation centre since 2003, and is currently supporting an interpreter working in a refugee camp with thre charity Medical Justice.

Anna Turner is a Manchester-based social worker, currently working for the NHS in an early intervention in psychosis service. She began her career working as a care co-ordinator in a community mental health team. Following this, she spent 10 years with a charity, working with refugees and people seeking asylum. Anna has developed and led on several projects and created a working model of therapeutic social work with torture survivors in exile. Anna guest lectures at universities and offers training to a range of professionals and students. She is currently studying for a diploma in transactional analysis in psychotherapy.

Katie Whitehouse works in Leeds for the Women's Counselling and Therapy Service, a voluntary sector organisation. Since 2014, she has co-ordinated and was the lead psychotherapist in a project that specialised in providing long-term psychotherapy for highly traumatised refugee and asylum-seeking women. She describes herself as a relational and integrative therapist and is qualified in EMDR. Katie has a background in adult mental health and social work, and has worked in health, statutory and voluntary sector settings.

Index

A

Abdelaziz Mousa 393
abuse(s) vi, viii, 21, 25, 28, 110–13, 117, 119–20, 122, 125–27, 129, 132, 135, 228–31, 315–16, 353, 371
    domestic, 9, 34, 55, 75, 94, 155, 220, 245, 286, 305, 368, 395
    human-rights, 48, 350, 352, 364
    sexual, 61, 111, 135, 399
acceptance 173–74, 182, 193, 209, 215, 225, 228, 232, 234–5
    societal, 4, 111
accommodation xi–xii, 97, 139, 147, 190, 208–9, 276, 358, 363, 392–3
acculturation 77–8, 85, 94
activism, political, 14, 61, 150, 202, 380
activists
    human-rights, 60, 325
    political, 4, 61, 388
Adam H, 137, 155, 290, 305
adjustment 72, 94, 182, 186, 200–1, 209–10, 212–5, 247, 259
adolescents 135–7, 142, 153, 221, 263, 289–1, 293–4, 297–8, 303–4, 306
adversity 25, 74–5, 131, 182, 187, 204, 211, 213, 215, 221, 252, 303, 367
Afghanistan 18, 140, 141, 142, 146, 153, 301, 389, 391
Africa 62, 65, 100, 101, 104, 276, 307, 320, 377
    West, 311
Afuape T 21, 33
age 36, 113, 120–1, 138–41, 144–5, 147, 149, 154, 162, 164, 236, 243, 263, 289, 295, 302, 352
    assessments 139–40, 299
Ahmed S 158, 159, 161, 175, 184
Ainsworth M 292
Akhtar S 176, 184
alcohol use 148, 259, 263

alienation 22, 26, 163, 187, 198, 218, 377
Alinsky S 359, 368
Alleyne A 89–91, 93
alliances, working, 314, 328
American Psychiatric Association 54, 219, 369
American Psychological Association 94, 132, 184, 395
Amering M 202, 219
Amnesty International 13, 26, 33, 112, 132, 210
Amris K 27, 33
Andersen T 259, 269
Anderson H 33
anger 29, 63, 73, 128, 131, 150, 152, 169, 172, 178, 181, 352, 362, 364, 366
Anthony WA 56, 75
anxiety 2, 21–2, 124, 141, 147, 197, 205, 209, 212–13, 219, 222, 308, 333, 344–5, 357–8, 383, 389, 391
appeal rights exhausted (ARE) 20, 147, 240
appeals x, 18, 33, 118, 215, 235
appointments 22, 27, 40, 44, 66, 101–2, 107–8, 115, 140, 150, 208, 279, 311, 359, 381
appraisals 167, 172, 176, 192, 201, 206, 212, 214
    post-traumatic, 173, 182
Arab(ic) 161, 324
Aroche J 11, 30, 33, 80, 93, 129, 132
arrival 12, 18, 20, 135, 139, 146–7, 272, 295, 299, 302, 317, 357
art 15, 58, 61–3, 257, 271, 274–6, 280–1, 286–7, 329, 283, 348
assault 80, 135, 229, 277, 300
    sexual, 149, 156–57, 200, 353
assessment 6, 15–20, 28, 40, 68–69, 14–5, 155, 196, 209, 211, 373–4
    holistic, 113–14, 139, 190, 371
    initial, 49, 144, 389–90

asylum x–xiii, 5, 7, 9, 63–4, 69, 72, 98, 104, 110–11, 116–19, 121, 127–8, 147–9, 230, 243, 245, 251, 326–7, 356–8, 380–81, 385, 389–90
  claims x–xii, 2, 23, 38, 60, 63, 117, 120, 122, 141, 147–49, 153, 230, 235, 242–3, 245, 247, 251, 356–8, 375, 389, 392
  interviews x, 117, 133, 166, 389
Asylum Aid 117, 122, 132
Asylum Gender Guidelines 117, 133
Asylum Policy Instruction (API) 117, 133, 225, 242, 245
Asylum Registration Card (ARC) xi
asylum-seeking v, ix–xii, 2, 11–13, 16–19, 23–4, 33–4, 58, 75, 79, 86–7, 91, 93, 97, 115–18, 127–9, 132–4, 139–0, 217–21, 250, 307, 325–6, 350–1, 356–9, 381
Asylum Tribunal x, 122, 153, 235, 312, 357
Atkinson DR 77, 93, 95
attachment 155, 181, 291–3, 295, 305–6
  and development 288–91, 293, 295, 297, 299, 301, 303, 305
  and trauma 295–6
  bonds 125, 177, 292–3
  figure 292–3, 295, 304
  primary, 177, 294
  reconsidered 305–6
  relationships 150, 291–3, 296
  systems 160, 205, 292
  theory 155, 291–4, 305–6
Austria 351
authorities, local xiii, 138–9, 146, 272, 295, 376
autonomy 20, 30, 198, 208, 257, 311
  relinquishing, 20, 311
avoidance 15, 59, 67, 69, 73, 84, 89, 172–4, 176, 182, 194, 197, 210, 212, 214–16

B

babies 128, 143, 247, 291–4, 296
Bager-Charleson S 345, 347
Bains S 261, 269, 326, 329
Baker A 32, 33

Baker R 278, 329
Balkan conflicts 120
Bashir C 33, 187, 191, 192, 200, 202, 204–7, 212, 213, 215, 219
Basoğlu M 61, 75, 191, 219, 221
Batchelor T 227, 244
Beacon House 95, 348
Bemak F 30, 33
Bennett SK 83, 95
bereavement 214, 327, 364, 398
  cultural, 14, 85, 94
Berkowitz N 110, 132
Bernard Van Leer Foundation 94
Berne E 335, 347, 395
Berry JW 85, 93
Berry K 155, 292, 305, 306
Bhavnani KK 161, 184
Bhui K 191, 219
Bion WR 87, 94
bisexual 127, 223–4, 239
Blackburn IM 190, 219
Blackwell D 185, 219, 274, 286
Boas S 93, 94
body 24, 27, 150, 152, 180, 183, 194, 196, 201, 204, 274, 277, 280, 284–5, 382
  language 179, 291, 327
  psychotherapy 34
  sensations 284–5, 362
Boiger M 158, 159, 184
borders 113, 140, 160, 230, 247, 269
Bosnian War 304–5
Boss P 142, 155, 216, 219
Bothne N 19, 33
boundaries 72, 79, 83, 92, 99, 129, 131, 175, 230, 249, 258, 333, 338, 359, 362
Bourke J 377, 395
Bowlby J 292, 304, 305
Bowley J 28, 33, 75, 187, 189, 191, 192, 200, 202, 204, 207, 209, 211, 212, 213, 215, 217, 218, 219
Boyles J 1, 9, 11, 20, 33, 97, 130, 132, 134, 185, 307, 315, 320, 329, 330, 355, 368, 396, 397
boys 62, 111, 126, 138, 237–8, 257, 259
Bracken P 6, 9, 15, 33, 59, 75

Bradford DT 321, 330
brain 41, 53, 101, 150, 193, 205, 213, 297, 306, 364, 382
breathing 22, 45, 99, 150–51, 214, 283–5, 364, 388
Brewin CR 195, 219
Briefing Guidelines for Interpreters in Psychotherapeutic Settings 219
British Association for Counselling and Psychotherapy (BACP) 339, 347, 397–9
British Psychological Society (BPS) 310, 330
British Red Cross 398
brothers 24, 38, 46, 140, 252, 255, 258, 301, 316, 342
Brown LS 94, 113, 132, 377, 395
Bryant-Jefferies R 15, 22, 33
Burck C 332, 347
Burman E 81, 94
Burnham J 248, 269
Burundi 5
bus 32, 66, 107, 114, 255

C

Calhoun LG 57, 58, 60, 75, 95, 204, 220
Cameroon 109, 147, 152, 226, 231, 294
camp guard 140, 301
camps 3, 32, 110, 239
captivity 27, 143–4, 290, 295, 299, 302
caregiver 137, 142, 158, 177, 283, 289, 292, 294, 296, 389
Carroll M 347
caseloads 366, 376, 397
case management 342–3
Ceneda S 117, 132
Central African Republic 355
Chang DF 94
Chaplin J 15, 34, 109, 132
Chartered Institute of Linguists (CIOL) 309
Chelvan S 242, 244
child 87, 103, 126, 139, 147, 149, 177, 254, 289–90, 296, 304, 381, 386
 age-disputed, xiii
 looked-after, 139, 295
 rehabilitation of, 155, 306

Child and Adolescent Mental Health Services 136
childcare 8, 115, 117, 247, 255, 293
childhood 4, 100, 120, 129, 187, 210, 274, 292, 352
 abuse 144, 351, 353
 trauma 296
child marriage 111
child soldiers 25, 126
children 67, 128–9, 135, 137–40, 142–3, 145–9, 246–7, 253, 256–8, 275, 288–9, 291, 293–4, 303–5, 389–90
 refugee, 273, 287, 399
 separated, 137–9
 torture of, 135, 155
Children Act 139
children's accelerated trauma therapy (CATT) 282
Christians 128, 321
Chun KM 94
Cienfuegos A 191, 220
class 30, 95, 160–5, 203
clinical supervision 73, 333, 336, 348–9, 359–61, 365
closure 142, 327–8
co-construction 89, 296
 cultural, 175
Code of Practice and Ethics for Interpreters and Practitioners in Joint Work 310
Coello MJ 11, 33, 80, 93, 129, 132
cognitive behaviour therapy (CBT) 7, 101–2, 185, 187, 189–95, 201, 204–5, 210–11, 215, 218–20, 283
cognitive models of PTSD 189
Cohen J 23, 34, 75, 220
Colzato LS 238, 244
communication 308, 330, 348
communities
 local, 272, 278–80, 381, 390
 refugee, 273–4, 309
compassion 33, 116, 193, 329, 337
 fatigue 368
compassion-focused therapy (CFT), 193, 220, 393
Complex Trauma Task Force (CTTF), 144, 155, 290, 305

confidentiality, 17, 121, 130–1, 207–8, 235, 247, 312–13, 338
Conservative Party Conference 269
contact, psychological 151, 231, 352
context marker, highest 249–2, 255
contextual authenticity 233, 235, 240
continuing traumatic stress (CTS) 21, 217
contracts, therapeutic 208
Cooper A 79, 132, 355, 368
Coram Children's Legal Centre 139, 155
core symptoms of PTSD 144, 290
Costa B 8, 310, 321, 332, 325, 330, 336, 340, 341, 344, 347, 348, 397
co-therapists 286, 341
 informal 275
counselling 7, 62, 80, 95, 98–9, 102–5, 107, 117, 217, 398
counsellor 98, 101, 104, 106–8, 125, 231, 325, 338
Cozolino L 299, 305, 364, 368
Crawley H 137, 155
creativity 63, 142, 151, 248, 271, 275, 276, 287, 340, 345, 372
credibility 17, 22, 28, 122, 170, 226, 229–30, 240, 318
 assessment 122, 227
Crenshaw K 161, 184, 377, 395
Cropper R 78, 94
Cuellar I 78, 94
culture 14–15, 26–27, 68, 85, 87, 124–5, 129–31, 159–62, 170–1, 202–3, 265–6, 268–9, 317–18, 324–6, 377–8
 collectivist, 64, 87, 159, 169, 202, 205
 individualistic, 64–5, 159, 169, 205
 western, 87, 129, 225, 231, 235, 238
culturally-adapted cognitive behaviour therapy (CA-CBT) 205, 220
Cvetkovic-Jovic N 354, 369
Czech Republic 230

D

Dalenberg CJ 78, 80, 94
Dallos R 30, 34, 76, 95, 206, 220, 253, 255, 256, 264, 269
Danquah AH 155, 305–6
Darfur 6, 38, 39, 44

daughters 61–2, 89, 128, 165–6, 175, 183, 248, 250–2, 254, 257–2, 281
David D 194, 220
Davies D 228, 244
Dearing RL 157, 169, 184, 186
death v, ix, 13, 38, 68, 71, 118, 122, 149, 154, 197, 227, 250, 257, 289, 295, 353, 358
debriefing 260, 315, 323, 324, 346, 359
defences 27, 85, 91, 177, 180–1, 183, 237
dehumanising 12, 196, 288, 380
deliberate infection viii, 322
Democratic Republic of the Congo (DRC) vi, 3, 14, 32, 73, 88, 142, 281, 291, 317, 351, 381
denial 44, 80, 92, 181
depersonalisation 198, 298
depression 11, 57, 157, 169, 177, 189–91, 197, 199, 205, 215, 217, 255, 319, 342, 394
despair 154, 177, 216, 233, 251, 327, 354
destitution 23, 49, 115, 147–8, 213, 232, 351, 358–9, 380, 384
detention viii, xi–xii, 2–3, 12, 14, 20, 23, 65, 119, 147, 150, 165–6, 215, 230, 233, 248, 295, 357–8
development 8, 138–39, 148, 150, 184, 288–93, 295, 297, 299, 301–3, 305
 adolescent, 289, 297
 adversity-activated, 75
diagnosis/es 17, 42, 39, 47, 144, 193–4, 319, 383, 387
dialectic behaviour therapy (DBT) 193
difference, stigma, shame, harm (DSSH) 242
Dillane P 226
Diploma in Public Services Interpreting (DPSI) 309
disability 30, 77, 164
disbelief 180, 229, 233, 235, 240, 243, 380
disclosure 3, 44, 117, 122, 149, 229, 232–4, 266, 313, 322–23, 337, 374, 384
disconnection 61, 132, 152, 299, 376, 393
discrimination viii, 56, 66, 83, 90–2, 109, 112–13, 116–17, 127, 187, 196, 377, 380

disempowerment 113, 132, 183, 251, 253, 262, 324, 338, 361
disfigurement viii, 229, 322
displacement 138, 144, 199, 201–2, 210, 213, 286
dissociation 57, 79, 84, 144, 169, 194, 198, 216, 290, 298–301, 323, 355, 381
dissonance 57, 82, 84, 169
documentation of torture and other xiii, 28, 35, 75, 155, 221, 245, 306
Doherty SM 336, 338, 341, 348
Doyle McCarthy ED 160, 185
Drakulic S 120
drama triangle 90, 335
dreams 124, 143, 271, 284
Drožđek B 12, 13, 34, 59, 65, 69, 75, 77, 79, 94
Diagnostic and Statistical Manual of Mental Disorders (DSM) 230
Diagnostic and Statistical Manual of Mental Disorders 5th Edition (DSM-5) 197
Diagnostic and Statistical Manual of Mental Disorders 3rd Edition (DSM-III) 47
Diagnostic and Statistical Manual of Mental Disorders 4th Edition (DSM-IV) 80
dual representation theory (DRT) 195–6

E

Eagle G 217, 220
education 4–5, 111, 120, 139, 205, 211, 214, 217, 227, 252, 255, 275, 375–6, 380, 400
 231
Eisenbruch M 14, 34, 85, 94
Ekman P 171, 185
Elias N 179, 185
Elsass P 11, 15, 18, 22, 34, 123, 124, 125, 126, 133, 227, 244
Emerson D 24, 34
emotion 62–3, 70, 73, 124–5, 158–9, 161, 169–2, 174–5, 177, 194, 197, 201, 212–13, 253, 285, 332, 341, 356, 364, 375, 377
empathy 32, 80, 92, 128, 213, 233, 254, 252, 263–4, 283, 329, 338, 363–4, 388
burnout 384
endings 31, 59, 68–73, 218, 327–8
engagement 18, 26, 31, 40, 203–4, 207–8, 210, 217–18, 272, 316–19, 336, 362, 367, 373
England 7, 66, 81, 85, 86, 87, 272, 301, 333, 396
Epstein D 233, 245
Erskine RG 44, 52, 55
escape 3–4, 62, 111, 113, 120–1, 140, 144, 200, 210, 257, 295, 388, 392
essentialism 171, 175, 189
ethics 42, 253, 310, 312, 337–9, 342, 344, 376
ethnic differences 6, 76–7, 79, 81, 83, 85, 87–9, 91, 93, 95
ethnicity 76, 110, 139, 161, 326, 377–8, 380, 391
Europe 4, 140, 239, 286, 301, 320, 332
 Eastern, 351
European Convention on Human Rights (ECHR) x, 381
European Refugee Convention (ERC) 381
European Court of Human Rights 381
European Union 243
Everton Football Club 278
Every Child Matters 386, 390
Every Child Protected Against Trafficking UK (ECPAT UK) 146, 155
executions 23, 152, 226
 mock, 4, 135
exile 1–2, 4–5, 7, 9, 13–14, 16, 24, 26, 30–1, 79, 86, 200–1, 203–4, 227, 302–3, 372
eye contact 15, 39, 71, 83, 172, 316, 319, 344
eye movement desensitisation and reprocessing (EMDR) 193, 282, 320, 399–400

F

faith 25, 36, 66, 71, 262, 269, 317
 groups 19, 272, 275
family 4–5, 24–26, 119–22, 128, 136–7, 141, 151–4, 182–3, 246–9, 273–5,

290-1, 293-4, 303-4, 385, 389-91 (*see also* brother, daughter, grandfather, grandmother, husband, in-laws, parents, wife)
therapy 247, 250, 253, 267, 269, 399
Fassin D 47, 55
father 46, 61, 86, 127, 129, 141, 147, 153, 257-8, 263, 294, 388, 390-1
Fazel M 12, 34, 221
female genital mutilation (FGM) 7, 111, 118, 138
Ferguson T 169, 185
Figley CR 362, 368
Fischer W, 168, 185
Fisher J, 123, 133
flashbacks, 150, 196-8, 300
Fletcher A, 7, 223, 398
Fontaine J, 168, 169, 170, 171, 185
food, v, xi, 4, 14, 50, 72, 111, 115, 136, 269, 277, 281, 359
football, 61, 276-79, 286
forced
 marriage 7, 111, 119, 124, 127, 260, 266
 separation 135, 137, 303
forensic evidence 97, 105, 206, 230, 247
formulation 47, 157, 169-70, 174-6, 179, 195, 200, 202, 204, 206, 212-13, 217-18
Foucault M 189, 220
Fox JL 86, 94
France 301, 320
freedom 65, 111, 129-30, 146, 163, 258, 339, 378, 386
Freedom from Torture 14, 56, 274
Freire P 359, 368
friendship 68, 250, 263, 305, 378, 380, 390

G

Garcia A 86, 94, 287
gay 4, 7, 97-8, 223-28, 231-3, 235-9, 241-4
Gaynor G 223, 245
general practitioner (GP) 22-4, 27, 65, 215, 272, 300, 312, 385
gender 30, 58, 111, 113, 116-17, 127, 131, 135, 160-3, 166, 225, 245, 310, 320, 377-8, 380 (*see also*, girls/boys)
-based abuse/persecution v, 7, 109, 110-13, 115-17, 119, 121, 123, 125, 127, 129, 131, 133, 138, 188
George House Trust 398
Germany 351
Giddings P 79, 94
Gilbert P 176, 178-9, 193, 220
girls 4, 110, 126, 135-6, 138, 236, 239, 247, 249, 257-8, 266
Girma M 110, 113, 119, 121, 133
Glenn C 130, 133
Goffman E 89, 94
Graessner S 12, 15, 34
grandfather 263, 284-5
Grandi F 111, 133
grandmother 284-5, 294
Gregg B 164, 185
Grey N 220
grief 14, 43, 46, 68, 70, 88, 128, 142, 144, 201, 216, 255, 327, 355, 376, 388
Griffiths P 325, 330
Grossman V 23, 34
Grotberg EH 90, 94
group/s 101, 273, 351, 366, 393, 399
 supervision 327, 338, 341, 372
guilt 24, 29, 62, 79, 84, 126, 128, 143, 168-71, 197, 206, 209, 216-17, 233, 244, 253, 261-2, 353-4, 362, 382
Gurris N 12. 14, 15, 34

H

hallucinations 22, 199, 302
Harré R 158,185
Harvey A 193, 220
Harvey MA 337, 348
Hassan A 263, 269
Hawkins P 340, 348
Hayes SC 193, 220
Hays PA 77, 94, 377, 395
headaches 26, 199, 280, 382, 392
healing 37, 48-9, 68, 125, 142, 200, 234, 272, 276, 282, 286, 393
health 5, 26, 50, 115, 145, 148, 209, 215, 275, 282, 378, 385-7, 390

psychological, 13, 22, 28, 43, 157, 189, 200, 225
healthcare 4, 14, 111, 139, 208, 247, 363
health services 49–50, 382
  mental, 114, 136, 145, 307
Held N 245
Helms JE 77, 83, 84, 94
helplessness 18, 79, 90, 92, 197–8, 273, 354–5, 361, 382, 286
Her Majesty's Courts and Tribunals Service (HMCTS) x
Herman JL 6, 13, 15, 19, 21, 45, 47, 49, 55, 57, 69, 75, 133, 144, 155, 177, 185, 188, 200, 207, 215, 217, 220, 234, 254, 271–2, 283, 286, 305, 354, 363, 367–8, 383–4, 395
Hernández P 367, 368
Hernández-Wolfe P 362, 369
Hetherington A 335, 336, 338, 341, 348
Hinshelwood G 121, 133
Hinton D 204, 205, 211, 220
human immunodeficiency virus (HIV) viii, 110, 224, 231, 239, 322, 398
holism 1, 12, 61, 113, 144, 174, 396
Holmes J 151, 155
Holocaust 352
home x–xiii, 2–3, 13–14, 104–6, 117–18, 122, 132–3, 139, 147–49, 225–7, 229–31, 233, 235–6, 242, 245
  culture 164, 226, 235, 257, 260, 267
Home Affairs Select Committee (UK Parliament) 2, 9
homelessness 2, 20, 23, 48, 51, 115, 147, 248, 375, 384, 386
  street 38–9, 41, 43, 148
Home Office x–xiii, 104–6, 117–18, 122, 132–3, 139, 147–49, 155, 225–7, 229–31, 233, 235–6, 242, 245, 299
  Presenting Officer (HOPO) 122
  Reporting Centre 66
homophobia 129, 233
homosexuality 224, 226, 230–1, 237, 239
'honour'-based violence 259, 260
'honour' killings 111, 138, 266
hopelessness 22, 43, 131, 197, 215, 233, 249, 251, 275, 350, 354, 364

horror 29, 89, 126, 256, 262, 295, 299, 303, 324
housing 1, 13, 18, 50, 65, 69, 144, 206, 375–6, 382, 386, 390, 392
  provider vi, 1, 19, 272
  support 18, 20, 50
Hudgins MK 274, 277, 286
Hughes G 277, 286
human rights vi, 5, 7, 9, 11, 14, 25, 28, 111, 113, 130, 135–6, 165, 188, 206–8, 353, 355, 36–8, 371, 376, 379–1, 384
  approach 32, 42, 50, 64, 136–37, 147, 219, 379
  violations 2, 26, 29, 37, 39, 136, 149, 189, 152, 358, 367
Human Rights Watch 26, 210
humiliation 2, 4, 18, 135, 162–6, 229, 289
  sexual, viii, 322
hurt vi, 41, 100, 144–5, 300–1, 396
husband 61, 89, 111, 113, 117, 119–20, 124–5, 127–8, 165–6, 257, 342, 388

I

identity 11, 60–4, 77, 79–81, 83, 86, 88–90, 161, 198, 200, 224–5, 227–9, 233–4, 239, 241–2
  cultural, 77, 376, 378, 386
  racial, 77–8, 82, 89
  sexual, 160, 224, 233, 240
If This is a Man 352
In Other Words 337
International Federation of Social Workers General Meeting 371
imagery/images 16, 28, 46, 158, 194, 197, 210, 212, 215–16
  intrusive, 303, 352, 362, 381
immigration xi, xiii, 18, 33, 104, 147, 326, 359, 377
  status 43, 48, 139, 375–6, 382
Immigration Act xii, 147
Immigration Appellate Authority 117, 133
Immigration Law Practitioners Association (ILPA) xiii, 137, 155
immigration removal centre (IRC) v, xii,

3, 147, 357–8
immigration reporting centre 18, 326, 357
imprisonment 4, 14, 24–5, 29, 59, 180, 183, 289, 295
Improving Access to Psychological Therapy (IAPT) 189, 396
individualism 6, 87, 158, 160, 164, 205, 211
Initial Accommodation Centre (IAC) xii
injuries 21, 27, 97, 99, 105, 113, 178, 199, 300, 303, 382
injustice 32, 42, 244, 253, 259, 308, 324, 332, 371, 384
in-laws 113, 165–6, 175, 180
Inskipp F 340, 348
insomnia 199, 215, 280
internalisation 89–90, 159, 163, 167, 177, 233, 291, 326
International Association of Schools of Social Work (IASSW) 371
International Classification of Diseases (ICD-10) 47, 197
International Criminal Court 42
international human rights law 13, 225
International Society for Traumatic Stress Studies (ISTSS) 144
interpreter 8, 16–17, 70, 72, 105–6, 121, 130–1, 140–1, 206–8, 229, 260, 291, 307–29, 331–7, 360
   male, 166, 322
   qualified, 309, 311, 319, 346
   therapist and, 309, 314, 317, 319, 341, 346
   -mediated therapy 308–9, 331–2, 336, 340, 341, 344
Interpreting and Communication Forum 308
intimacy 19, 62, 87, 177, 232, 234, 261
   sexual, 242, 382
Iran 1, 19, 24, 25, 140, 161, 165, 179, 226, 231, 233, 301, 321, 361
isolation, 23, 26, 92, 142, 165, 177, 187, 226, 258, 275, 304
   social, 60, 215
Istanbul Protocol xi, 28, 60, 148, 196–7, 240
International Society for Traumatic Stress Studies (ISTSS) 144
Complex Trauma Taskforce 155, 290, 305

J
Janet P 45
Janjaweed 38, 49–50
Jewish 352
Jones L 303, 304, 305
Joseph S 59, 71, 75, 368
Jovic V 354, 369
justice 5, 37, 57, 111, 192, 244, 251, 353, 376
   social, 9, 32, 187–8, 370–1, 384

K
Kadrić M 336, 348
Kalmanowitz D 282, 286
Karcher S 26, 34
Karpman SB 90 94, 335, 348
Kastrup MC 113, 115, 128 133
Kazembé, Jonathan vi
Kinouani G 161, 185
Kira IA 12, 34, 58, 75
Klass D 142, 155
Kohli R 383, 395
Kohut H 90, 95
Korzinski M 354, 369
Kurd(ish) 24, 25

L
Laub D 21, 34
Lavik NJ 12, 34
Law Society Immigration and Asylum Accreditation Scheme xii
Lee D 179, 185
Leeming D 158, 185
legal aid 118, 148–49
Legal Aid Agency (LAA) xii, 147
lesbian 4, 104–6, 127, 223–4, 226, 228, 398
Lesbian, Gay, Bisexual, Transgender (LGBT) 9, 102, 163, 223–8, 230–1, 241–2
Lesbian Immigration Support Group 398
letters, clinical 28, 60, 148, 240, 243
Levine PA 21, 26, 34, 125, 133, 299, 305

Levi P 27, 34, 352, 369
Lewis HB, 179, 180, 181, 185
Liberation Tigers of Tamil Ealam (LTTE) 79
Liddell B 159, 185, 204, 211, 216, 220
Linehan M 193, 220
Lingala 143, 317, 320
Lingala interpreter 317
loneliness 22, 43–4, 142, 153
loss 68, 70, 73–74, 85, 137, 141–4, 149, 151, 202–3, 211, 213–14, 216–18, 296–8, 376, 378
Lyotard JF 189, 220

M

Maatta Simo K 338, 348
Malchiodi CA 271, 275, 287
Malloch MS 16, 34
Mann N 136, 155
Mansell W 200, 220
marginalisation 85, 161, 239
marriage 4, 62, 113, 119–20, 138, 239, 260
    arranged, 391
Maslow AH 64, 75, 356, 369
Masocha S 383, 395
Mason B 246, 248, 249
May T 269
McFarlane AC 19, 35
McFarlane CA 190, 220
McIntosh P 91, 95, 261, 270
McLeod J 19, 35
medication 39–41, 94, 100–1, 110, 208–9, 393–4
Mediterranean 301
Meehan CL 293, 305
Meichenbaum D 362, 369
memories 26, 28–9, 44, 62, 65, 122, 141, 172–4, 194–5, 212–15, 262, 267, 301–2, 382–83
    autobiographical, 160, 196, 205
    intrusive, 189, 197
Mendez JE 1, 5, 9, 13, 35
mental health 17, 20, 24, 56, 82, 99, 118, 122, 148, 151, 248, 300, 319, 342, 354, 356, 358, 381
    interpreters 340–1, 397
    team 24, 101, 106, 300, 391, 400

mentoring 339, 342–3
Middle Eastern 161
migration 77, 85, 170, 183, 202, 214, 217, 276, 351, 393
Miller KE 316, 330, 341, 344, 346, 348
Milner M 333, 348
mindfulness 22, 214, 216
    -based cognitive therapy (MBCT) 193
Misheva V 158, 186
money 23, 61, 67, 136, 140, 281, 352, 359–60, 392
Montgomery A 138, 155
Montgomery E 249, 250, 257, 270
Moorey S 200, 201, 220
Morelli GA 293, 294, 305
Moreno JL 86, 88, 95, 273, 274, 293, 294, 286, 344, 348
Morling E 169, 186
mother 39, 67, 127–8, 141–3, 145, 165, 180, 183, 248, 251, 253–4, 256, 265, 293–5, 298, 301–2
    single, 128–9
Mothertongue 8, 310, 332–3, 336–9, 341–3, 345–7, 397
    interpreters 336–7, 343
mourning 41, 45, 57, 123, 137, 188, 201, 216, 234, 383
Mudarikiri MM 318, 330
Mueller M 192, 220
Munt S 158, 162, 163, 186
Murray LK 217, 220
music 58, 269, 271, 275, 280–1, 286
Music G 297, 306
Muslim 84, 86, 128, 304, 321
    non-, 261
mutilation viii, 322 (*see also* female genital mutilation)

N

narrative exposure therapy (NET) 191–93, 196, 212, 214, 217, 282–84
Nathanson DL 95, 171, 173, 186
National Asylum Support Service (NASS) xi
National Health Service 4, 6–7, 114, 189, 224, 272, 275, 333, 336
National Referral Mechanism (NRM) 146

Netherland, the 59, 239
Neuner F 192, 196, 220, 221
neurobiology/science 158, 176, 303, 364
neuro-expression 159, 204
Nickerson A 191, 221
nightmares 22, 89, 124, 142, 145, 150, 153, 209, 211, 214–16, 278, 355, 362, 381, 388, 392
Nijdam MJ 195, 221
normalise 167, 212–13, 351, 336
norms 159, 189, 167–68, 261, 268, 293

O

Office for the Immigration Services Commissioner (OISC) xii
Office of the High Commissioner for Human Rights (OHCHR) xi, xiii, 5, 9, 11, 35, 56, 75, 133, 135, 221, 245, 288, 291, 306
Onufer Corrêa S 225, 245
oppression 25, 30, 42, 48, 77, 82–4, 90–2, 109, 187, 189, 261, 325, 331, 333, 371, 376–8
Ortega RM 80, 95, 318, 330

P

Page S 340, 348
Pakistan 231
panic 22, 122, 124, 152, 213
Papadopoulos RK 14, 20, 21, 25, 35, 57, 35, 133, 153–5, 204, 221, 265, 270, 306, 330, 368
parallel processes 71, 188, 335
parents 8, 62–3, 135, 137, 148–9, 247, 257–61, 263–6, 289–91, 293, 296, 298, 303–4, 383, 389–91
partners xi, 62, 97, 106, 239, 241, 382, 392
pathologising 21, 201–2, 387
Pearlman A 336, 348, 353, 361, 369
Pedersen P 92, 95
peri-traumatic 166, 174, 176, 182, 195–6, 213
Perkins UE 88, 95
perpetrators xi, 32, 90, 92, 176, 179, 182–3, 198, 353
persecution 93, 110, 196, 214, 226, 268, 315–17, 325–26, 364, 301, 335, 380–2, 386

Persian 161
Persons JB 209, 221
phone cards 23, 392
photographs 97, 229, 242, 388
pictures 1, 15, 46, 64, 268, 281
PinkUK 239
poetry 271, 279–82, 286
police 65–6, 97–8, 113, 119, 129, 146, 259, 267, 326
  stations xii, 140, 229
Pope KS 17, 35, 350, 369
post-traumatic 175, 200, 202–3 (see also trauma)
  growth (PTG) 57–8, 60, 71, 90, 204
  stress disorder (PTSD) 47, 58, 144, 290, 383
poverty 13, 26, 43, 146, 214, 257, 265, 356, 358–59, 380
power 30, 76–7, 80, 88, 90–2, 113, 129–30, 218, 260–1, 277, 314, 321, 324–5, 351, 361, 377–8
  structural, 30, 130, 325
  and oppression 91–2, 109, 189, 333, 371, 376–7
  differentials 91, 162, 315, 325, 343
  dynamics 78, 91, 113, 218, 313, 361, 388–9
  relations 93, 333, 377
powerlessness 23, 89–90, 131, 179, 196, 227, 234, 295, 298, 327, 358, 361, 367, 376, 384
practice, anti-oppressive 84, 326, 343
prejudice 20, 83, 91, 136, 228, 230, 315
prison 3, 4, 23–4, 38, 97–9, 106, 119, 121, 179, 228, 257, 295, 342, 355, 392, 394
  officers 165, 231, 302
privilege 84, 91–2, 113, 129–30, 325, 351, 377–8
Proctor G 132, 340, 348, 368
prostitution 110, 119
protection v, x–xi, 11, 29, 32, 36, 39, 136, 139, 223–24, 231–2, 235, 240, 242–3, 375–6
  seeking, v, 14, 28, 226, 230, 233, 253, 256
psychiatry 57, 100–2, 107, 158, 188 –90, 338

psychodrama 273, 278, 344, 398
psychoeducation 21, 64, 69, 123–4, 150, 166, 210, 212–13, 217, 384–5, 388
psychological
  distress 2, 26, 57, 78, 359
  therapy 22, 24, 60, 62, 72, 74, 208, 223, 354, 368, 389, 399
  interpreters in, 310, 330, 347, 397
  survivors of torture for, 11, 13, 15, 17, 19, 21, 23, 25, 27, 29, 31, 33, 35
psychotherapy 7, 87, 110, 114–15, 124–25, 127, 131, 141, 157, 190, 232, 292, 298, 332, 366, 399–400
  interpreter-mediated, 331
post-traumatic stress disorder (PTSD) 11, 21, 47, 57, 114, 144, 157, 173, 179, 185, 189–92, 195, 197, 199–200, 210, 290, 358, 383
  flashbacks 179, 205, 213
  symptoms 12, 114, 123–4, 159, 201, 204, 209
punishment x, 28, 56, 129, 229, 267, 353

Q

qualia/experience of shame feeling 174, 176
Quinn N 293, 294, 305, 306

R

race ix, 76–79, 81–85, 90–2, 112, 129, 131, 161–62, 187, 326, 377
racism 30, 77, 82–4, 91–2, 129, 131, 182, 209, 215, 261, 278, 325–6, 329, 364, 386
rage 18, 162, 177, 354–5
Raghuvanshi L 191, 221
rape 3–4, 32, 88–90, 110–11, 119–22, 127, 135, 138, 157, 163, 165–6, 179–80, 228, 295, 298, 374–5, 392–3
Rape Crisis Centre 397
Ratner C 158, 175, 186
Raval H 309, 325
Reader Organisation 281
reconnection 6, 41, 45, 56–61, 63–7, 69, 71, 73, 75, 123, 152–3, 200, 215–17, 234

recovery 48, 56–9, 62–4, 66–7, 69–70, 200, 214–15, 223, 225–7, 245, 247, 375–6, 383–5, 387–8
  and reconnection 56–7, 59, 61, 63, 65, 67, 69, 71, 73, 75
redress ix, 37, 56, 112, 119, 135–6, 206, 226, 229
reflexivity 36, 76, 184, 206, 218, 252–53
refugee(s) 3–4, 11, 13–14, 18, 31, 36–8, 43, 110, 154, 181, 190–2, 271–3, 325–6, 330, 363–6, 370–1, 378, 380–1, 393
  status ix–xi, 2, 6, 33, 43, 51, 63, 69, 97–8, 153, 199, 243, 355, 358, 376–7, 380, 386
Refugee Convention x, 110, 112, 226, 380–1
Refugee Council 18, 111, 138, 140, 235
Refugee Women's Resource Project 117
Regel S 191, 221
rehabilitation ix, 5, 11, 21, 25, 29, 37, 41, 56–7, 136–7, 155, 189, 199, 217–18, 223, 226–7, 288–90, 306, 329
relationships
  intimate, 196, 199
  professional, 338, 378–9
  three-way, 307–8, 325, 330, 349
religion ix, 25, 71, 145, 161, 377, 380, 388
remembrance 41, 45, 57, 123, 188, 201, 234, 383
Remen RN 362, 369
Remer R 77, 95
removal xii, 12, 20, 43, 51, 63, 119, 147, 209, 215, 217, 248, 250, 357–8, 384, 389–90
reparation 5, 111–12, 121, 169, 189, 342
research 43, 111, 187, 239, 293–4, 296, 304, 336, 339, 341, 380
resettlement 202, 258, 384
resilience 57, 60, 184, 187, 196, 199, 200–4, 211–12, 214, 216, 227–8, 303–4, 367, 370, 391–3
  young person's, 149, 288
rights-based approach 5, 80, 136, 318, 387, 399
  human, 113, 115, 343, 379–80

risk assessment/management, 23, 145, 258, 371, 386, 390
Rober P 262, 270
Roberts E 7, 246, 399
Robjant K 192, 221
Rogers CR 80, 95
Roland A 87, 95
Rothschild B 82, 95, 123–4, 126, 133, 382, 383, 395
Rousseau C 273, 287

S

Saakvitne K 336
Saari S 274, 284, 287
Safe in Our Hands? 23
safety 18–19, 57–8, 60, 64, 79, 127–8, 149–51, 188, 194, 200, 207, 212–15, 231–4, 251, 266–8, 278, 291, 350–2, 375, 383–4, 387
    cultural, 80, 96, 265
Salaets H 333, 338, 348
Salans M 280, 287
Salcioğlu E 191, 219, 221
Samaritans 106
Same City, Different Journeys 281
Sampson EE 91, 95
sanctuary 35, 123, 180, 369–70, 380
Sande H 337, 349
Sarup M 89, 95
Schauer M 191, 221, 283, 287
Scheff T 156, 158, 172, 179, 180, 181, 186
Scheurich J 87, 95
schools 136, 247, 258, 275, 277, 281, 380, 390, 400
Schore AN 177, 186, 292, 296, 297, 306
Scotland xii
Scottish Legal Aid Board xii
Scottish Translation 308, 330
screening interview x–xi, 105, 122
    initial, 117, 229
Segal ZV 193, 221
self-
    attack/hate 89, 172–4, 178, 185, 197, 382
    care 22, 218, 244, 337, 363, 369
    disclosure 81, 88, 318
    harm 24, 145, 300, 314, 323, 357

Seligman M 203, 221
separation 13, 22, 85, 137–8, 151, 210, 265, 290–1, 311, 315, 355
sex 120, 149, 224, 226, 236–42
sexual
    exploitation 61, 144, 146, 259–60, 358
    minorities 224–8, 232, 238, 242, 398
    organs viii, 322
    orientation (*see also* LGBT) 7, 30, 36, 61, 66, 77, 161, 164, 224–7, 235, 242, 377
    violence viii–ix, 3–4, 62, 110, 114, 117, 119–22, 127, 135, 247, 322, 381
sexuality (*see also* LGBT) 65, 99, 127, 131, 162, 187, 223–3, 235, 237, 239, 241–3, 245
    clandestine, 228, 232, 235
sexually-transmitted diseases (STDs) 26
shame 22, 62, 88–91, 122, 149, 156–85, 205–6, 209, 216–17, 228–9, 233, 237–8, 365
Shapiro F 193, 221
Sherif C 189, 221
Siegel D 363, 369
silence 29, 42–3, 121, 140, 156, 180–1, 311, 316
Silove D 79, 95
Sinason V 296, 306
sisters 32, 38, 46, 82, 128, 131, 258, 301, 394
slavery 38, 322, 380
sleep 22, 47, 79, 100, 197, 211, 214–15, 277, 279–80, 392–3
Smale G 374, 395
Smith E 4, 9, 56, 75, 111, 112, 116, 119, 122, 134, 307
Smith HC 319, 330
smuggling 136, 140, 257, 301–2
Snodgrass LL 191, 221
social
    withdrawal 176, 182, 197
    work 8–9, 101, 108, 129, 136, 149,184, 211, 259, 275, 370, 372, 374, 376–9, 382, 385–7
soldiers 4, 142–3, 381
solicitor xii, 166, 211, 229, 355
Somalia 248

son/s 61–2, 110, 120, 258, 263, 392
space
  confidential, 124, 247, 341
  safe, 45, 282
  therapeutic, 15, 85, 180, 188, 232, 311
spirituality 86, 202, 214
Splevins K 64, 65, 75
sports 61, 271, 274–5
spouses xi, 61–2, 196, 291
Sri Lanka 79
stabilisation 13, 45, 57, 90, 114, 123, 133, 234, 354, 356, 363
Stammer N 164, 186
Stedmon J 76, 95
Steele K 292, 293, 297, 306
Sternberg P 279, 287
Stockport Ethnic Diversity Service 400
stress 5, 26, 91, 215, 293–4, 333, 347, 387
  acute, 197, 200–201, 208–9, 290, 292, 390
  extreme, 47, 213, 295
Strosahl KD 193, 220
St Thomas B 279, 281, 287
Stutheridge J 46, 55
Sudan 6, 38, 46, 49, 226, 386, 393
Sue DW 93, 95
suicide 23–4, 145, 249, 251–2, 314, 323, 360, 390
  bomber 140, 301
  risk 23–24, 197, 209, 215, 314, 352, 360,
Summerfield D 14, 21, 32, 35
supervision 8, 87, 184, 218, 232, 263, 274, 276, 310, 315, 324, 331–7, 359–60, 364–5, 399
  reflexive, 331, 340–2, 343
supervisor v, 3, 343, 350, 360, 365, 399–400
  clinical, 347, 366
Supreme Court (UK) 226–7
Syria 150
Syrian Vulnerable Persons Resettlement Programme 397
systemic therapy 246–9, 251, 253–5, 257, 259–61, 263, 265, 267, 269

T

Takano Y 64, 75
Taliban 140–42, 146, 152, 153, 301, 302, 389
Tamil 6, 78, 79, 81, 87
Tangney JP 168, 169, 184, 185, 186
Taylor M 363, 364, 365, 369
Taylor T 171, 172, 173, 179, 186
Teasdale JD 193, 221
Teater B 385, 395
Tedeschi RG 57–8, 75, 90, 95220
Tehran 1
Telvi J 343, 349
terror 18, 51, 124, 135, 177, 246, 265, 298, 301, 303, 354, 380
testimony 28, 32, 57, 122, 191–2, 237, 240, 243, 284, 352
therapeutic
  alliance 8, 15, 20, 43, 45, 92, 150, 308, 315, 389
  approaches v, 32, 74, 166, 187, 192, 276, 308, 323, 354, 363, 365–6, 395
  practice 92, 155, 188, 206, 350
  process 37, 76, 88, 114, 153, 294, 316, 329, 341, 354
  relationship 53, 58, 60, 63–4, 71–2, 74, 76, 79–80, 82, 149–51, 223, 225, 253, 267–8, 374
  settings 30, 248, 308, 363, 398
  social work 370–71, 373, 375, 377, 379, 381, 383, 385, 387, 389, 391, 393, 395, 400
therapist and interpreter 3, 16, 131, 307, 310, 318–19, 321, 339, 344–6, 360
The Reader Organisation 281
The Reflecting Team 255
threat 147, 149, 165–6, 174–5, 178, 180, 183–4, 189, 191, 194, 196–7, 202, 205, 212–14, 217
Time Magazine 33
Tomkins S 171, 172, 186
torturers 22, 27, 29, 63, 152, 227–8, 291, 302, 335, 355–6
trafficking 111, 138, 146, 380
transactional analysis 55, 335, 347–8, 400

transdiagnostic model 194, 200, 205, 209, 212, 215, 217, 219
transference 80, 232, 334, 341–2
 counter-, 39, 79, 80, 85, 131, 232, 334, 342, 354, 356, 367, 382
translation (*see also* interpreting) 50, 309, 314, 349, 400
trauma 42–44, 47–50, 57–59, 76–80, 122–3, 149–51, 195–7, 200–2, 204–5, 213–14, 283–5, 295–9, 354–5, 381–5, 387–9 (*see also* post-traumatic)
 processing 63, 67, 69, 71, 72, 150–1, 320, 354–5
 symptoms 21, 57, 59, 72, 91, 121, 125, 150, 223, 280, 283, 354, 356, 361, 372
 memories 57, 63, 122, 124, 172, 216, 303
 transference 374, 382, 390
 vicarious, 8, 60, 131, 323, 336–7, 351, 361–2, 366, 369
re-traumatisation 3, 12, 59, 140, 180, 210–11
Travis A 230, 245
triad/triangle (therapist-client-interpreter) 17, 307–8, 309–11, 315, 318, 321–2, 324–5, 327, 331, 333–6, 340, 345–8
Tribe R 307, 309, 310, 315, 318, 319, 320, 325, 330, 333, 337,
Turner S 12, 35

U

Uganda 6, 97, 98, 100, 105, 231
United Kingdom asylum process 13, 18, 116, 245, 247, 251
United Kingdom Council for Psychotherapy 397–99
United Kingdom government v, 32
United Kingdom Lesbian and Gay Immigration Group (UKLGIG) 226, 245
United Kingdom Visas and Immigration (UKVI) xi, 117, 1 United Nations 34
United Nations Convention against Torture (UNCAT) viii, xi 5, 9, 35, 56, 75, 112
United Nations Convention on the Rights of the Child (UNCRC) 139
United Nations High Commissioner for Refugees (UNHCR) 4, 9, 36, 39, 55, 110–12, 118, 134, 395
United Nations Expert Group Meeting on gender-based persecution 133
United Nations Security Council 120, 134

V

validation 32, 44, 70, 225, 231, 233–5, 384
van der Kolk BA 25, 28, 30, 31, 35, 55, 151, 152, 155, 275, 277, 278, 282, 285, 287, 296, 297, 303, 306, 329, 330, 364, 365
Van Parijs P 308, 330, 332, 349
Verfaellie M 221
verification 223, 225, 229–31, 233, 235
Verkuyten M 77, 95
vicarious trauma (*see* trauma, vicarious)
victims ix, 5, 11, 17, 29, 32, 48, 56, 66, 90, 93, 136, 138, 156, 335
Victim Support 66
Vine, John 230
violence 4, 14, 112, 126, 129, 146, 167, 184, 247, 259, 274, 290, 305, 353
 domestic, 7, 61, 111, 138, 157, 166, 200, 351, 353, 397
visualisation 45, 214, 285
Vontress C 80, 81, 95

W

Wales 66, 396
Wallin D 292–94, 306
war v, 32, 53, 61, 112, 120, 157, 166, 269, 276, 278, 280–1, 290, 307, 380–1
 civil, 53, 110, 126
Wells A 193, 216, 222
white racial identity models 83, 95
White WA 287
wife/wives 38, 46, 61, 120, 128, 165, 180, 183, 239, 256–7, 355, 386
Wilkin L 377, 383, 395
Williams JMG 193, 221
Wilson JP 11, 35, 59, 65, 69, 75, 93–5

Wilson KG 193, 220
Winnicott DW 87, 96, 275, 287
women viii–ix, 4, 7, 9, 14, 32, 35, 62, 109–31, 133–4, 138, 156–7, 166–7, 180–1, 239, 241, 247, 263, 329, 393
Women's Aid 397
Women's Counselling and Therapy Service 400
women survivors of torture and gender-based abuse 109–11, 113, 115, 117, 119, 121, 123, 125, 127, 129, 131, 133
Work GB 78, 96
Working with Interpreters in Health Settings 310
Working with Interpreters in Psychological Therapy 310
World Health Organization (WHO) 47, 55, 57, 75
Wraparound Approach 12, 58

X

xenophobia 3, 16, 325, 381

Y

Yarlswood removal centre 119
young people xiii, 136–39, 142, 144–9, 151–53, 272, 275–6, 283, 288–91, 293–4, 296–300, 302–5
  age-disputed, 139
  separated, 141–2, 148, 15

Z

Zanen DE 339, 349
Zimányi K 335, 336, 349